THE BEAST IN THE M

THE CORRESPONDENCE OF RONALD ROSS AND PATRICK MANSON

THE WELLCOME INSTITUTE SERIES IN THE HISTORY OF MEDICINE

Forthcoming Titles
Constructing Paris Medicine
edited by Caroline Hannaway and Ann La Berge

Drugs On Trial:
Experimental Pharmacology and
Therapeutic Innovation in the 18th century
Holger Maehle

Academic enquiries regarding the series should be addressed to the editors W. F. Bynum, V. Nutton and Roy Porter at the Wellcome Institute for the History of Medicine, 183 Euston Road, London NW1 2BE, UK

THE BEAST IN THE MOSQUITO: THE CORRESPONDENCE OF RONALD ROSS AND PATRICK MANSON

Edited by
W. F. Bynum and Caroline Overy

Rodopi

Amsterdam – Atlanta, GA 1998

First published in 1998
by Editions Rodopi B. V., Amsterdam – Atlanta, GA 1998.

Design and Typesetting by Alex Mayor, the Wellcome Trust.
Printed and bound in The Netherlands by Editions Rodopi B. V.,
Amsterdam – Atlanta, GA 1998.

British Library Cataloguing in Publication Data
A catalogue record for this book is available from the British Library
ISBN 90-420-0721-4 (Paper)
ISBN 90-420-0731-1 (Bound)

Bynum, W. F., and Overy, Caroline
The Beast in the Mosquito: the Correspondence of
Ronald Ross and Patrick Manson
– Amsterdam – Atlanta, GA:
Rodopi. – ill.
(Clio Medica 51/ ISSN 0045-7183;
The Wellcome Institute Series in the History of Medicine)

Front cover:
Portraits of Ronald Ross and Patrick Manson,
courtesy of the Wellcome Trust Photographic Library.
Background image: a composite of sketches from the Ross and
Manson correspondence, original manuscripts courtesy of the
London School of Hygiene and Tropical Medicine.
Design by A. Mayor.

Printed in The Netherlands

Contents

List of Plates

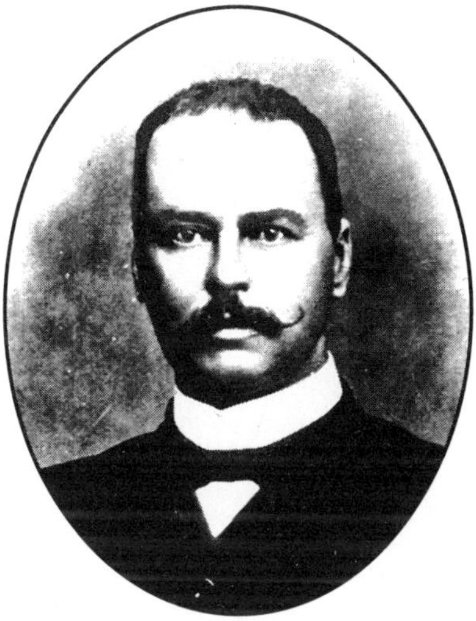

Figure 1
Ronald Ross

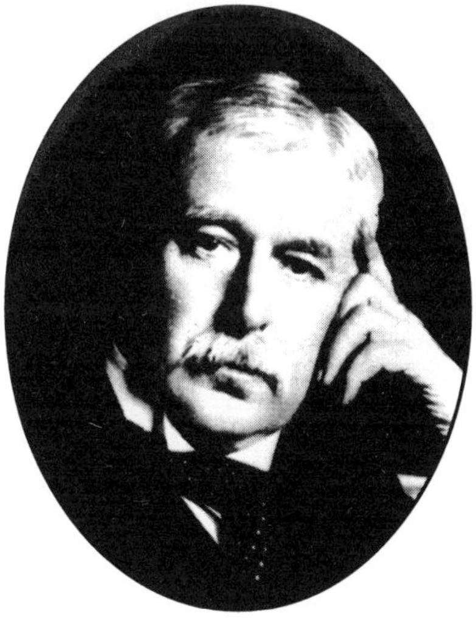

Figure 2
Patrick Manson

Introduction

When Ronald Ross (1857-1932) and Patrick Manson (1844-1922) began systematically to exchange letters in May 1895, neither could have known that their correspondence was to acquire such historical significance. Its purpose was strictly practical. Ross faithfully reported the results of his enquiries into the possible role of the mosquito in the transmission of malaria; he was, Manson wrote, looking for 'the beast in the mosquito.' (Letter **13**) For his part, Manson acted not only as sounding-board, he gave advice, encouraged Ross in his frequent, darker moments and became a kind of London agent for this disciple of his, cut off by three weeks' post or a two-pound telegram from the capital of the British Empire. By the time Ross returned home from India, in February 1899, both knew that their epistolary record (they had then exchanged 173 letters) was something special. 'I shall have your replies bound in a volume!'(Ross enthused), 'The solution of the great malaria problem is history you know!' (Letter **171**) For the older, more laconic Manson, writing a few years later, their correspondence will 'have an interest and value in years to come to some medical Dryasdust writing the history of malaria when we are dead and gone – the bugs hunting us & not we the bugs'. (Letter **240**)

Ross himself used the correspondence in his later obsessions about the priority of the discovery of the role of the *Anopheles* mosquito in the transmission of malaria, and included generous portions of it (with the emphasis on his letters to Manson) in his *Memoirs*,[1] published two years after Manson's death. Most subsequent historians, dryasdust or otherwise, have relied on the *Memoirs*, though Edwin Nye and Mary Gibson's recent biography of Ross[2] has admirably returned to the archives. But there is much more to the correspondence, including almost a hundred surviving letters which the two men exchanged after Ross returned to England.

Their correspondence is rich in both scientific and human terms. It describes, in great detail, research which won Ross a Nobel Prize for medicine and physiology, in 1902, only the second year of its award. It analyses malaria work, and tropical research more generally, during the crucial years of the formation of the medical speciality. There is a good case for 1898 as the year in which the discipline was born. It witnessed the moves towards establishing the schools of Tropical Medicine in London and in Liverpool, the appointment of a lecturer in tropical diseases at Edinburgh University, the formation of a section on tropical medicine by the British Medical Association, the appearance of the first issue of *The Journal of Tropical Medicine* and the publication of the book which helped define the field: Manson's *Tropical Diseases*. Although malaria is quite naturally the principal theme of Ross's Indian years, the correspondence touches many other diseases as well, including kala-azar, ankylostomiasis,[3] filaria, cholera, plague, and pellagra. Ross and Manson analysed not only diseases; they also dissected the achievements and foibles of men. This volume's Biographical Appendix includes most of the leading figures in the formative age of tropical medicine.

At a human level, too, the correspondence has its fascination. Their relationship quite naturally evolved over the years. It began as one of teacher and pupil, with the younger Ross deferential to the already established Manson. Even when Ross returned triumphantly from India in 1899, having proved what he still called Manson's 'Grand Induction', that mosquitoes are agents of malaria transmission, Ross still considered himself as largely Manson's agent, his hands and eyes in the tropics. Already in the early correspondence, however, the darker side of Ross's personality is evident, as are the avuncular characteristics which made Manson such a loved and respected figure. It is easy to sympathise with Ross's exasperation with the stultifying bureaucracy of the Indian Medical Service, but also easy to observe that, as his confidence in his own scientific worth grew, his tolerance shrunk for those whom he perceived as obstructing him, or who disagreed with him. Eventually, Ross included Manson among that ever-growing group, and the stiff coldness of some of the later letters is still poignant. Their relationship did not deteriorate as swiftly or completely as that of Sigmund Freud and Carl Gustav Jung, but the two correspondences do share some striking similarities, not least in detailing the declaration of independence of a pupil/son from a teacher/father.[4] Ross seemed to thrive on controversy and loved a fight; Manson hated controversy and was, emotionally, a pacifist. Neither man could have had an inkling of how it would all end when Manson found Ross's calling card at his London residence on 9 April 1894.

I. Manson before Ross[5]

Although Patrick Manson was a Scot, only the occasional Scotticism in this correspondence betrays his origins. His fervent patriotism is couched in terms of England and her empire. He was born on 3 October 1844, at Cromlet Hill, Oldmeldrum, Aberdeenshire, the second son in a family of nine children. His father, John Manson, was a substantial local figure, being laird of an estate near the town and the manager of a bank. Originally destined from the age of fifteen for that second great Scottish profession, engineering, Patrick Manson turned to medicine after discovering during his engineering apprenticeship that his physique was not up to its rigours. He developed a curvature of the spine and slight weakness of one arm, infirmities which never left him. His family had already settled in Aberdeen for the education of the children, and Manson passed his final Aberdeen medical examinations in 1864, still too young to take his degree. He thus spent a year in London, reading and attending the teaching hospitals, returning to Aberdeen in 1865, to receive his M.B., C.M. An appointment as Assistant Medical Officer in the Durham Lunatic Asylum gave him the opportunity to perform post-mortem examinations, to write his first paper, on carotid artery aneurysms, and to use that publication as the basis of his Aberdeen MD thesis, which he was awarded in 1866.

His elder brother already being in Shanghai, Manson used family influence to obtain the post of Medical Officer to the Chinese Imperial Maritime Customs for Formosa. This move determined the whole structure of his career. He remained in Asia for twenty-three years: in Formosa from 1866 until 1871, in Amoy until 1883, and from then until 1889 in Hong Kong. In 1875, while on furlough in Britain, he met and married Henrietta Thurburn, with whom he had 5 children.[6] Throughout these years Manson maintained a busy medical practice, among both resident Europeans and Asians, and was attached to missionary hospitals in both Formosa and Amoy. He also became an effective teacher, and in his Hong Kong days was instrumental in founding (and served as the first dean of) a school of medicine which eventually became the Victoria University and Medical School of Hong Kong. In 1890 he established a highly successful consulting practice in London, where his reputation in tropical diseases served him in good stead. By the time he met Ross, he had become Physician to the Seamen's Hospital Society,[7] and thus had the opportunity of seeing many of the 'tropical' cases in London.

Manson is best seen as a scientific clinician, in the mould of Sir William Jenner (1815-1898), or Manson's almost exact contemporary, Sir William Osler (1849-1919). He became adept at microscopy, made frequent dissections in the deadhouse and was at home in the laboratory. But he was never really very far from the bedside, where he was in his element and where most of the scientific problems he investigated originated. The most important of these early problems was filaria, a chronic parasitic infection which through lymphatic obstruction can lead to massive swelling of the legs and genitalia. Manson acquired competence at surgically removing the resulting elephantoid tumours, (he once described himself as an 'indifferent surgeon but a good carpenter'), and on hearing in 1874 that Timothy Lewis (1841-1886) had discovered the filaria embryos in the blood and urine of patients, he turned his attention to the worm's life history, by then named *Filaria bancrofti,* and its relation to human disease. He established that the filaria embryos could frequently be found in the blood of individuals who were not suffering from elephantiasis, and that in many patients, the parasites were present in the blood at night but not in the day. Arguing, somewhat dubiously, that the parasites could not carry out their entire life-cycle in the human host without killing their victim, he began to search for the intermediate host. Mosquitoes had already been suggested as a possible alternative one, and through feeding experiments, whereby patients with the filarial embryos in their blood were bitten by mosquitoes, he was able in 1877-8 to show that parasite development did take place in that insect. Further work by Manson and others established that only certain species of mosquitoes could thus act. Manson speculated that the dead mosquitoes contaminated drinking water with the parasites, and that this was how filaria re-entered the human chain. He thus argued that the mosquito was a necessary agent within the filaria's developmental cycle, but only an incidental one in the parasite's passage to human beings.

Manson did original work on a number of other human and animal parasites, but his filaria research highlights several features which influenced his attitude towards malaria, and, hence, the nature of the advice which he offered Ross. The first might be summarised by the old adage 'Nature does nothing in vain'. Although Manson does not appear to have been an especially religious man, his thinking was imbued with teleological reasoning. He was in awe of the way in which biological adaptations (to use a phrase equally applicable to Darwinian and natural theological explanations) were so subtly efficient. His concern with what he called the 'law of periodicity' in filaria is but one example, for he argued that the day-night variation in the presence of filaria in human blood was an adaptation whose purpose was to increase the likelihood of further filarial development within night-biting mosquitoes. He used an analogous argument with Ross about malaria. More generally, he advised Ross to remember that every biological function has significance, and that this dictum must ever guide the investigator's reasoning. 'Nothing walks with aimless feet.' (Letter 32)

That the filaria underwent part of its life-cycle in the mosquito was also highly significant. Just as Manson was not the first to postulate that the mosquito might be incriminated in the transmission of filaria, so, too, several authors argued, principally on epidemiological grounds, that mosquitoes were involved in malaria-transmission. While Manson accepted the general weight of these early hypotheses, his own reasoning was more biological: when the blood of a human malaria sufferer is drawn, the malaria parasite can continue to develop. For him, this bespoke an extracorporeal phase in the Plasmodium's life-cycle, analogous to that of *Filaria bancrofti* and other parasites which he had studied. He wanted Ross to follow this process in the tissues of the mosquito, just as he had done for the other parasite. That Manson still believed that mosquitoes bite only once and then die, and that water was the intermediary vehicle of filaria transmission, complicated the issue, but did not invalidate the general basis of Manson's hypothesis, or 'Grand Induction'.

Finally, Manson's Chinese career provided the foundation for his approach to the whole field of tropical medicine. It was not, he argued, simply the application of old-world bacteriology to the diseases of warm climates. While it was true that bacteria caused many important diseases in the tropics, among them plague, cholera and leprosy, these were not the quintessential tropical diseases. Manson called these bacteriological diseases 'cosmopolitan' rather than tropical,[8] arguing that they had been largely banished from Europe and the temperate parts of North America 'by the spread of civilisation, and the improved hygiene that has followed in its train'. They were essentially diseases of social and hygienic deprivation. Most of the real 'tropical diseases' were parasitic, caused by organisms other than bacteria and dependent on complicated chains of transmission which often involved intermediate hosts. Tropical medicine was thus to be built on disciplines such as parasitology, entomology and helminthology, and had to be distinguished from bacteriology. This was to be the essential message of Manson's classic textbook, *Tropical Diseases* (1898), and would undoubtedly have been communicated to his younger colleague, Ronald Ross, when they first met in London in April 1894.

II. Ross before Manson

Like Manson, Ross was Scottish, though he was born (on 13 May 1857) in Almora, in the foothills of the Himalayans, where his father was serving in the Indian Army. Ross's mother was English and he was the eldest of ten children. The family had connections with India which stretched back five generations, and like so many other children of the Raj, Ross retained vivid memories of his early years in India, before being sent back in 1865 to England for schooling. He stayed with various relatives, though his mother returned for an extended visit in 1867, his parents both came in 1873, during his father's two-year furlough. Ross enjoyed his boyhood, engaging in the usual outdoor pursuits and acquiring a love of literature, music and drawing. Given the choice, he would have made his way in art or literature, and he always valued highly the novels and poems he later published.

His father, however, determined that he should become a doctor, so Ross, who commented that he 'had no predilection at all for medicine' (*Memoirs*, 29), entered St. Bartholomew's Hospital Medical School in October 1874. He was only an average student who seemed to have enjoyed the social and cultural life of London more than his medical studies. In 1879 he passed his MRCS examinations, but failed the examination for the Licentiate of the Society of Apothecaries (LSA), then the standard dual qualification of most rank-and-file medical practitioners. Although technically only the surgical qualification was necessary for entry into the Indian Medical Service, Ross chose to bribe his way into a post as a ship's doctor, where he made four or five voyages, continuing his medical reading and collecting material for what he planned as his first novel. He successfully retook the LSA in early 1881, and then passed the entrance examination for the IMS, though his seventeenth place did not qualify for the most desirable postings in Bengal. Ross was attached to the Madras branch of the Service.

Ross's first tour of duty lasted from 1881 to 1888, where he was stationed in Madras and Bangalore, saw active service in Burma and spent a period in the Andaman Islands, one of the major convict stations of the Raj. In many ways, he was an ordinary medical officer, playing golf, fishing and shooting, and largely uninterested in his medical duties. He did, however, continue his literary pursuits, completing a first novel (*The Child of Ocean*, published in 1889) and writing verses and a couple of playlets, and he also threw himself into mathematics, a subject which had fascinated him as a boy, and which he was later to use in his malarial work. For some reason, he never bothered to apply for the civilian branch of the IMS, which Medical Officers were eligible to do after two years' service. This branch was generally thought more attractive than the military side, since the work allowed more time for private practice, and, hence, a larger income. Ross's lack of interest in practice may have been the reason, but the lapse came back to haunt him when, in 1897, he was attempting to carve out a more stable and well-paid niche as a researcher in India. (Letters 74, 76, 78)

In 1888, Ross finally obtained his first furlough. He returned to England, leaving the ship to see Italy, Switzerland and France for the first time. He also returned determined to make more of himself professionally, and bacteriology had matured considerably during his eight-year absence. Accordingly, he took the newly-established conjoint Diploma of Public Health (DPH) run by the Royal Colleges of Physicians and Surgeons, and studied bacteriology with E. E. Klein at St. Bartholomew's. He returned to India on 1 August 1889, with microscopical and bacteriological equipment, and a new bride, Rosa Bloxam, whom he had married in April. His next five years in India were somewhat more settled, especially when he was in Bangalore. His first three children, two daughters and a son, were born, he continued with his mathematics and literary work, and he began to publish a few papers in Indian medical journals. He searched in vain for the plasmodium parasite of malaria which the Frenchman C.L.A. Laveran (1845-1922) had first identified in 1880, arguing instead that malarial fevers were rooted in intestinal infections. He even sought out his fellow IMS officer, Patrick Hehir, who was also working on malaria but was equally unable to find Laveran's organism. It took Patrick Manson 'a few minutes' to show him some crescents in a blood stain, after Ross called on him in April 1894, during his second furlough home.

III. Ross and Manson in India and Britain

Manson easily convinced Ross of the existence of Laveran's parasite in the blood of malaria patients. Seven months later, at about 2.30 on a November afternoon, on Oxford Street, as the two men were walking together from Manson's home in Queen Anne Street to the Seamen's Hospital, Manson told Ross that he had formed the theory that 'mosquitoes carry malaria just as they carry *Filariæ*'. Ross tells us that he immediately replied that Laveran had made a similar conjecture, and, unbeknownst to either of them, so had several other individuals, including Joseph Nott, Louis Daniel Beauperthuy, and A. F. A. King. Manson's line of reasoning was well summarised in Ross's *Memoirs*:

We knew the function of the *asexual* forms of the [malaria] parasites, but were ignorant of the functions of what were later proved to be the *sexual* forms – the so-called crescents and flagellate bodies. Shortly after blood containing these forms is drawn from a patient's finger the crescents swell up, become oval, and then spherical, and lastly sometimes emit the long and actively motile filaments which were then wrongly called flagella, and these may sometimes be seen under the microscope to break away from the parent cell and to wriggle about rapidly in the fluid of the blood. They had long been subjects of discussion. Some observers, chiefly of the Italian school, held that they represent only the dying struggles of the parasite; others, including Laveran and Danilewsky thought that they are really living bodies, and Mannaberg even suggested that they may be connected with the life-history of the parasites outside the human body – though he did not explain how this could be. Manson now offered an explanation. He thought that when the mosquito sucks the blood, these sexual forms enter its stomach, and there, in a few minutes, emit their motile filaments just as they do under the microscope. The motile filaments, he thought, were *flagellated spores* which next pass through the walls of the mosquito's stomach and take up their abode in its tissues, where they must develop further into some unknown state and then enter drinking water. (*Memoirs*, 128-9)

This in essence was Manson's 'Grand Induction' which Ross set out to prove, and it highlights the reason why Manson's advice was frequently: 'Follow the flagellum'. (Letters **27**, **34**, **48**, **82**) Ross was, he himself confessed, badly equipped for the task he had set himself. He knew little about mosquitoes (a volume on tank angling was one of the few sources he could find back in India); he had never heard of Romanowsky's stain; and he had to teach himself how to dissect the insects. The terminology of protozoa, and of the several phases of the complicated life-cycle of the malarial protozoan, was not standardised, and Ross was to discover that mosquitoes harbour a variety of parasites which, early on, he often assumed to be part of the malaria cycle. The letters need to be read with the aid of a glossary, for which purpose we have reproduced, with the kind permission of the BMJ Publishing Group, the excellent one prepared by the late Leonard Bruce-Chwatt, with the assistance of the late P. C. C. Garnham, FRS. (pp. xxx-xxxv)

The story of Ross's three-year search for proof of the mosquito transmission theory has been told several times and is a central feature of his *Memoirs*.[9] Returning to Secunderabad in April 1895, he quickly became adept at diagnosing malaria from blood smears and became a proselyte for his patron, hoping to persuade the Indian Government to buy copies of Manson's Malaria Chart for instructional use. (Figure **3**) He also set to work attempting to infect subjects by giving them water with the debris of mosquitoes which had fed on malarial patients. Ross worked before the requirement of informed consent, and in a colonial setting; nevertheless, both he and Manson were aware of ethical considerations, including the ethics and dangers of self-experimentation. (Letters **2**, **11**, **13**, **14**) Malaria was different from many diseases, in that quinine was available, and Ross once joked that he would rather have malaria than the head cold from which he was suffering. (Letter **189**) For the most part, Ross believed that extra payment, from his own pocket, was sufficient reward for the native soldiers who were the principal subjects of his human experiments, and Manson, of course, famously and successfully infected his own son with malaria, just days before Patrick Thurburn Manson's final medical examinations. (Letters **203** and **204**) On at least one occasion Ross resorted to deceit, when he remarked to Manson that he had told a patient that the mosquitoes biting him were good for him, in that they sucked out the malaria parasites. (Letter **114**)

Ross's excitement with his 'certain experiments' (Letter **6**) on Abdul Kadir and the mysterious Lutchman (Letters **6** and **8**) was considerable; although they proved inconclusive, he had not discounted the possibility that malaria is transmitted through mosquito-infected water two years later, when he was in the Sigur Ghat, and attributed his own case of malaria to drinking tea made with improperly boiled water. (Letters **66** and **67**) At the same time, he was busy observing the development of the malaria parasite outside the human body, even if the significance of the various forms he could observe remained unclear. He puzzled that 30 or 40% of the parasites do not throw out flagella, since he had no appreciation of the sexual nature of the reproductive process in *Plasmodia*. His penchant for mathematics also surfaced early, in his attempt to use a haemocytometer to estimate the number of

DEC. 1. 1894.] DR. PATRICK MANSON'S MALARIA CHART. [THE BRITISH MEDICAL JOURNAL

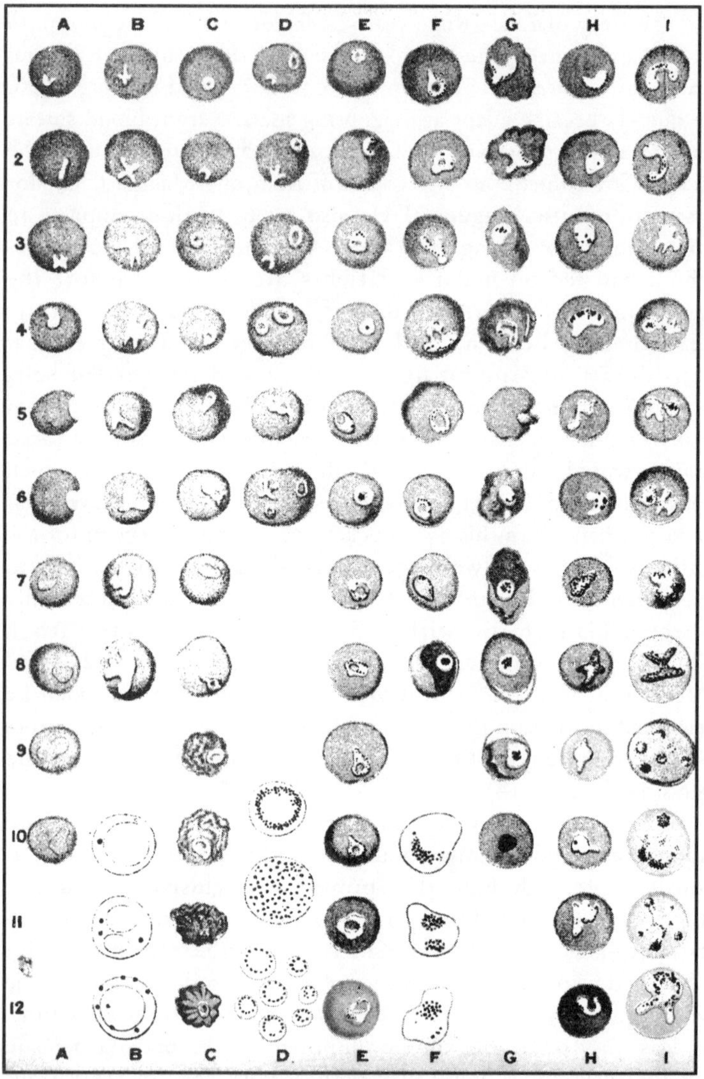

Figure 3 (this page and across)
Dr Patrick Manson's Malaria Chart which appeared
in the British Medical Journal, 1 December 1894.

DEC. 1, 1894.] DR. PATRICK MANSON'S MALARIA CHART. [THE BRITISH MEDICAL JOURNAL

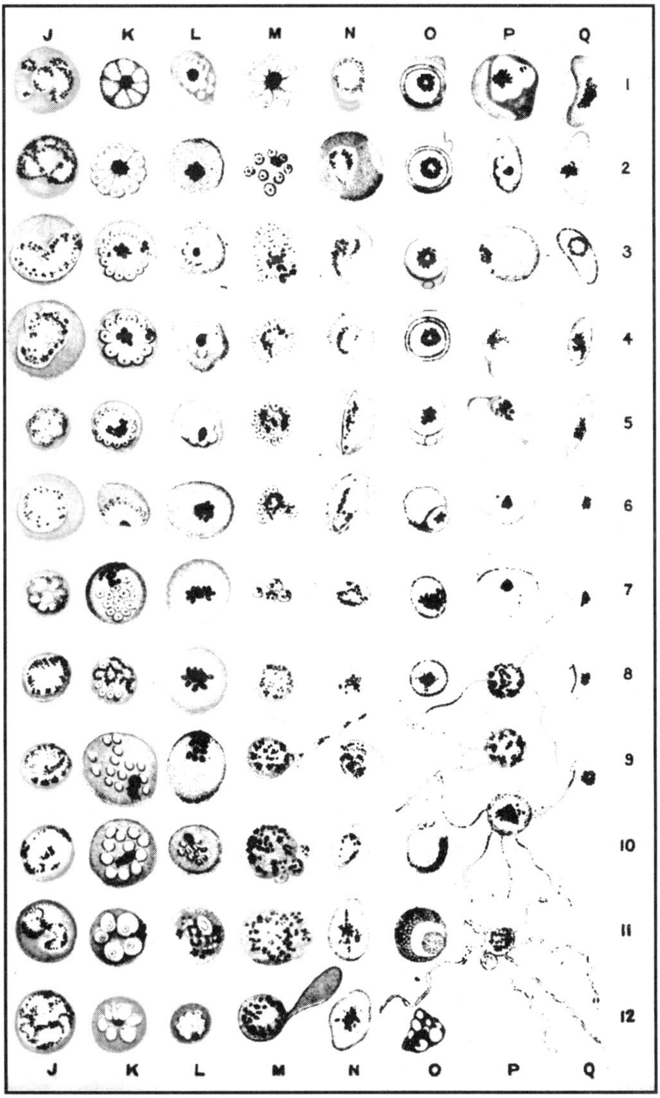

parasites in malarious blood. (Letters **4** and **5**) At Sigur Ghat, where he encountered *Anopheles*, probably for the first time, he returned to his mathematical ways of thinking, in estimating how many malaria germs he must have breathed, should infection come through the air. (Letter **67**) Other parasites of mosquitoes complicated matters for Ross, and for a time, gregarines much occupied him, as probably part of the malaria cycle. (Letters **18**, **20** and **22**)[10] By the time of his adventures at Sigur Ghat, in April 1897, Ross was sufficiently expert in the dissection of mosquitoes, and the identification of their parasites, as to be able to report to Manson on half a dozen, which, with typical Rossian tenaciousness, he wrote up years later, to claim priority on some of them. (Letter **73**)

Ross's early malaria work at Secunderabad was interrupted by an outbreak of cholera at Bangalore.[11] He remained in Bangalore from September 1895 until March 1897, engaged primarily in sanitary activity. He enjoyed the 'plenary powers' which the temporary posting gave him (Letter **24**) and the fact that his family could join him in a relatively settled life. He was proud of the sanitary report which he wrote, and even hoped that the post would be made permanent. At the same time, he resented the fact that the demands of the job left little time for malaria research, even if it was during his Bangalore period that he first suggested to Manson that malaria might be conveyed by the bite of the mosquito (Letter **43**), a notion which Manson doubted. (Letter **48**) Throughout this period, however, Manson was a source of strength for his younger friend and colleague (though Ross was now forty years old); he acted as a sounding board, gave advice, encouraged Ross during his increasingly frequent dark moments, helped with the publication of Ross's papers and communicated Ross's findings through his own publications. Manson also exerted his influence in an effort to have Ross seconded for malaria research, a task which proved formidable in the bureaucratic atmosphere of the Indian Medical Service.

Towards the end of his stay in Bangalore, facing an uncertain future and increasingly confident of his research capacities, Ross became disenchanted with his lot in India. The rest in the hill-station of Ootacamund, and the adventures at Sigur Ghat, did little to soften his attitudes towards his superiors in the Indian Medical Service, made worse by the fact that no good position in the Service seemed to be possible. His letters in June 1897 (Letters **74**, **75**, **76**, **78**) were those of a man close to desperation, and, in Manson's opinion, at least, of a man with an exaggerated notion of his capacity to earn a living by his literary endeavours. Manson's advice

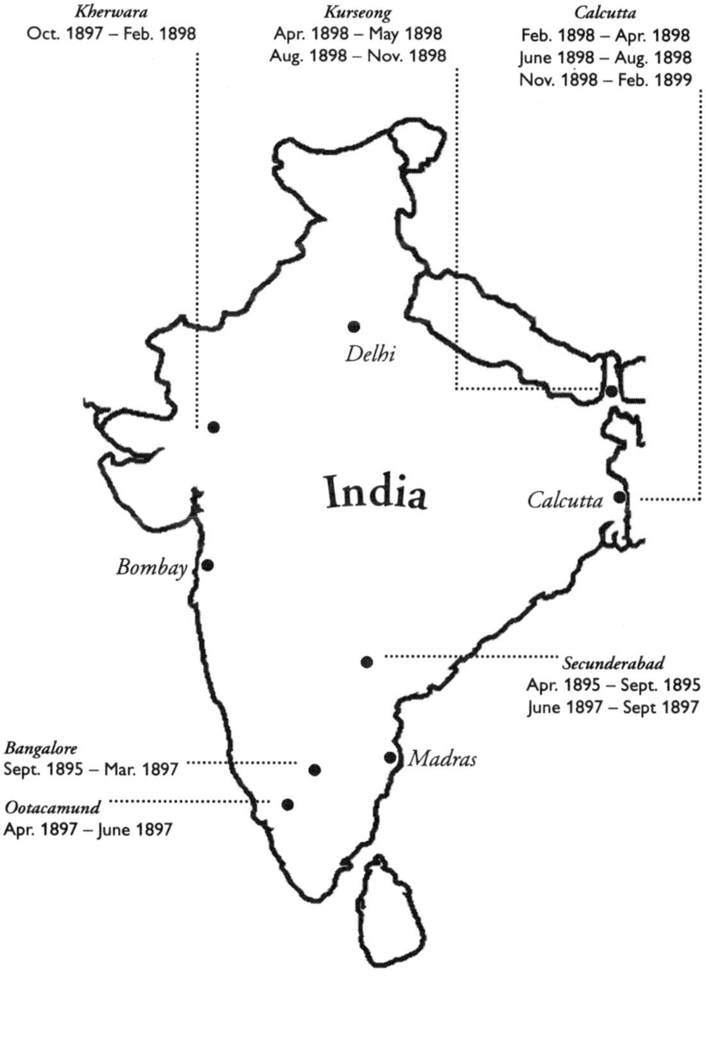

Figure 4
Map of India depicting Ross's movements
between 1895 and 1899.
Outline adapted from © Mountain High Maps.

to Ross's petulant threats to abandon malaria for a career in literature are pointed, the more so when contrasted with the patience Manson usually showed to his highly-strung protégé. (Letters **82** and **194**) It can be inferred that Manson had a relatively low opinion of the imagination; there is no reference in the entire correspondence to any cultural event, or any novel, poem or play which either man might have read during a quarter of a century. Since we know that Ross counted among his friends a number of literary and artistic individuals, the absence of a cultural dimension to their friendship was probably Manson's doing.

Nevertheless, Ross's own culture of complaint was one theme which Manson had to deal with during Ross's last years in India; nor was Ross to find inner peace in Liverpool. What he did find, however, now back in Secunderabad, on 20 August 1897, was the malaria parasite ('some cells') in the stomach wall of a 'brown' mosquito (probably *Anopheles stephensi*) he was dissecting after it had fed on a malarious patient. (Letter **89**) His letter of 22-4 August, describing the observations of what he ever afterwards called 'Mosquito Day' is a classic of controlled emotion ('wonder if I am really on it at last!'), the outcome of more than two years' investigation. In the subsequent letters, (Letters **91-4**) the cautious scepticism Ross had imposed on himself disappeared, as he saw the pigmented cells develop, discovered that only certain kinds of mosquitoes contained them, and argued cogently that the cells were pathological, not physiological. 'In reality - *pigment* - it is almost proof already! What else can the thing be? Mosquito's cells don't contain pigment or anything like it. I am not mistaken - it is *pigment*, absolute, unmistakable *pigment*! I have hardly restrained myself from wiring "pigment" to you, but fear you would think I had gone mad. Well, I know pigment by this time. *I am on it*'. (Letter **91**)

The vagaries of the postal service between India and Britain meant that Ross had to keep his excitement to himself, and by the time he received Manson's reply of 1 October, wishing Ross had tried chemical tests on the pigmented cells, Ross had been transferred on duty to Kherwara, where there was little malaria. The next months were especially frustrating for Ross, who thought another month's work would resolve the malaria problem definitively, and instead a frontier war, a plague epidemic and an unsympathetic Service hierarchy created a new set of difficulties for him. (Letter **103**) He became even more anxious to secure a place in one of the new medical institutes then being planned, or at least to have his request granted for malaria research leave. Retirement from the Service also became an increasingly attractive option. Despite the uncertainties, Ross continued intermittent work on the malaria parasites, and the relative scarcity of human cases in Kherwara had the positive effect of turning his attention to birds, which were subject to infection by a parasite (*Halteridium*, now called *Haemoproteus*) closely related to that which causes malaria in human beings. (Letter **107**) In the meantime, Manson could report on the discovery, by W. G. MacCallum, of the sexual nature of *Plasmodium* reproduction, though it was some months before Ross could obtain the paper itself.

The long-awaited news finally came in late January 1898, when Ross could report to Manson that he had been granted six-months research leave. It was later extended for a further six months, although part of it had to be spent in Assam, investigating kala-azar, then thought probably to be a kind of chronic malarial infection. Ross removed to Calcutta in February 1898, and since malaria was not very common there, he concentrated on bird malaria. Within a month, he could write to Manson, 'My one wish is that you were here to share with me the pleasure which I have experienced yesterday and today in seeing your induction being verified step by step'. (Letter **120**) Despite plague and the distractions of kala-azar, Ross's work proceeded rapidly, especially after he traced the malaria parasite into the salivary glands of the mosquito, a discovery which strongly supported the inoculation mode of transmission. (Letter **136**) In July 1898 Ross was able to telegraph his triumphs to Manson, who was President of the newly-formed Section of Tropical Diseases of the British Medical Association. One of the telegrams seems to have disappeared, but there is evidence that they were read out, and Manson's address summarised Ross's work. (Letters **136** and **141a**)

The importance of Ross's work was recognised in Britain and catalysed the establishment of a Malaria Committee by the Royal Society as well as the formation of the Schools in Liverpool and London. By the end of 1898, C. W. Daniels had been sent by the Royal Society to work with Ross, who was by then counting the days before he could return to Britain. He left India in February 1899, returning only twice to the country of his birth and greatest triumph.

IV. Two Public Men

In one of his many encouraging asides to Ross, Manson assured him that he would be 'lionised' when he returned from India to Britain. (Letter **161**) Seen historically, he was: an immediate post at the Liverpool School of Tropical Medicine, FRS within two years, a

CBE the next year and a Nobel Prize six months later. Unfortunately, Ross's perception was different, and his later honours never seemed to bring him any real satisfaction.

There are, perhaps, some objective circumstances. Liverpool was, in Ross's own evaluation, the 'second city of Empire' (Letter **176**), but it was not London. Nor was the Liverpool School of Tropical Medicine quite so successful, or visible, as the London School, with which Manson was so closely associated. Ross tried London once, briefly, before settling there permanently in his later life. (Letters **225** and **226**) But that final translation to the first capital of empire came too late for Ross ever to be the figure within the London medical establishment that Manson had enjoyed. Even the foundation of the Ross Institute, eventually within the heart of Manson's School, came too late to give Ross anything but too little, too late. Ross's medical practice never flourished like Manson's, for reasons which seem clear now, but the result was that Ross was never so comfortable financially as Manson, at least by his own reckoning.

The later correspondence reveals other, subtler, signs that Ross and Manson had difficulty being equals. The gaps in the correspondence make it difficult to be certain, but the absence of a letter of condolence after Patrick Thurburn Manson's death is strange. Manson found out about Ross's Nobel Prize by reading the newspapers, and Ross had known about it for three weeks. (Letter **229**) Manson's letter after Ross's abortive attempt to establish himself at the Jenner Institute is curiously abrupt. (Letter **226**) By the time of Ross's second trip to Freetown, Sierra Leone, there is no evidence that he still considered himself Manson's 'pupil'. The references to staying with each other ('your bed is waiting for you') when visiting their respective cities disappear fairly quickly. (Letters **188**, **214**, **219** and **228**) Eventually, they disagreed fundamentally about the worth of the researches of Louis Sambon. Ross had the better line of argument, but it may also have been a subtle disagreement about London and Liverpool, since Sambon was attached to the London School. (Letters **250** and **251**)

Nevertheless, Ross remained psychologically the older man's pupil for some time after he returned to Britain. Communication from the first journey to Sierra Leone was much more frequent than that of the second, and Ross gaily announced before going that Manson could 'expect to get weekly letters from a pupil again'. (Letter **182**) Ross appreciated Manson's efforts on behalf of his election to the Fellowship of the Royal Society (to which Manson had been elected only the previous year), and the exchange of specimens, curricula and information about the two fledgling schools continued on a regular basis for some time. So did the two men's efforts to increase public support for tropical medicine, and their identification of urgent problems in the field which could be efficiently and economically tackled. (Letters **245** and **246**) They were in almost complete agreement about the latter, even if Ross's preoccupation continued to be malaria, and Manson was visibly slowing down during the early years of the new century.

Ross's preoccupation was not simply with malaria, but, increasingly, his own role in the elucidation of its transmission mechanism. Ross's priority dispute with G. B. Grassi is well known and is one of the least attractive episodes in the whole history of malariology. Neither man emerges with garlands from the affair, though both of course made fundamental contributions to the subject. It was Grassi's cheek at dedicating a second book to Manson which was the most obvious reason for the late cooling of the relationship between Ross and Manson; and the act was made worse by the book itself, which was Grassi's own, rather partial, historical account of his role in the mosquito-transmission discovery. (Letter **230**) Manson had already urged Ross to 'Leave him [Grassi] alone', before Ross responded with a vitriolic letter, even while admitting that he had not read Grassi's second book. (Letter **232**)

Manson had had some responsibility in Ross's preoccupation with laurels, for his letters to Ross in India were filled with nationalistic sentiment, and sharp asides about the underhanded behaviour of 'furrineers' (Letter **159**), to say nothing of the fact that Americans, Frenchmen, Italians and Germans were all hot on the malaria trail. (Letters **19**, **27**, **48**, **77** and **105**) His mode of encouraging Ross in his Indian researches simply reinforced the younger man's sense of his own worth and achievements. Manson had even cautioned Ross to beware of Laveran, a malariologist Ross came to admire even more in his later life. (Letter **125**) Grassi, on the other hand, became for Ross the incarnation of duplicity and intellectual thievery, a man he could not refrain from assaulting time and again in his later publications on malaria.

There is not much point rehersing the relative contributions which Ross and Grassi made to the malaria problem.[12] The present correspondence offers an interesting version of events, though of course one seen only through British eyes. In addition, Manson had his own reasons to feel grieved at Grassi's behaviour, though he acted with much more restraint. (Letters **196**, **199**) The correspondence also throws light on two further incidents which alienated Manson and Ross. The first concerned the inaccurate reports which the English newspapers carrried of a visit Manson made to Italy, and which Ross himself had to correct. (Letter **190**) In the second, Ross joined with Rubert Boyce and Charles Sherrington in supporting Everett Dutton's claims to the discovery of the organism causing sleeping sickness, implying that Manson had claimed too much for himself and C. W. Daniels. (Letter **239**) At one level, this can be seen as simply an instance of London-Liverpool rivalry, but the tone of Manson's letter, in which, ironically, he also congratulated Ross on his Nobel Prize, shows the hurt which this most generous of men felt.

These episodes killed the intimacy between them, although these two men, now both eminent, continued to cooperate in more general matters relating to the development of their discipline. While there are occasional signs of missing letters, they are probably rare, and the increasing time between communication symptomatic of the psychological distance between them. Appropriately, the dominant theme of the last years was the fate of the correspondence from the Indian years.

Manson died in 1922, the year before Ross published his *Memoirs*. Grassi, however, was still alive and threatened to sue for libel for Ross's handling of their priority dispute. The matter never came to court, but it resulted in one final raking over of the old, old coals, before Grassi's own death in 1925.[13] Ross was by then obssessed with his own past, and his late publications almost invariably returned to fight old battles.

One of the very last of these was Ross's *Memories of Sir Patrick Manson*, privately published in 1930.[14] By then Ross himself had had a stroke and was confined to a wheelchair. Whether his stroke had affected his judgment is another matter, but the mean-spirited little volume certainly did Ross little credit. Insisting that he still held Manson in the 'warmest affection and regard', Ross proceeded to belittle Manson's filaria work, to suggest that Manson's ideas had often hindered Ross's own Indian researches, and to dismiss him as 'nothing but a medical man'. Even Manson's election to the Royal Society was 'chiefly, I think, because of his induction, and of my work on malaria'. (p. 21) This was a sad gloss on both the friendship and the consequent correspondence, which were integral to Ross's most significant achievement.

Manson once said that his role in the malaria story was to have discovered Ross. (Letter **180**) He did much more, of course, and deserved better of his pupil and colleague. There were plenty of spoils to be had in malaria research. In the end, Ross became his own worst enemy, and his inappropriate obsession with his place in history threatened to overwhelm the waning years of a gifted and creative scientist.

Notes

1 Ronald Ross, *Memoirs with a Full Account of the Great Malaria Problem and its Solution* (London: John Murray, 1923).

2 Edwin R. Nye and Mary E. Gibson, *Ronald Ross: Malariologist and Polymath. A Biography* (Basingstoke: Macmillan, 1997).

3 In the correspondence we have retained Ross and Manson's spelling, anchylostomiasis.

4 William McGuire (ed.), *The Freud/Jung Letters: The Correspondence between Sigmund Freud and C. G. Jung*, translated by Ralph Manheim and R. F. C. Hull (London: Hogarth Press, 1974).

5 See Philip H. Manson-Bahr and A. Alcock, *The Life and Work of Sir Patrick Manson* (London: Cassell and Company Ltd., 1927) and Douglas Haynes, 'From the Periphery to the Center: Patrick Manson and the Development of Tropical Medicine as a Medical Specialty in Britain, 1870-1900', (PhD Thesis: University of California, Berkeley, 1992).

6 Information supplied by Dr Gordon Manson-Bahr. Published sources are inconsistent as to the number of Manson's children: the *Dictionary of National Biography* states he had 3 sons and 3 daughters; *Who was Who,* 1 son and 3 daughters; Obituaries in the *BMJ* and *Lancet,* 2 sons and 3 daughters.

7 See G. C. Cook, *From the Greenwich Hulks to Old St. Pancras: A History of Tropical Disease in London* (London: Athlone Press, 1992).

8 Patrick Manson, *Tropical Diseases: A Manual of the Diseases of Warm Climates* (London: Cassell, 1898), xvi.

9 Gordon Harrison, *Mosquitoes Malaria and Man: A History of the Hostilities since 1880* (London: J. Murray, 1978); Mary E. Gibson, 'Ronald Ross and India', *Indian Journal of Malariology*, 34 (1997), 56-70; Nye and Gibson (1997); Paul F. Russell, *Man's Mastery of Malaria* (London: Oxford University Press, 1955); H. H. Scott, *A History of Tropical Medicine*, 2 vols, (London: Edward Arnold, 1939).

10 See **Glossary**, xxxii.

11 See Figure 4 for Ross's movements in India between 1895 and 1899.

12 See Scott (1939), Russell (1955) and Harrison (1978).

13 See G. B. Grassi, 'Twenty-five years after: a chronicle of the discoveries relating to the transmission of human malaria', *Parasitology*, 16 (1924), 355-64; *idem*, 'The transmission of human

malaria', *Nature*, 113 (1924), 304-7; R. Ross, 'The transmission of human malaria', *Nature*, 113 (1924), 353; Nye and Gibson (1997).

14 Ronald Ross, *Memories of Sir Patrick Manson* (London: Harrison, 1930).

Editorial Note

We have arranged the letters chronologically in the order which Ross would have written or received them, allowing approximately 2/3 weeks for the shipment of the mail. The number below the Letter number is the Ross Archive number in the Library of the London School of Hygiene and Tropical Medicine.This was catalogued by Mary Gibson. Towards the end of the correspondence are a few letters which are held in the Ross Collection at the Royal College of Physicians and Surgeons of Glasgow - these have numbers preceded by 'L'. The Collection was catalogued by B.E. Beaumont. There are also three letters in the possession of Dr Gordon Manson-Bahr - these have been noted in the footnotes.

The layout and punctuation of the letters have been standardised to follow the norm for the authors: addresses have been justified to the right and commas added after the salutation and removed after 'yours sincerely'; Ross tended to sign his name ending with a stop, Manson without - this format has been adopted throughout. Slight variations in line spacings at the beginning and end of letters have been necessary to accommodate the drawings and sketches within the body of the text.

General errors in punctuation, spelling and occasionally grammar have been corrected, although the varied spelling of words such as mosquitos / mosquitoes, Goulstonian / Gulstonian and the former spelling of ankylostomiasis (anchylostomiasis) has been left as written. We have also corrected many proper names which were frequently misspelt, notably Leuckart, Lawrie, Lutchman and MacCallum. Although Ross's hand writing is for the most part clearly legible, (Figure 5) proper names of patients may have been transcribed incorrectly and indeed it is likely that Ross himself wrote them phoenetically and never saw them written; likewise, Ross frequently spelt place names phoenetically and these have in general been left as such. Kalhutti and Punkarbari for which Ross varied his spellings have been standardised; we have also changed Ross's *Edinborough* to the modern spelling. Manson's hand writing was, quite frankly, appalling especially in the later years when he was suffering badly from gout. (Figure 6) We have noted in the text such

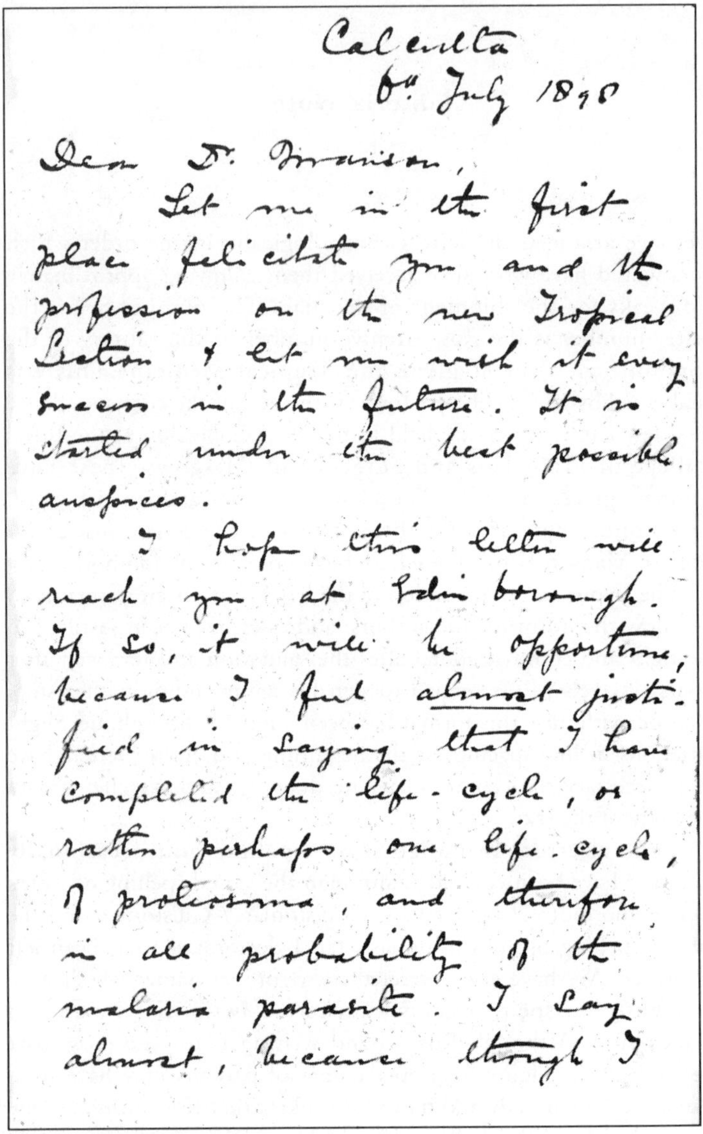

Calcutta
6th July 1898

Dear Dr. Manson,

Let me in the first place felicitate you and the profession on the new Tropical Section & let me wish it every success in the future. It is started under the best possible auspices.

I hope this letter will reach you at Edinborough. If so, it will be opportune, because I feel <u>almost</u> justified in saying that I have completed the life-cycle, or rather perhaps one life-cycle, of proteosoma, and therefore in all probability of the malaria parasite. I say almost, because though I

Figure 5
Sample letter from Ross to Manson.

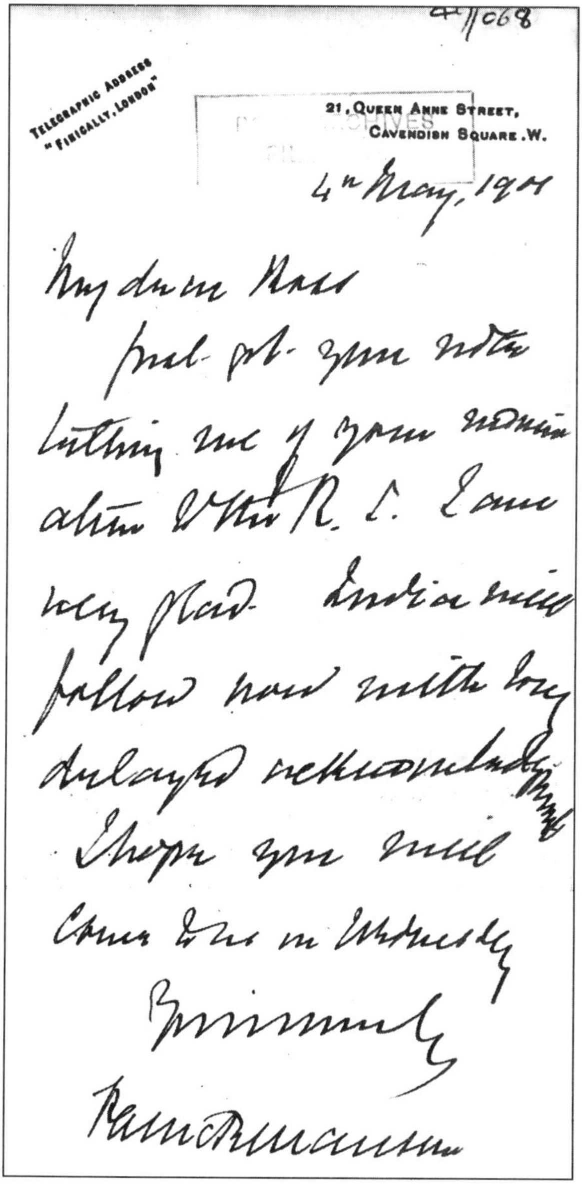
4/1068

TELEGRAPHIC ADDRESS
"FIBICALLY, LONDON"

21, QUEEN ANNE STREET,
CAVENDISH SQUARE. W.

4th May, 1901

My dear Ross

Just got your note telling me of your return after the R. C. I am very glad. India will follow now with long delayed acknowledgment. I hope you will come to us on Wednesday.

Yours sincerely

Patrick Manson

Figure 6
Sample letter from Manson to Ross.

words as we have been unable to decipher - in all cases, however, the sense of the sentence is clear.

References in the footnotes are given in full at the first mention and thereafter in abbreviated form with surname and date; all references with the exception of anonymous reports have been listed in the bibliography. Individuals when first mentioned are, whenever possible, given birth and death dates, a brief description and reference to the biographical appendix; they are not referenced again unless there has been a considerable time span since the first mention. In the footnotes references to items in the Ross Archives are preceeded by 'RA'.

Acknowledgements

We have acquired many debts in our excursion into the worlds of Ronald Ross and Patrick Manson. Our special thanks go to two of their descendants, David Ross of Ross and Dr Gordon Manson-Bahr for permission to publish this correspondence. Dr Manson-Bahr also kindly supplied us with copies of documents still in his possession. Our transcription of the letters was facilitated by the permission of Brian Furner, Librarian at the London School of Hygiene and Tropical Medicine, to have the correspondence deposited in the Wellcome Institute Library, under the care of Richard Aspin. Mary Gibson's retirement as Assistant Librarian at the LSHTM will be a loss to Ross scholars everywhere. She has patiently answered all our queries and lent her expertise in deciphering difficult passages. Chris Hilton at the Wellcome has also shared with us his palaeographical skills. James Beaton, Librarian of the Royal College of Physicians and Surgeons of Glasgow, also kindly supplied us with copies of some correspondence there.

At the Wellcome Trust, Alex Mayor has been wonderfully efficient at laying out the text and scanning in the many drawings. Our thanks go to him, as well as Chris Carter and Mohsina Somji. Lise Wilkinson and Gordon Cook have supplied much expert information which has been incorporated into our footnotes, Helen Power kindly supplied us a manuscript copy of her history of the Liverpool School of Tropical Medicine, and Chandak Sengoopta was a valuable resource for Indian names. Roy Porter and Helen Power read and improved the introduction. Mistakes are ours.

The late Eli Chernin was just beginning to plan an edition of this correspondence when he unexpectedly died. It was through him that one of us (WFB) became convinced that it was an exciting and worthwhile endeavour. We like to think that he would have been pleased with our own efforts.

As always, the support of the Governors of the Wellcome Trust must be acknowledged.

Glossary

Reproduced from L. J. Bruce-Chwatt, Glossary in *The Great Malaria Problem and Its Solution* (London: The Keynes Press, 1988), xvii-xxii, with permission from the BMJ Publishing Group. Some of the terms do not occur in Ross's correspondence with Manson.

....

A number of scientific terms used by Ross in the *Memoirs* are either those invented by him during his work in India or those generally used in scientific writings between 1890 and 1920 but obsolete now. Some of Ross's original suggestions concerning the terminology for the different stages of the development of malaria parasite can be found in the addenda to the book *The Prevention of Malaria*, 2nd edition, published by him in 1911, but few have been generally adopted.

The brief glossary given below follows much of the terminology of malaria as quoted by P C C Garnham in his authoritative *Malaria Parasites and other Haemosporidia* (1966).

Amoeba coli	A protozoon occurring in the intestine. The taxonomy of the genus is complex. It seems that Ross referred to the pathogenic form known as *Entamoeba histolytica.*
Anopheles costalis	*Anopheles gambiae* Giles.
Anopheles fuliginosus	*Anopheles annularis* V d Wulp.
Anopheles rossi	*Anopheles subpictus* Grassi.
Bioplasm	Cytoplasm.
Black spores	Dark banana shaped or round bodies, occasionally observed on the midgut wall of anopheles mosquitoes and probably caused by the secretion of chitin in response to an irritant.
Blasts	Synonym used by Ross for sporozoites.
Blastophore	Ross's term for the appearance of radial islets of cytoplasm ("sporoblasts") in a

	growing oocyst from which sporozoites are formed by budding.
Blood plates	Blood platelets or thrombocytes.
Brindled (mosquitoes)	Brownish or tawny with streaks of other colour. (*Oxford English Dictionary*).
Cercomonas	A genus of flagellates present in faeces and in faecal cultures.
Chromatin	Nuclear body of cells that stains strongly with basic dyes.
Coccidia	Loose term for a group of protozoa of the order of Coccidia, parasites of the intestinal tract of animals and humans causing various forms of coccidiosis.
Coccidium	A term often loosely used by Ross in his letters and *Memoirs* (1923) for the oocyst stage of the development of malaria parasite in the gut of mosquitoes. He also applied this term to the gregarines. In reply to Nuttall's criticism Ross explained that these terms were provisional.
Coelome	Main body cavity of insects.
Crescents	Common term for gametocytes (sexual forms) of *Plasmodium falciparum* owing to their semilunar shape.
Crescent-sphere-flagella metamorphosis	Growth, maturation, and release of gametes (exflagellation) of male sexual stages of plasmodia.
Culex sylvestris	Probably *Aedes* (*Aedimorphus*) *vexans* Meigen.
Dacoits	Armed robber bands (Anglo-Indian (A-I)).
Dak bungalow	Travellers rest house (A-I).
Dappled-winged (mosquitoes)	Variegated with spots or patches of colour. (*Oxford English Dictionary*)
Dhooley bearer	Litter bearer (A-I).
Durwan	Porter or gatekeeper (A-I)
Exflagellation	The extrusion and liberation of microgametes by male gametocytes (microgametocytes).
Flagellates	Loose term for protozoa of the class of Mastigophora, which includes organisms that move by the help of specialized ectoplasmic structures, the flagella.

Flagellum (flagella)	A Whip. An organ of locomotion of a number of protozoa. An early and common term (in plural) for microgametes released by male sexual cells (microgametocytes). Hence flagellulae, exflagellation, flagellated body, for the phenomenon of release of microgametes by the male gametocyte.
Gametids	Gametocytes, sexual forms of malaria parasites.
Germinal rods or threads	Ross's terms for sporozoites, the final stage of development of the plasmodium in the mosquito. These are the infective forms of the malaria parasite released the mature oocyst and invading the salivary glands of the mosquito.
Gregarines	Protozoa of the subclass of *Gregarinina*, intestinal parasites occurring in some insects, including mosquitoes.[1]
Grubs	Mosquito larvae.
Haemamoeba	Obsolete generic name for malaria parasites of primates but applicable to a subgenus of plasmodia in birds.
Haemomenas praecox	Obsolete name of *Plasmodium falciparum* causing the "aestivo-autumnal" (malignant tertian) fever.
Haematozoin	Malaria pigment produced by the digestion of blood by the parasites. Haemozoin is the correct term. Melanin is a wrong and obsolete term.
Haematids	Erythrocytes, red blood cells.
Haustellation	The process of sucking.
Imago	Adult mosquito, after emergence from the pupal case.
Karyokinesis	Mitosis, the process in which the nucleus divides.
Laveranity	Colloquial reference to Laveran's discovery of malaria parasite and its mosquito transmission.
Leukids	Leucocytes, white blood cells.
Malariated or malarialised	Infected by malaria parasites.

Malpighian tubules	Tubular glands connected with hind gut of insects. Their function is excretory.
Mere	Term used for a division of whole cell. Hence merozoite: product of division of a blood schizont (or of a tissue schizont).
Merozoite	Product of segmentation of erythrocytic and exo-erythrocytic schizonts.
Metaxeny	Change of hosts in succeeding generations of parasites.
Microsporidia	Protozoan organisms of the order Microsporidia, parasites of mammals, insects, crustacean, fish, and reptiles transmitted by spores.
Murrain	Infectious disease of unknown origin, often in cattle, imprecise term. (*Oxford English Dictionary*)
Nagana	Trypanosomal disease of cattle in tropical Africa, transmitted by tsetse flies.
Nosema	Genus of microsporidia causing disease of insects.
Oocyst	An encysted zygote in the mosquito stomach.
Panoplites	Former name of the mosquito genus *Mansonia.*
Piroplasma	Former name for the genus *Babesia*, parasites of cattle, sheep, horses, dogs and occasionally humans, which invade blood corpuscles and cause specific diseases (piroplasmosis or babesiosis).
Polar bodies	Small round bodies at the edge of a mature female gametocyte (macrogametocyte), formerly believed to be due to the reduction division of the nucleus; now known to represent part of the membrane of the erythrocyte after the escape of the *macrogamete.*
Proteosoma relicta	This avian malaria parasite, the sporogonic development of which was demonstrated by Ross in 1897, is *Plasmodium* (*Haemamoeba*) *relictum.* The former name Halteridium was a synonym of *Haemoproteus* of avian parasites in birds - for example, *H columbae*

	of pigeons.
Protospore	Ross's synonym for sporozoite.
Psorosperms (or pseudonavicellae)	Encysted forms of *Lankesteria culcis* found in the bodies of mosquitoes. Both Manson and Ross believed at first that they represented some stage of the development of malaria parasites, and Ross carried out a few experiments in humans (including himself) in 1895.
Schizont	Asexual parasite after the division of the nucleus. Hence schizogony.
Sperms or spermatozoa	Ross's occasional term for flagella (male gametes).
Spore	Single celled or multicelled reproductive body that becomes detached from the parent and gives rise, directly or indirectly, to a new individual. Occurring in plants, bacteria, and protozoa. Ross used this term rather freely for the trophozoites in the red blood cells and for the daughter cells (merozoites) formed by the segmenting schizont.
Sporocytes	Obsolete name for merozoites, products of the division and multiplication of mature erythrocytic schizonts (schizogony).
Sporogony	Process of development of the malaria parasite occurring in the mosquito after the union of male and female gametes and ending with the formation of sporozoites.
Sporulation	The process of spore formation.
Stegomyia calopus	Former name of *Aedes aegypti*, a mosquito responsible for transmission of yellow fever and other viral diseases.
Terai	A large stretch of marshy or overgrown land with underwood or tangled vegetation (A-I).
Vermicule	Also "travelling vermicule," a motile stage of the zygote, before the formation of the oocyst on the gut of the mosquito.
Undulant fever	Also called Malta fever, a disease now known as brucellosis, caused by *Brucella melitensis* and other species of this bacterium in humans and also (*B abortus*)

	in cattle, swine, sheep, goats, and horses.
Zygote	The product of the union of male and female gametes.

I am grateful to Professor P C C Garnham, FRS, for his comments on this glossary.

1 In 1895 Ross found parasites, which he believed to be some Coccidia, in the intestine of a *Stegomyia* (Aedes) mosquito. He then found them in the malpighian tubules and recognised them as encysted gregarines containing "psorosperms." These parasites were so common in larvae and adult mosquitoes in Secunderabad that Ross suspected them of representing a stage of the developing malaria parasite; however, he soon realised that they were of a different nature. The name *Gregarina culicis* given by Ross was changed to *Lankesteria culcis* in 1898. The remarkable cycle of development of this parasite related to the stages in the life of the insect was fully described in 1926 by Wenyon in his *Protozoology* (**2**: 1120-24). (See also Manson-Bahr P. The story of malaria - the drama and actors. *International Review of Tropical Medicine* Vol 2, Lincicome D R, ed. Academic Press, New York and London, 1963: 329-390.)

Letter 1

21, Queen Anne Street,
Cavendish Square. W.
9th April 1894

Dear Surgeon Major Ross,

I am very sorry I was out when you called this afternoon.

I read your papers some time ago in the Indian Medical Gazette[1] with much interest. As against Hehir[2] & some others your position is perfectly correct. They see only physiological phenomena. But I am certain, judging from the minuteness and accuracy of your observations, that you have not seen the plasmodium malariae, otherwise you would never have failed to recognise its pathological character. And the reason you have not seen it is the technique you employ. It will give me great pleasure to be of any service to you for I am quite sure you can do good work and have the patience to do it. The first forenoon (tomorrow if possible) you have leisure call on me and we can arrange to make the most of the malaria cases I have access to.

Yours very truly

Patrick Manson

1 R. Ross, 'The true nature of the plasmodium and the malaria parasite', *Indian Medical Gazette* (Oct. 1893), 329-336; *idem*, 'The third element of the blood and the malaria parasite', *Indian Medical Gazette* (Jan. 1894), 5-14.

2 (Sir) Patrick Hehir, (1859-1937), had shown Ross a 'spheroidal body' which Ross rejected as a cause of malaria. For Hehir, see **Biographical Appendix**.

Letter 2
02/064

Secunderabad – Deccan
1st May 1895

Dear Dr Manson,

I write to report progress, and hope you will excuse size of paper. After leaving Malta I examined the blood of all likely cases on board ship (and none were anything but remotely likely) without any result. The day after reaching Bombay I went to the Civil Hospital and immediately found a woman with tertian from Ahmedabad with splenitis but not treated with quinine. The parasites were rare but I found one in the marginal clot in five minutes. There were only about six in the first specimen, crescents & mature spheroids very deeply pigmented. The same evening & next morning I found the same forms apparently, & in same state, but had not time to work properly as I had to get luggage through the customs. I have been here now less than a week & though I have been very much occupied in calls and business have spent four days & more with the microscope and out of 11 cases have found 5 due to the parasite. Carter[1] found 9 only during some months. The heat is awful and the wind like the blast of an engine-furnace. There were only convalescent cases drenched with quinine in my hospital, so I had to drive three miles to the Civil Hospital in the heat of the day. There were five cases in one ward in three of which, though they all had had quinine, I found the parasite in 30 seconds (2nd & 3rd fields) each – crescents & large spheroids deeply pigmented. The two cases in which I did not find it were convalescent and were discharged next day. I immediately made a push for the mosquito. By bad luck hardly one was to be found, the air being *fiery* and the three I caught & put into bottles were too *frightened* or otherwise un-willing to bite; I had no mosquito net. Up to date I have failed in getting a single mosquito to lay hold, which I think is because I have had to catch them. I am now breeding numbers & have a net ready for use. The three cases were examined carefully the whole day next day & I found one of the reasons why I could not find the parasite before. Above 90° phagocytosis is so quick that all free forms are gobbled up in *twenty minutes.* I used to take my specimens home generally. I found two beautiful forms ready for flagella & had logged their position & moved off to study some crescents; on coming back *10 minutes* after making the specimen they were both inside phagocytes. Next day in my hospital I found two cases of intraglobular parasites with very fine pigment. Malaria was diagnosed in both cases within one minute each. I am sorry that I foolishly packed your chart in the wrong box, now coming by goods train; so that I cannot quote numbers of forms.[2] Four cases in my hospital have hitherto given negative results; but I am at present engaged in looking at the parasite rather than for it. I am delighted & surprised at number of cases & ease with which they have been found. My microscope is invaluable. Have you read Crombie's speech in Indian Medical Gazette for March.[3] He (and all the doctors in the country) are furious with Dr Hart's speech.[4] He is trying to throw cold water on the microscopic diagnosis of malaria & says that he found the parasite in only 4 cases out of 50 in Calcutta in January. My results within a week & before the fever season give 50%! He talks too of half an hour being required, as if that was the average time – so I am keeping careful notes for time taken for each diagnosis. When present, the parasites generally swarm – 1 or 2 in three fields about. Today however the two cases in my hospital show not a trace of any, but I am off to them again after sundown. Both are fresh cases with very low fever & much headache. Evidently the laws of these sudden appearances & disappearances must be made out if possible. All the cases are beautiful! and I am wild with excitement; but these mosquitoes! They *will not* bite. I tried them on myself for experiment,[5] but having been caught they are frightened I suppose. I expect a crop of new ones in one of my bottles this evening & hope a fever case will show itself to suit. No flagella been seen as yet; but I certainly saw a spent crescent in one specimen. I believe (or rather think) from what Carter says that they are released almost immediately in a high temperature – but we shall see. The finely pigmented bodies seem to belong to quite a different species from the others. I am touting round the country for cases. The doctor in charge of the policemen refused to transfer them to me for experiment & there are difficulties in the way of my experimenting at his hospital. By bad luck I am engaged for tomorrow.

2nd May. All my mosquito grubs have been killed owing to my foolishly putting the bottles in the sun. I have consequently started a new lot; but it is vexatious. My two cases were examined again today. In one the parasite remains absent (no fever). In the other (fever, vomiting & headache) there are a very few which however are much more deeply pigmented than before. I have had two more negative cases. Unfortunately the principal medical officer here seems to be putting me on every duty conceivable; but I shall go & look for cases at the civil hospital again tomorrow. In case examined today the parasite is so delicate that it breaks up apparently in half an hour; & otherwise appears too *young*, as it were, to form flagella. I fancy it

must get a good hold in the system before being ripe for mosquito. Its presence in blood does not seem to be necessarily connected with fever, because one of my cases had fever yesterday without parasite being visible. Please excuse scrawl; & give my kind regards to Mrs Manson & your son.[6] I should like Hunterian lecture.[7] Will write about the charts as soon as my boxes come. Don't trouble about reply to my verbosity.
Yours truly
Ronald Ross.

1 Henry Vandyke Carter, (1831-1897), Deputy-Surgeon-General, IMS, Bombay. H. V. Carter, 'Note on some aspects and relations of blood organisms in ague', *Scientific Memoirs by Medical Officers of the Army of India* (1887 part III), 139-167. See **Biographical Appendix**.

2 Manson's chart is reproduced, Figure 3. See also Letter 3, note 3.

3 Alexander Crombie, (1845-1906), I.M.S. (Bengal). A District Surgeon in Calcutta. See **Biographical Appendix**. A. Crombie, 'Scientific research on India', *Indian Medical Gazette* (Mar 1895), 116-119.

4 Ernest Hart, 'An address on the medical profession in India. Its position and its work', *BMJ* (29 Dec, 1894), 1469-1474. Ernest Hart (1835-1898), Editor of the *BMJ*, had strongly criticised the medical services in India in an address delivered before the Indian Medical Congress at Calcutta, December 1894, excepting only Carter in the area of malaria studies.

5 Self- and human experimentation are recurring themes in the correspondence.

6 Patrick Thurburn Manson, (1877-1902), was the subject of Manson's famous experiment with Italian mosquitoes. Educated at Aberdeen and the London School of Tropical Medicine, he died on an expedition to Christmas Island. See also Letters 203 and 218.

7 Patrick Manson, 'The annual oration, 1894. Malaria and its associated parasite', *Hunterian Society Transactions* 76th session (1894-1895), 19-50.

Letter 3
02/065

Secunderabad
15th May 1895

Dear Dr Manson,

The fortnight since I wrote to you has been made up partly by disasters & at last by success. I had a bad case (officer) requiring constant attendance; the two ague cases in my hospital ceased to show parasites; when with much difficulty I had got two cases out of the bazaar, all my mosquitoes died again; and next day when I had got a fresh crop of mosquitoes, my two cases ran away, because I pricked their fingers, in spite of my giving them a rupee a prick! I now saw that it was necessary to get a Sepoy case & so spent a day at another regimental hospital. I examined a number of cases in vain (all being soaked with quinine); but at last cast my eye on a case just come in for dysentery: success – two crescents in specimen – case transferred to my hospital. Next day there were a fair number of crescents (11th May) and nothing else – just the sort of case required – but the mosquitoes would not bite. The temperature was between 90 and 100°F and as dry as a furnace; so that the mosquitoes died shortly after being released from the bottle. Nothing I could do persuaded them to bite. The same happened on 12th, the crescents *swarming*, three or four in a field, the mosquitoes as obstinate as mules and myself nearly frenzied. I watched specimens however and saw that at this temperature the crescents show but little change, only a very few becoming spherical. I did not see a single flagellate body though I must have looked at hundreds of parasites on 11th & 12th; and I saw only a few doubtful spent crescents.

Next day (13th May, my birthday) there was better luck. It had rained at night & the morning 6.30 a.m. was cool – I obtained four full mosquitoes. I also found out how to make the insects bite; that is by wetting the bed & mosquito-net with water – this makes them hungry in a moment. The finger blood was swarming with crescents and crescents only. By an accident I did not know that a mosquito had bitten till an hour after he had done so. I bottled him, smoked him (or rather *her*) and separated the abdomen just as you had described; but it was now so hot & dry again that the blood dried almost as soon as squeezed out so that I had to moisten with normal salt solution. Results at once –

1. Parasites present. This was interesting as owing to exceedingly pointed ends of crescents ( ) I thought they might stick in proboscis.

2. Numbers apparently same as in finger blood (very numerous).
3. Forms, *apparently* nearly all spherules, many spent crescents (?) & very few distinct crescents.

With regard to (3) however I saw that there were many elements of doubt, requiring experiment. I examined the other three mosquitoes within five hours with identical results in all; and then set to work to experiment. First the salt solution which it was necessary to add in all the cases, does, I find, turn a large number of crescents into spherules in a minute at this temperature (I believe Laveran says so,[1] but have not had time to look him up). In the spherules produced in this manner the pigment granules *swarm* of course for a time; but only once did I observe (in salt solution) a flagellate form & that was unsatisfactory. This showed however that the spherules in the mosquitoes might be due only to the salt solution. Moreover I noticed that in pure blood, in the marginal clot, the crescents change much more frequently than elsewhere; so I thought that the change in the mosquito might be due to the clotting of the blood (as is likely). As for the *spent* crescents, they seemed very numerous, but I was not certain that they *were* spent crescents. The three forms are 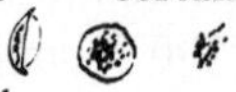 . In the obscurity of the exuded haemoglobin I could never make out satisfactorily whether the  spent-looking form had not really a cell wall round it. I noticed no flagellate bodies.

Next day 12th I spent over six more mosquitoes; much hindered by the rapid drying; trying water, glycerine, canada balsam, salt solution &c. In none of the mosquitoes could I get the specimen in the same condition as my control specimens from the finger; and I remained unsatisfied both about spherules & spent crescents; though I was forced to confess that these *appeared* much *more* numerous & the crescents much *less* numerous than in my control specimens. Today I have been at work on three mosquitoes. One had no parasites by which I could see that he had got into the net after biting someone else outside (the moisture of the net is attracting outside gentry). The other gave no more certain results, though I got him twenty minutes after biting & examined the blood pure. I have been trying control specimens on ice, too, and found one good flagellate form with *very* delicate flagella, scarcely visible, nothing like the thick flagella I saw with you. I find both spherules & spent crescents in different conditions of the same control specimens; which is irritating because I cannot satisfy myself as to cause. At last this evening, however, my dull brain suggested the proper course – to try *dry smears.* I got a $^{1}/_{2}$ hour mosquito & *smeared* his blood with the needle on cover glass, inverted the same after drying in air & simply laid on slide, using oil immersion but no medium. *Nothing but spherules.* Not a single crescent & only one or two masses of spent pigment (?). A control finger blood made in same way, gave, of course, *all crescents* & *no spherules*; while a finger blood, which had been kept for two hours & was then opened & dried, gave *mostly crescents* & *a few spherules.*

This last experiment then seems to me to *prove* that the crescents undergo change into spherules in the stomach of the mosquito as outside; and to *suggest* that they do so faster than in control specimens. I must satisfy myself much more however, before I state so much definitely. I am, as it were, touching the matter with my soul before my intellect has reached it; just as a phagocyte touches a microbe with its bioplasm while the nucleus lumbers up behind(!) Talk of phagocytosis! I have seen things these last three days; but have no time to write about them. I am dead beat now & the lids of my right eye are swollen & painful – at work from 7 a.m. to 7.30 p.m. with snatches at breakfast & tea.

16th May. Four more hours work but no good results & have to break off to write mail letters. Certainly crescents are very rare in mosquitoes' stomach after half an hour, but remain in numbers up to 12 hours in finger blood. Have tried a thick film (to avoid pressure) kept for 2 hours & then smeared & partly stained. Numbers of crescents, many spherules and some clusters of pigment. I hope by degrees to improve my manipulation and get a clear certainty whether crescents do or do not transform more quickly in mosquitoes than in specimens.

I mentioned that two men in my hospital had different looking parasites to other cases. These on reference to Marchiafava[2] turn out to be exactly like his tertian, while the others are quartan seemingly; but I must work it out when I have time. I sent your charts[3] to government the other day, with letter asking them to buy for hospitals.

A few days ago I saw Lawrie[4] who read me part of a letter from Hehir, in which he said that he found 30% of the corpuscles infected in a case of malaria! One third! I saw Hehir,[5] too and can't make him out. He seems to stick to his vacuoles, and was very short with me. I should not wonder if he will have out a full verification of your mosquito theory in a little. To close, I want to try an experiment – keep an infected mosquito for a week in a bottle containing water, and then drink mosquito & water together. But it ought to be tried systematically. I shall get a number of mosquitoes in bottles

tomorrow. Case still swarming with crescents – no fever.
Believe me,

Yours truly

R. Ross.

1 A. Laveran, *Paludism* trans. by J. W. Martin (London: New Sydenham Society, 1893), Chapter 4. See **Biographical Appendix.**
2 E. Marchiafava and A. Bignami, *On Summer-Autumn Malarial Fevers* trans. by J. Harry Thompson (London: New Sydenham Society, 1894), 9ff. See **Biographical Appendix.**
3 Manson invented and had printed malaria charts which comprised numbers of coloured drawings of malaria parasites taken from various books mounted onto a single sheet. Reproduced in Patrick Manson, 'A Malaria Chart', *BMJ*, (1 Dec. 1894), 1252-1254, and here as Figure 3.
4 Edward Lawrie, (1846-1915), Lieutenant-Colonel, IMS. From 1885 until retirement Residency Surgeon at Hyderabad. See **Biographical Appendix.**
5 Letter 1.

Letter 4
02/066

Secunderabad
22nd May 1895

Dear Dr Manson,
On the 17th (the day after I finished my last letter) I made another dry smear of mosquito blood, which, like the former one showed spherules & pigments only. On staining it with water solution of methylene blue without fixing, the cellular structure of the spherules was shown more clearly; and they looked very different to similarly stained specimens of (a) fresh blood & (b) blood that had been kept liquid for two hours & then smeared & dried; the former of which gave, as before, only crescents & the latter mostly crescents & a few spherules and pigment masses.

This confirmed me in the view that crescents are transformed much more certainly into spheres in the mosquito's stomach than in specimens. I now determined however to make another attempt at liquid specimens, because I hate dry smears; so I thought it out, and gave the patient instructions to let the mosquitoes fill themselves completely, while I provided myself with a small pair of tweezers with which I could squeeze out the mosquito's stomach with one hand, while I held the cover glass with the other, ready to clap on. The result was my first perfect specimen of mosquito blood. About twenty minutes (?) had elapsed since the mosquito had begun sucking, and the haemoglobin was of course much diffused. The blood swarmed with perfect spherules, not very large (about 6μ in diameter) but showing an almost eruptive movement of the pigment as if flagella were about to burst forth in a moment. I looked in vain for flagellated organisms; not one was to be seen, to my surprise. In a very few minutes the pigment-oscillation (the intensity of which was much greater than in control specimens) began to quiet down. Many of the spheres were *shaking*, but as I have said, not one was flagellate. The general view however was very different from an ordinary specimen. All the spheres had *perfect* circular contours & I now noticed that they seemed to be in much larger numbers than in finger blood (contrary to my first impressions). Here are my notes in *thin* fields mostly -

$$7 . 3 . 9 . 7 . 1 . 2 . 3 . 2 . 2 . 0 . 2 . 2 . 1 = \frac{41}{13} = 3.1$$

the fields were consecutive ones & the numbers will give you some idea of the quantity of parasites. I made a specimen of a second mosquito at ¾ hours after beginning to suck & the results were precisely the same.

On counting the numbers of crescents, spheres & masses of pigment respectively, I obtained

	crescents	spheres	pigment
1st specimen	7	80	8
2nd	14	30	9
2nd specimen next day after 19 hours	0	8	32(?)

In both these the number of crescents is a great deal too favourable because it was possible to examine field after field without finding one. Of course the blood last sucked by the mosquito would contain most crescents.

Next day (18th) I began with a finger blood specimen, which gave when fresh

Crescents & ovals	Spheres	Pigment masses
39	10	1

Then I made two more liquid mosquito specimens at about $^1/_2$ an hour, my 18th & 19th mosquitoes.

Up to date I had observed only two flagellate bodies, both in finger blood. I was astonished that I did not meet more. Always the spheres seemed ripe for flagella, but they did not come (temperature of air 95°F). Now, directly I looked at mosquito 18 I saw flagellate organisms in every field; I saw 9 altogether in a few minutes, but instead of counting them I wasted my time looking at them. Two fields held two each & I could have found numbers, I do not doubt, if I had looked at once over the specimen. As it was the spectacle afforded by mosquito 18 was amazing. All the spherules seemed bursting with excitement & were exceedingly numerous. In contiguous fields I noted

$$6 . 10 . 8 . 7 . 10 . 14 . 12 . 16 = \frac{83}{8} = 10.0$$

But when I came to examine special fields I found

Sixty parasites in one field
Seventy two in the next!

all swarming & ready to burst. I think you will confess that no one has had such an experience as this in finger-blood. On looking through mosquito 19 I found the same swarms of spheres, but no flagellate organisms. I lit a cheroot, went home (though it was only 12 noon) & slept for three hours; the spectacle of flagella had ceased after about 10 minutes.

Next day (19th) I began with mosquito 20 of yesterday. Mostly pigment masses but about 20% still cellular. At 11.50 I made specimen of a fresh mosquito (21) at $^1/_2$ an hour, with a presentiment of what I was going to see.

4 flagellates in 1st field of 20 spheres
5 " a field of 12 "
3 " " 10 spheres

Flagellate organisms everywhere; one or two in every field. I must have seen over 30 or 40 though I examined only a few fields, being hardly able to tear myself away from individual organisms. The flagella were excessively fine, quite invisible in open spaces & seen in haemoglobinous serum & clot; but the flagellate organisms were unmistakable because they were being dragged about all over the field generally, or were quivering & being shaken as a dog shakes a rat. The manifestation ceased in a few minutes, though I saw flagellates for $^1/_2$ hour afterwards. Mosquitoes 22 & 23 at 70 & 90 minutes gave no flagellates & but few parasites comparatively. The patient was put under the net again. Mosquito 24 gave same results at 1/2 an hour as mosquito 21. 5 flagellates in one field of 12 parasites. Flagellate organisms everywhere, especially in open parts (?). Manifestation lasted in its intensity only for about five minutes.

On 20th & today I did not observe anything new, & I did not work yesterday. I have been engaged in studying the following questions. 1. Are all the masses of pigment met with *spent* spherules or merely broken ones? 2. Why do spherules often seem to become spent after a little, *without* the escape of flagella? 3. How is it that I have never been able to observe a swarming spherule become flagellate, all flagellate organisms seen by me having been so when I came upon them? 4. Is the greater number of parasites in mosquito only apparent?

I am not satisfied about any of these but have killed only 4 more mosquitoes. With respect to last question I have tried haemacytometer with results of 6000 parasites in cubic mm. in finger, & 316000 corpuscles only; and much the same in mosquito. But results not trustworthy. A comparison of ordinary specimens gives -

Finger 6 . 2 . 0 . 1 . 2 . 2 . 0 . 3 . 4 . 2 . 3 . 3 . 1 . 0 . 3 . 1 . 5 . 1 . 1. 2 in ordinary fields = 3.3, on average, a field

Mosquito 5 . 4 . 7. 4 . 10 . 10 . 9 . 9 . 7 . 3 . 4 . 8 . 3 . 5 . 5 . 7 . 4 . 4 . 5 . 5 . in ordinary fields, some very thin = nearly 6.0 on average.

The patient has had a little fever lately & I am obliged to give quinine; but have observed no fever parasites (not looked carefully).

23rd May. Another disaster among my mosquito grubs owing to heat I suppose. All dead, but a crop of small mosquitoes which seem *all to be males* & won't bite!

As mail goes today I will close with summary of results. I am inclined on the whole, after examining 28 mosquitoes, to gather that the stomach of the mosquito is very probably the natural *locus* for the crescent-spherule-flagella metamorphosis; & I base my opinion on the following five reasons -

1. The number of parasites in mosquito appears to be greater than in finger-blood (especially in some mosquitoes). In mosquito 18 I found fields of 60 and 72, as I have said; but in a control of the same time the largest number found in a field was 14. Further study is required.
2. It is certain (& very important) that in mosquitoes, at half an hour after beginning to suck, practically all the crescents have turned into perfect spheres; whereas in control specimens which have been kept for 1/2 an hour & much longer 70% of the parasites remain crescents & ovals (90 - 100°F).

3. In the mosquito the pigment of the spheres seems more scattered & much more active than in finger-blood; while almost all the spheres are in this swarming condition when the specimen is first made, whereas in controls many motionless spheres are seen.
4. In the large number of controls examined carefully by me I have only seen 3 flagellate organisms (1 yesterday) (temp. 90-100°F); whereas out of 11 good mosquito specimens I must have seen sixty or seventy at a modest figure, & these, all but one, in three mosquitoes 18, 21 & 24; & might have seen many more had I rushed through the specimens quickly enough. On two occasions I saw five flagellates in a field.
5. The phenomenon of ex-flagellation appears to be going on when the specimen is made & certainly ceases a few minutes afterwards. I have not yet watched a single spherule becoming flagellate however ripe it has appeared for that development.

I must now cease, Dr Manson, as I have numbers of letters to write; but cease with regret because I could write much more. I propose for the present to go over & over these points as opportunity affords, but alas! the wonder case which fortune has sent me is *drying up*, and I may be ordered off to Patiala in a day or two. I may tell you that after seeing mosquito 18, & much more after mosquitoes 21 & 24, I *felt* that practically the first step was assured; but I don't care to be incautious. You can imagine my excitement during the week; yet as I have been able to make step after step I have had a presentiment of what was coming. Of course the principal excitement was over the flagellate organisms. I *knew* that I would get them in 18 & still more in 21. The *first* mosquito of a batch examined will I think nearly always yield flagellates, the rest none - why? But the mosquito ought to be killed within half an hour. I leave you to judge as to value of evidence; but must state that every point you predicted seems to come true; certainly there is nothing contrary to the theory & certainly neither iced nor deep control specimens show any thing like the same degree of crescent-sphere-flagella metamorphosis as is seen in the mosquito. I look upon these observations to be as much yours as if you had made them; & if you think they will in any way advance the first steps of the mosquito-malaria theory please make use of them. They are facts but require sifting. Presently I shall give infected mosquitoes, & the water they have died in, to natives on payment & see result; then for seeing where the flagella go to. You will be very pleased with the following. The Maharajah of Patiala[1] in the Punjab (whose medical officer Surgeon Major Owen C.I.E., C.M.G.[2] I wrote to) has written officially to government asking for my services from 1st June to 1st Nov to investigate the fevers which abound in this country! What an opportunity. But government may possibly object; in which case I will ask you to help me in the B. M. J. I received a very nasty letter from head-quarters which knocked me over on 21st. I have found another typical spring tertian in my hospital. I laughed at Hehir for his 30% infected corpuscles; but see that Marchiafava notes 50%.[3] Kind regards to Mrs Manson

Yours truly

R. Ross.

Are you trying gnats[4] at home? Is anyone else working at mosquito?

1 Maharajah of Patiala - head of the Sikh nation in Northern India.

2 Surgeon-Major Charles William Owen, (1853-1922), IMS, CIE had persuaded the Maharajah of Patiala to approve a scheme whereby the latter would apply for Ross's services in a special malaria survey in the region. It was vetoed however by the Lieutenant Governor of the Punjab on the grounds of expense - see Letter 9, and R. Ross, *Memoirs with a Full Account of the Great Malaria problem and its Solution* (London: John Murray, 1923), 162. Henceforth, *Memoirs*.

3 Marchiafava and Bignami (1894), Chapter 9.

4 Mosquitoes were commonly called gnats until the late nineteenth century.

Letter 5
02/067

Secunderabad

28th May 1895

Dear Dr Manson,

I think that my last letter missed the post owing to the date of sailing having been advanced one day without sufficient notice; I am not sorry, because my former observations were somewhat erratic, and I have now been able to put in five days of more methodical and satisfying work. I have been going over & over the same ground and have been able, I think, to reach some definite conclusions respecting the first step of the metamorphosis inside the mosquito.

After writing I determined to follow your advice exactly, get a batch of full mosquitoes & examine one after the other at short intervals. On the 24th I obtained a batch of six mosquitoes all of which had begun biting nearly at the same moment, that is, directly the patient was put into the net. They were now dissected &

examined with the utmost rapidity possible at intervals of 8, 22, 40, 60, 120 & 180 minutes after they had begun to bite. The results were.

Mosquito 29, Examined at 8 minutes. Many crescents; mostly swarming spheres; one or two pigment masses in specimen. No pigmented leucocytes. No flagellate organisms seen either at first or 12 minutes afterwards.

Mosquito 30, Examined at 22 minutes. No crescents; all swarming spheres; some pigment masses, One flagellate organism.

Mosquito 31, at 40 minutes, all spheres & spent pigment masses - no flagellates - parasites comparatively few in number.

Mosquito 32, at 60 minutes. All spheres & many pigment masses. 2 nearly spent flagellates. A very few crescents.

Mosquito 33, at 2 hours. Spheres & pigment masses. No crescents. The pigment masses are certainly much more common than in mosquitoes 29-32. Out of 53 parasites, 30 were pigment masses & 23 spheres; but the spheres are almost all quiet without pigmentary movement, the pigment sometimes scattered 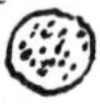 but generally collected motionless at a point near the circumference. 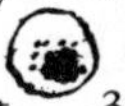

Mosquito 34, at 3 hours. About 30% of the parasites remain spheres; the rest 70% are pigment masses. The spheres are quite motionless with pigment collected near circumference. Some are swelled up & others present an irregular outline . Numbers of phagocytes containing 1, 2, 3 parasites each.

The above is taken from notes made between each mosquito. Before beginning the process I made a sealed control specimen from the finger which, together with mosquitoes 29-32 I reexamined whenever I had time in order to watch & compare progress, *pari passu*.

25th May. The process repeated

Mosquito 35, at 8 minutes. Crescents 30%. The rest spheres; one or two almost flagellate. No pigment masses.

Mosquito 36, at 20 minutes. A few crescents; mostly spheres with very active pigment; a few pigment masses. No flagellates.

Mosquito 37, at 30 minutes. Many crescents; mostly spheres; some pigment masses; no flagellates.

Mosquito 38, at 40 minutes. No crescents; swarming spheres; many pigment masses.

Mosquito 39, at 50 minutes. 35% only, spheres; 65% pigment masses. Many of the spheres still swarming. No flagellates. Pigment & parasites in phagocytes. No crescents.

Mosquito 40, at $2^1/_2$ hours. Spheres 43%; pigment 57%. The pigment in most of the spheres is collected motionless to one side; in some continues to oscillate slowly; while in many the bioplasm is swelled & irregular.

The above, with all my former experiments had now given me a very good idea of what occurs in mosquito's stomach. Sunday, 26th I set aside for experiments with haemacytometer - of which later. On 27th & 28th (today) the whole course of the 24th & 25th was repeated to make absolutely sure.

The result is that I can now make a definite statement of the life history of the parasite from its being drawn in to some hours later; and this with the greater certainty because the experiments invariably confirm each other with but trifling differences. You will observe that I found but few flagellates on 24th & none on 25th; these appeared again on 27th in a mosquito at 7 minutes, when I counted six, two in three fields each, all close together; also in the next mosquito but one, at 27 minutes, when I counted 11 flagellates, all close together in a few fields. I saw none today.

The progress of things, then, is this.

1. Almost all the crescents are converted into spheres very shortly after they enter the mosquito's stomach. Sometimes a fair number may be found at 10, 15, 20 minutes or even more; but these are almost always *seen in the same part of the specimen* and therefore belong probably to the *last intake of blood*. It is very rare to find more than *one* or *two* crescents in a whole specimen made at a longer interval. *Ovals* are not often seen. Untransformed crescents are I believe injured or *aborted* ones.

2. The spheres are always found. They have a perfect contour & contain a clear fluid which distinguishes them markedly from the masses of corpuscles in the midst of which they are generally found. At first their pigment is clustered together; then the outermost pigment particles begin to oscillate; lastly all the pigment particles commence *swarming* while the whole cell may take on a slight jerking rotatory movement.

3. Flagellate organisms may be found from 7 to 35 minutes or more. When seen, they lie almost always in great numbers in *contiguous fields* suggesting that they belong to the *same intake* of blood and have *ripened* at the same time. They are always, so far as I have experienced, found within a minute or two of the lens being brought into focus (my first survey being very rapid). The whole manifestation ceases in a very few minutes. Owing to this last fact & possibly owing to the *process of making the specimen allowing the*

flagella to free themselves, they are sometimes not to be found (?).
4. The spent pigment masses may sometimes be seen very early, even at 8 minutes, but then are *very few* in number. This number steadily increases, almost without fail, in successive mosquitoes; until, as in mosquito 39, they may reach 65% of all the parasites (not enclosed in phagocytes). Their appearance is quite characteristic, simply because they are not enclosed in the clear cells of the spheres compare  &  or  or 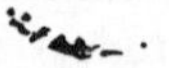. They are easily seen to be mere dead clusters of pigment, (sometimes with very feeble oscillations). They may be masses, rings, or *drawn-out* clusters. Their absence in the earliest mosquitoes & their large numbers in the latest show conclusively that they are due to a progressive metamorphosis inside the mosquito & not to *crushing* in making the specimen. But many of these may be *pigment rejected* by phagocytes which have swallowed spheres; I think Mannaberg[1] allows this.
5. Phagocytes containing spheres and pigment begin to be seen later than the spent pigment, at about 20 minutes or so; & increase in number up to about 2 hours.
6. About 30 or 40% of the parasites *fail* in *throwing out flagella* & remain as spheres, the pigmentary movements gradually becoming slower & slower, the pigment collecting in a heap to one side & then (2 hours) the bioplasm beginning to swell up irregularly (Laveran's old corps No 3).[2]
The above developments may be shortly stated in two sentences -
A. Practically *all* the crescents become spheres a few minutes after being taken into the mosquito's stomach.
B. From 30 to 40% of the spheres *die* after 1 or 2 hours; the rest having either given out flagella, been eaten by phagocytes, or having simply broken up (?).

29th May. These observations, then, prove conclusively that the crescent - sphere - flagella metamorphosis *does* go on inside the mosquito; which I think you said was to be considered as the first step in the theory. But it may now be said with reason that this does not prove that the stomach of the mosquito is the *natural locus* of the metamorphosis, because a similar metamorphosis may be seen to occur whenever the blood is drawn from the patient & allowed to remain still for a sufficient period. Against this objection, I will state that *the metamorphosis proceeds to a much greater degree in the mosquito that in control specimens of finger-blood.*

1st. The number of crescents which, in a finger-blood specimen, become spheres varies much in different specimens made at the same time & also in different parts of the same specimen. I think you will agree with me that from 10 to 70% of the parasites remain crescents. Thus this morning I made two good controls; in the first of which the crescents were only about 10% after 35 minutes; while in the second made shortly afterwards the crescents numbered from 50 to 70% after half an hour. In short it seems that the crescent-sphere metamorphosis is greatly influenced by certain local conditions of the specimen; but it may be stated confidently that a very fair number of undeveloped crescents are always to be found in finger-blood, even after the lapse of many hours. This is not the case in the mosquito; here, practically *no crescents* are to be found after half an hour or so. In fact I am prepared to state that I can distinguish at sight between a specimen which has been made directly from the finger and one in which the blood has passed for 5 or 10 minutes through the mosquito's stomach.

2ndly. I have remarked already on the greater violence of pigmentary movement in the mosquito.

3rdly. Since my last letter I have found flagellates in control specimens much more readily because I now know exactly the period when to look for them (10 to 20 minutes). Still I have never seen anything like the numbers witnessed in mosquitoes 18, 21, 24, 44 & 46.

4th. A curious proof from the *effect* of *quinine*. Patient has 15 grs on 27th & 10 grs yesterday morning. In my preliminary control of yesterday I was astonished to find hardly any of the crescents transformed, and, since I had seen the same before, after quinine, I thought that all the crescents had been killed. On examining my first mosquito at 10 minutes, I again found all the parasite *crescents*. This was quite contrary to all former observations; & I was now getting certain that the crescents were indeed dead, until, on examining my next mosquito at 20 minutes, I observed that the proportion of spheres was much greater, though crescents were still much commoner than they ought to have been. Successive mosquitoes gave fewer & fewer crescents, until after 69 minutes there were only three in the whole specimen, while the sphere-pigment metamorphosis had gone on as before. Returning now to my original control, I found all the crescents still there & no pigment masses. From which I conclude:-

Quinine *checks completely* the crescent sphere evolution in finger-blood; but only *delays* it in the mosquito. In other words, the mosquito's stomach has the power, apparently, of resuscitating parasites paralysed by quinine. Of course the effect of quinine on flagellate organisms has long been given; but it is generally stated that it has no effect on crescents.

On Sunday 26th I made some laborious attempts to estimate number of parasites in mosquito blood with haemacytometer. These all failed owing to difficulty of obtaining *enough* blood & dryness of air. I estimated parasites in finger blood at 1 to 410.3 corpuscles; that is 8000 parasites to 3,282,400 corpuscles in cubic millimetre of blood (my first attempt was computed wrongly). Number of parasites still appears to me to be generally much greater in mosquito; but I cannot get proof.

I have seen only one free flagellum, but some curious things. Do you think it possible that all the flagella are coils of a single long animal inside the sphere (?) Hardly possible. Tomorrow I begin second step - watching the flagella. Please send me advice. I watched a sphere this morning break up & become spent pigment apparently without exit of flagellum. Parasites continue decreasing slightly in numbers. Have dissected 54 mosquitoes up to date. My Parkes gold medal arrived.[3] No further news from Patiala. Three more cases of Tertian parasite in my hospital. On 25th I made a *certain experiment* on two men; of which you may hear later. Every one of your predictions has come true

With kind regards
Yours truly
R. Ross.

1 Julius Mannaberg, *The Malarial Parasites. A Description Based upon Observations Made by the Author and Other Observers*, trans. by R. W. Felkin (London: New Sydenham Society, 1894), 245. See **Biographical Appendix**.

2 Laveran's old corps no 3, in A. Laveran, *Traité des Fièvres Palustres avec la Description des Microbes du Paludisme* (Paris: Octave Doin, 1884), 177.

3 Ross won the Parkes Gold Medal of the Army Medical School, Netley, for an essay which he wrote in March 1895, while still on furlough. It analysed the epidemiology of malaria but remained unpublished. 'Malarial fevers; their causation and prevention. Da nobis lucem', Hand written manuscript, **RA** 05/019.

Letter 6
02/068

Secunderabad

5th June 1895

Dear Dr Manson,

I am in a state of great excitement & have no time to write you a full letter this week as the post goes out today. One of my "certain experiments" which I mentioned has come off.

On 17th May I took four full mosquitoes from the crescent case, Abdul Kadir, & put two in one bottle & two in another with a little water. They were kept in a cool place until the 25th June, when they were found dead on the surface of the water. In one of the bottles very small mosquito grubs were found, showing that the mosquitoes' eggs had been hatched. The contents of this bottle, minus the dead bodies of the mosquitoes, was given to a native Lutchman on 25th June [sic - May] at 8.0 a.m. on payment, after full explanation of the nature of the experiment.[1] The contents of the other bottle was given to another native in a similar way. I think myself justified in making this experiment, because of the vast importance a positive result would have & because I have a specific in quinine always at hand.

Lutchman is 20 years old, a healthy looking young fellow who *says* that he has never had fever. Yesterday he was all right. This morning at 8. a.m. (exactly 11 days from drinking the water) he came to the hospital-assistant complaining of head-ache. Temp. 99.8. Looking ill. Temperature has been taken every half hour & rose to 101.4 at noon, since when (1.30) it has been declining. This looks very promising. Incubation agrees closely with former experiments. The type ought to be either quotidian or summer tertian according to Marchiafava, &c. (crescents), which do not necessarily begin with rigor. There has been no rigor. Headache considerable. Three specimens carefully examined give no results; but such are not yet to be expected. If temperature rises again this afternoon it may be summer tertian. Chances are greatly against accidental fever, because out of the whole regiment I am getting only 3 or 4 cases weekly; these are always either spring tertians or *no parasite* (not carefully examined). Anyway, even if the attack is quite ephemeral, the result will be interesting. A third man drank mosquito water on 31st May.

The day after I wrote last the crescents in Abdul Kadir's blood began to cease abruptly & there were only 3 or 4 in specimen on 3rd June, when I was compelled to send him back to his regiment. I went through the whole "course of 24th May" again on 31st & 2nd June &

was able to make out the interesting fact that as the crescents decreased in numbers they became less able to turn into spheres in control specimens, while the whole metamorphosis was *delayed* in mosquitoes' stomach, but not *abrogated* as in finger blood. This gives the same result as obtained from quinine; but the patient had no quinine after 28th May. In short, after quinine or during convalescence, very few crescents become spheres in controls; but they all become spheres in mosquito's stomach about $^1/_4$ hour later than usual, that is in about $^1/_2$ hour from beginning to suck. I have seen no flagella since 29th. I forgot to tell you before the result of reexamination of mosquito blood at 10 minutes. If this contains a fair number of crescents & we examine again about 50 minutes afterwards, we find a large number of these crescents still remaining. If however we examine blood which has been kept in mosquito's stomach for one hour, we find practically no crescents at all. This I have seen over & over again; in fact, *making the specimen checks to a large degree the metamorphosis which was going on in the mosquito.* The same is true, I will venture to say, of ex-flagellation.

I must now break off as I have to write to my wife; but I hope to send you next mail a summary of results obtained from Abdul Kadir. Surgeon Major Owen (Patiala) wrote me a very nice letter about the Patiala investigation.[2] He is very keen about it, but apprehends delay from government. I ought to have begun this letter by congratulating you (or rather St George's) on the new course of lectures.[3] I am sure they will do wonders.

Yours truly

R. Ross.

Lutchman's temperatures today

8.0	8.30	9.0	9.30	10.0	10.30	11.0	11.30
99.8	100.4	101.2	101.2	101.4	101.4	101.4	101.2
12.0	12.30	1.0	1.30	2.0	2.30		
101.2	101.4	100.8	101.8	101.8	101.8		

|
(100.8)
R.R.

1 Although Lutchman disappears from Ross's correspondence with Manson after this early group of experiments, he remained in Ross's employ. Ross, *Memoirs*, 360, recounts leaving Lutchman on the Calcutta quay as he left for England in 1899, and of advertising unsuccessfully to try to locate his whereabouts in 1911. Lutchman features in a recent fanciful novel about Ross and the discovery of the malaria transmission cycle, Amitav Ghosh, *The Calcutta Chromosome* (London: Picador, 1997).

2 Letter from Charles Owen to Ross dated 28 May 1895, **RA** 01/071.

3 Manson first started giving public lectures on tropical medicine in 1894, at Livingstone College in Leytonstone, for missionaries. He was then appointed to both St. George's and Charing Cross Hospital Medical Colleges to offer them to medical students. Philip H. Manson-Bahr and A. Alcock, *The Life and Work of Sir Patrick Manson* (London: Cassell, 1927), 112.

Letter 7
02/003

21 Queen Anne Street,
Cavendish Square,
17th May 1895.

My dear Ross,
I was delighted to get your letters from Malta[1] and from Secunderabad[2] and to gather from them that you pursue the plasmodium with enthusiasm. You do not lack for material and energy and though you may get many a check I firmly believe you will work out some important result; you cannot fail to do so. Let this conviction fill your mind when inclined to despond, and look on a stone wall as a stimulant rather than as an insuperable barrier to progress. I have run my head against them often enough but somehow if I kept hammering at it and thinking about it sooner or later I got over or under or through when I had set my mind to it; and so will you.

I read Crombie's speech[3] and thought none the better of him for it. He is wrong in his facts and as a leader of the profession he is wrong to preach difficulty. I wonder what they asked Hart[4] out to India for. Was it to pat them on the back and to say they were wonderful fellows and to give them leather medals all round. Already you have proved that Crombie is wrong and that a diagnosis of malaria can be made with the microscope in less than five minutes. You must set them right about this in the first place. Crombie's speech will tend to undo all that Hart's speech might have done. Men are lazy enough at the best and are only too glad to get an excuse to persist in their laziness. If Crombie had sung a song of triumph and determination to overcome all difficulties he would have done much more good than this note of despair and "good enough for us" he has chosen to sound. 'Qui s'excuse s'accuse', seems applicable to the case. I was amused at his allusion to Hehir's work on the amoeba, etc...[5]

Soon I expect to hear that you have followed the plasmodium into the mosquito or some other suctorial insect. If you succeed in this you will go up like a shot and get any facilities you may ask for in the way of leisure for investigation and laboratory appliances and assistance. I only wish I were with you.

I am full up with preparing lectures for my course on tropical diseases at St Georges. I hate the labour of writing but I am in for it and have got to get it done somehow. My first lecture is next Tuesday. I have promised twenty - two a week - but so far have only some 8 or 9 ready. I wish they were all written.

In consequence of this work and a good deal to do in the way of practice I have not had much chance for further work at malaria. Indeed patients have been few for the last two months. I got a guinea worm case some time ago and have on hand a rare lot of infested cyclops.[6] It is really a very pretty experiment. I had some photomicrographs made of the cyclops by Pringle.[7] They show the embryos in the interior of the cyclops very well indeed. I shall try to get a spare one to send you one of these days. Pringle is very good natured but I dont like to ask too much from him.

The Hunterian speech[8] I have not got yet. There seems to be a hitch about the proofs. Why, I don't know.

Bakers' are going to lend me six of your microscopes[9] for my lectures. They will be well advertised therefore and I shall show my gratitude to you and to Baker by giving them a puff. He has already sold a considerable number and is now making a dozen.

Hoping to hear again from you soon and assuring you of my sympathies in your work and willingness to help you in any way I can.

I remain
Yours very truly
Patrick Manson

1 Letter missing.
2 Letter 2.
3 Crombie (1895).
4 See Letter 2, note 4.
5 P. Hehir, 'The amoeba coli; its relations to dysentery and tropical supurative hepatitis', *Indian Medical Gazette* (Nov. 1892), 321-326.
6 *Cyclops*, or the water-flea, is the host for the guinea-worm. Manson published a paper on this work, 'On the guinea worm', *BMJ* (30 Nov. 1895), 1350-1.
7 Andrew Pringle, whose photograph of these embryos was used in Manson's *Tropical Diseases: A Manual of the Diseases of Warm Climates* (London: Cassell, 1898), 514.
8 Manson (1894-1895).
9 Before returning to India, Ross had invented a small portable microscope which was brought out and sold by Mr H. C. Baker of Holborn. For details, see Edwin R. Nye and Mary E. Gibson, *Ronald Ross: Malariologist and Polymath* (Basingstoke: Macmillan, 1997), 231-4.

Letter 8
02/069

Secunderabad

10th June 1895

Dear Dr. Manson,
Many thanks for your letter of 17th May – but first about the man Lutchman. He had three days fever, but I failed entirely in finding any parasites in his blood. His temperatures were –
no rigor 5th June

8a.m	9	10	11	12	1	2	3	4
99.8	101.2	101.4	101.4	101.2	101.8	101.8	102.2	102.4

5	6	7	8	9	10	11	midnight
103.0	102	101.2	100.8	100.8	100.6	100.6	100.4

6th June

2.30a.m.	5.30	6.0	7	8	9	10	11
100.8	101	101	101.6	101.4	101.4	99.8	99.8

			no rigor					
12	1 p.m.	2	3	4	5	6	7	8
98.4	98	97	98.8	100	100	99.8	100	100
9	10	11	12					
100	99	99	98					

7th June

						no rigor		
4 a.m.	6.0	7	8	9	10	11	12	1 p.m.
98	98.4	98	97	97	96 (sic)	99.8	99.8	98.6
2	3	4	5 ...	9				
98.6	98	97	97	96.6				

normal

This gives three rises — at 8 a.m. on 5th, at 3 p.m. on 6th & at 11 a.m. on 7th. The first attack lasted 20 hours. Clearly it was intermittent fever possibly of a mild *postponing summer tertian* type. There was headache, but neither rigor nor splenic tenderness. Bowels constipated first day. No medicines given. Repeated examinations of the best possible fields of flattened smooth round corpuscles failed to show any parasites at all.

Remarks. The type, according to Mannaberg, should have been either summer tertian or quotidian because the original case contained syzygies.[1] I diagnose summer tertian because the first attack of fever lasted so long & there was something like a pseudo-crisis. With respect to the absence of the parasite I can only say that though I saw many ring-forms & pseudo parasites I never saw one which I was convinced was a parasite or which resembled in any way the young spring tertian forms with which I am now familiar. Compare Mannaberg or Marchiafava[2] (for instance p. 380). But I am examining the blood daily & may soon find *crescents.* The case certainly did not contain the common tertian type nor did the fever resemble one of the *spring* fevers. Perhaps there will be a relapse in a few days. On the whole I think that this result, occurring in my first case, is very encouraging. The second ~~case~~ man has not had fever; & it is only 10 days since the third drank the infected water.

12th June. No parasites in Lutchman's blood & no more fever. Neither of the other men has had fever. I am at present, as ill-luck has it, getting no cases of parasites & so have been dissecting a mosquito or two, pricking fingers at random and playing golf. The rains have broken, thank heaven, & it is only 88° in the verandah at noon. I found a beautiful double tertian some miles from here; but the man was too ill to be moved. The doctor asked me to look at the blood as he thought it was a *funny case.* During the last two days however I have examined six fever cases without seeing a single parasite. They were all fresh infections but were examined only before noon - golf in the evening - festina lente. Not even pigmented leucocytes. Yet the specimens were good with thousands of perfectly round smooth corpuscles (field B below).

The following is a summary of results from Abdul Kadir's case. I am pretty well confident of the truth of all the facts (so far as may be judged from one case) except fact 7, and of that - I should bet heavily on it. Nearly 70 mosquitoes were examined under microscope.

Summary from Abdul Kadir's case

The crescent-sphere metamorphosis

mosquito	**control specimens**
1. Almost all the crescents become spheres	1. Only a percentage of crescents become spheres
2. After quinine or during convalescence the transformation is delayed for about 1/4 hour; but eventually almost all the crescents are changed.	2. After quinine or during convalescence (?) a very few of the crescents only become spheres, the rest remaining unchanged for hours.
3. The act of making the specimen of a mosquito at 5 or 10 minutes checks the metamorphosis in a number of crescents.	

The sphere-flagella metamorphosis

4. The pigment movement is very active in nearly all the spheres from 10 to 20 or 30 minutes.	4. The pigment movement does not appear quite as vigorous as in mosquito.
5. Crowds of flagellate organisms may be seen in fresh-made specimens from mosquitoes up to 35 minutes or even more after their beginning to bite. I have twice seen 5 in a field.	5. It is rare to find more than two or three flagellate organisms in a specimen.
6. After 1 or 2 hours about 70% of the parasites have become spent pigment or have been devoured by phagocytes. The rest remain as dead motionless spheres. In these last a secondary brownian pigment oscillation may start again when the bioplasm swells after many hours.	6. Much the same as in mosquito, except that crescents which do not change at first rarely change afterwards; also many spheres may be watched breaking up without emission of flagella. The unchanged crescents appear to shrivel up simply after some hours

7. (?) The parasites are more numerous in the stomachs of some mosquitoes than in the finger-blood.
8. Out of three men to whom mosquito-water was given one contracted fever on 11th day.

On looking through my notes of the case & recalling the various observations it seems to me that when the crescents were most numerous in the blood, that is on about 20th May, they were also the most vigorous, that is, most capable of giving out flagella. What makes me so confident of the results is the fact that the experiments supported each other *without fail*, while I went right through the "course" on six different occasions, getting the same results on each occasion (except delay of metamorphosis due to quinine & convalescence). In fact I can tell in a minute (a) whether the blood has been through the stomach of mosquito or not & (b) how long it has been in the mosquito; and that by looking at the *parasites* alone.

I have now I think given you almost all the facts I have observed in connection with this case; but please send me any questions you would like to ask. My resolves for the future are:-
a. To try mosquitoes on all cases of parasites, not only crescents, which I get. I ought to have done this before, but felt that I would or might mistake intracorpuscular forms for spent-pigment.
b. To dissect & study anatomy of all mosquitoes.
c. To try infection by mosquito water methodically.
I should like to get your advice.

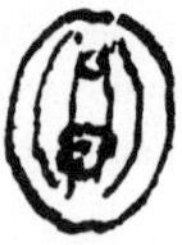

In several mosquitoes I find bodies like this which seem to me to be parasites, perhaps coccidia. They were about 20μ in length & were very numerous.

Very many thanks for your letter & especially for your patronising my microscope. Please suggest to Baker any improvements. I found my fine adjustment to be *execrable*. It will *never do*. The mirror mechanism is bad, & the oil-bottle ought to have a long stopper. I shall endeavour to reply to Crombie[3] when I have a little more experience. Certain it is that there is something funny about the non-appearance of the parasite in many of the cases, which requires to be worked out. Hehir is a curious man; he doesn't seem inclined to confess his errors. There was an article by him on malaria in March or April number of the Indian Medical Record[4] which you can see at the libraries. The photo of the cyclops I should like very much. Haven't got a case of guinea-worm.

My wife will send you a leading article from the Allahabad

Pioneer,[5] our principal paper, commenting on the Rajah of Patiala's application to government for my services for malaria investigation. I wrote to editor mentioning it & he is evidently taking it up. Would the B.M.J. like to touch upon it? but perhaps better wait for a mail or two; or only just mention it in the briefest way. I fear that government won't give my services without some such notice. Owen is very keen upon it & wants to work himself at mosquito. I have sent him directions. The Rajah gives me R1200 a month, travelling expenses & assistance; & we shall make a big thing of it, I hope, & do good work. The investigation lasts from 1st June to 1st November only; & I can't think why government is causing so much delay. I wanted to be up before the beginning of the rains. Do you think that you would like to come out to Patiala instead of Demerara?[6] I should like to sound Owen about it, if I go there. The final tracing of the flagella will be a difficult job, I fear; but we could have things ready for you. Of course I shall begin to try at once, but doubt my capacity in spite of your encouraging letter.

About Daniels' article in B.M.J. for April 27th,[7] I should like to reply later. The way not to mistake intracorpuscular forms for vacuoles is to look in a part of specimen where vacuoles are rarely found. In specimens made after your method we get five different kinds of fields which I find it very useful to distinguish thus:-

Field A. Very thin. The haemoglobin is crushed out of the corpuscles & forms a thin homogenous yellow field containing only shadows of corpuscles.

Field B. A little deeper. All the corpuscles are smooth, not crenated nor vacuolated, lying separate or tessellated; the serum is clear. This is the best field for intracorpuscular forms.

Field C. The corpuscles lie fairly separate but are crenated and vacuolated owing to no pressure being exerted on them by the cover-glass.

Field D. The corpuscles are in rouleaux. Good for crescents and crescent-sphere-flagella metamorphosis

Field E. The marginal clot of drying blood. Good for all sorts of pigment masses.

Have you ever seen a phagocyte take in a whole swarming sphere & *burst it*, as we burst grapes between the tongue and palate? I have, several times. It is done in an instant. Another point - the quinine & fever forms described by Mannaberg[8] occur, I think, only after the specimen has been made for some 20 minutes.

With kind regards, believe me

Yours truly

R Ross.

I shall write again when I have *something to say.*

1 Mannaberg (1894), 329-372.

2 Marchiafava and Bignami (1894); Mannaberg (1894). Mannaberg comments, p. 380, that in fresh infections, during the first days of illness, 'the parasite is sometimes missed'.

3 Letter 7, note 3.

4 P. Hehir, 'Plasmodium malariae, its importance in the diagnosis of tropical diseases', *Indian Medical Record*, 8 (1895), 326-328.

5 Untraced, *Pioneer* unavailable.

6 Manson had applied to the British Medical Association for a grant to enable him to go to Demerara, British Guiana, to test his malaria-mosquito hypothesis. Although he secured some money, he was unable to obtain any further support from the Royal Society, so the expedition foundered. Manson-Bahr and Alcock (1927), 113, 129-30, and below, Letter 16.

7 C. Daniels, 'The demonstration of malarial organisms', *BMJ* (1895), 920, argued that staining slides helped prevent mistaking vacuolated cells seen in anaemia for intracorpuscular parasites.

8 Mannaberg (1894), 401-411.

Letter 9
02/302 [postcard]

Dear Dr Manson.

I have had a trying week & have examined over twenty fever cases some carefully, without finding one parasite. The Spring Tertian seems to have ceased since the 31st May. At last, yesterday, one case of crescents, unfortunately a prisoner, in another hospital. Will try to get mosquitoes off him tomorrow. Don't know what to make of the cases. Fields B show perfect corpuscles.[1] No pigment nor pigmented leucocytes. Yet some high fever distinctly intermittent at times. Studying further. Second crescent case slight dysentery again & very little fever. Like Abdul Kadir's case. Yours R. Ross.

Sec'bad 19th June.

Lieutenant Governor of the Punjab objects to Patiala investigation.[2]

Fear it is done for.

Rains set in.

1 See Letter 8.

Letter 10
02/070

Secunderabad
26th June 1895

Dear Dr Manson,
The day after I sent my last post-card I found another crescent case in an out-hospital, again in a case of slight dysentery. But the authorities would not allow him to be transferred to my hospital because he was a prisoner. This is very annoying because I want to confirm my results from Abdul Kadir by means of another case of crescents. I took my mosquitoes however to the out-hospital, but they refused to bite, owing to the cold wet monsoon wind, I think. However, I shall try again perhaps.

I brought back Abdul Kadir to my hospital since he still has a few crescents but I was allowed to have him for only two days. I went through the "course" twice however. It appears useless to repeat this process on the man (I have done it eight times now) because the results are invariable in every experiment. The man has been having much quinine lately & consequently the crescents scarcely transform at all in finger-blood specimens. They remain unchanged for an hour or more (temperature of air 75°F) & then perhaps one out of four or five becomes a sphere. I saw one flagellated body with *8* distinct flagella. What now is so remarkable is that in the mosquitoes they are *all* transformed in 20 minutes at most. In six mosquitoes containing about 15 to 20 parasites each, I found only *one* crescent - all the rest were spheres or spent pigment. In these cases I examined the mosquitoes as well as the controls most thoroughly & deliberately & I am absolutely *certain* now of the great effect produced by the insect's stomach on the crescent-sphere transformation, at least so far as I can judge by one case alone (Abdul Kadir). It is a remarkable & significant fact.

There is much to be studied in the ex-flagellation process (shall we call it *ecdysis*?). In the prisoner I watched a sphere throw out flagella which almost immediately curled up round the cell & stopped moving (certainly within 120 seconds). Mannaberg describes this somewhere.[1] The extreme brevity of the stage in this case shows why one so often misses flagellated organisms. I saw none in my last mosquitoes though spent pigment masses abounded & showed that the process was occurring. When they *are* found I think they are generally found in *clear* serum. This suggests that in viscid blood the flagella are able to leave the cell so rapidly & easily that scarcely a movement is seen - what do you think? I remember that in mosquitoes 18, 21 & 24 nearly all the flagellate bodies were in pretty clear serum. But why do the flagella sometimes curl up so quickly? Also why do the cells sometimes break up without any flagella at all? Have you seen this? Why have I seen so few free flagella in the mosquitoes?

After examining my 20 negative cases I began to think that I was too stupid to recognise the small amoeboid intracorpuscular forms. On 19th June however I looked at a fresh fever case & immediately spotted them without difficulty. They were the typical annular forms. Since then I have had another case - both had *exactly* the characteristics of the *summer* tertian, & the parasite was quite different from the *spring tertian*, which has ceased here since 31st May. The case in Bombay I see now must have been summer tertian from the chart & presence of crescents; so that in May & June I have found altogether 6 spring tertians, 2 quartans, 3 summer tertians, 5 crescent cases & 1 with an undetermined fever form = 17 cases. What has made me rather conceited is that most of my 20 negative cases mentioned in post-card[2] turned out to have a curious *continued* fever lasting 4 or 5 days. They all began in a batch after the first heavy rain. On the whole I don't think I can have actually missed the parasite in more than 4 or 5 true malaria cases – & this though I made no persistent search. In fact I am inclining to the view that when the parasites are present they can usually be found in 2 or 3 minutes at most.

In an infected mosquito kept over one week I found some bodies like this [DRAWING][3] like those I mentioned before only much smaller – about 7μ in length. They look like coccidia. I wish I could get some literature on the pebrine corpuscle. Blanchard[4] only touches on it.

On 21st & 22nd we had two cases of cholera in the regiment. Both died in 9 hours; & they gave us a scare indeed. Examined blood for Hehir's organism & wired him to come & show me; but he replied that he had no time.[5] Fortunately no more cases. Hope to get some more crescents to work on soon. With kind regards,

Yours truly

R. Ross.

Have got six mosquitoes from Abdul Kadir maturing in order to give to a man. About 15 or 20 parasites in each. I shall give them all together. No crescents in Lutchman, nor any more fever.

1 Mannaberg (1894), 270-273.

2 Letter 9.

3 Drawing missing from hole in letter.

4 Raphael Blanchard, *Traité de Zoologie Médicale* 2 vols (Paris: J.-B

Ballière, 1889-1890), II, 540. See **Biographical Appendix**.

5 P. Hehir, 'Microscopical observations on the blood and excreta in cases of cholera', Special supplement to the *Indian Medical Gazette*, (1892). We have not been able to examine this article. Hehir's early views on cholera do not appear to have been especially influential. See, more generally, Jeremy D. Isaacs, 'D D Cunningham and the aetiology of cholera in British India, 1869-1897', *Medical History*, 42 (1998), 279-305.

Letter 11
02/004

21 Queen Anne Street, Cavendish Square,
21st June, 1895

My dear Ross,

I am exceedingly obliged for your letters. I look forward to receiving them with the greatest interest and when a mail passed without getting one the other day I was terribly disappointed for I thought you had fallen sick, or that you had got a check, or that you had given up the quest. Above everything don't give it up. Look on it as a Holy Grail and yourself as Sir Galahad and never give up the search, for be assured you are on the right track. The malaria germ does not go into the mosquito for nothing, for fun or for the confusion of the pathologist. It has no notion of a practical joke. It is there for a purpose and that purpose depend upon it is its own interests - germs are selfish brutes.

Your finds are most interesting and encouraging. The mere fact that the parasite is not digested is enough to prove to my mind that it is in its proper habitat and the fact you have discovered that it advances in development more rapidly and more frequently in the mosquito's stomach is confirmatory of this inference. But now the struggle to advance the next step begins. What next to look for and where to look.

I think you would do well to prepare a series of stained preparations from mosquito blood illustrative of what you have already done. I think that such as series of preparations would show the progress of development better than anything else as they could be made so rapidly at a few minutes interval and could then be stained and examined at leisure: If you have time to do this and if you are generously inclined send me a series either in bottle or stained or both. I am appointed to open a debate or something of that sort on the malaria germ at the next meeting of the British Medical Association at the end of July[1] and if I was armed with a series of such preparations I could speak with an authority of your work which could not be contraverted and you may be sure I will give you a good shove and help you so far as I can to get the ear of the authorities in India who may be in a position to forward your investigations. That Rajah is a brick. Tell him he is a public benefactor and ring his name out for the oriental loves publicity of that sort and likes to play the game of tit for tat.

About the next step. Among other things examine the dung, the little yellow specks you see on the glass the insect is kept in, for evidence of malarial products. It may contain nothing but it is easily examined. Then I should examine the ova of the mosquito from time to time before and after they are deposited in the water for I have an idea the beast gets into them and so into the larva and becomes a more or less permanent parasite not only in the individual mosquito that sucked him in but in the progeny of this mosquito. This will be a more difficult matter. Then I should keep mosquitos to maturity and tease them up in salt solution and examine their tissues one by one searching inside all cells for something like the plasmodium. I question if he will be pigmented but I am fairly sure he is intracellular. This too will be a long and difficult task. But it is not without hope. Look about the kidney tube or the analogous structure, about the long caecal tubes, about the little corpuscles representing the blood corpuscles in the walls of the stomach / in the muscles of the thorax. Compare malaria fed mosquitoes with non malaria fed mosquitoes and compare their progeny.

If you would experiment create an artificial marsh by allowing the water in which the mosquito has died and laid her eggs and in which her progeny have been swimming about to dry up / then pulverise this and get someone to inhale the dust you stir up from it. Or drink it suspended in water. The experiment would be interesting but perhaps not altogether safe. *Dulce et decorum est pro patria mori.*[2] But don't do it yourself.

My guinea worms are still alive in the cyclops and slowly undergoing changes.[3] It is now over six weeks since they entered the crustacean and they are still quite lively only casting their skins and dropping their tails according to last report three days ago. I hope you will have a chance of a fling at this subject as well as at malaria and filaria.

I must close my letter now as I have a lot to do this afternoon and I don't want to miss the post or to let you suppose I don't take a great interest in your work and give you an excuse of not writing to me.

With all good wishes for continued success I remain
Yours very sincerely
Patrick Manson

I give you a new tip I have I think arrived at. In looking for amoebae in liver pus look not in the pus coming from the centre of the abscess but in the pus arising from the abscess wall — that is in the pus that comes from the drainage tube 2 or 3 days after operation. The amoeba lives in the breaking down liver & not in the mature pus.[4] I have now found it, & in profusion, in the drainings of two liver abscesses, in the pus of which at the time of exploratory aspiration & operation I failed to find it. This is a reason why the amoeba is so often missed.

1 Sixty-third Annual Meeting of the British Medical Association held in London, 30 July to 3 August 1895. Manson gave a paper in the Section of Pathology on 'Some facts in the life history of the malaria parasite', reported in *Lancet* (3 Aug. 1895), 302. He incorporated much of this material in his Goulstonian Lecture, below Letter 32, note 3.

2 Horace, *Odes,* book III, ii, 13.

3 See Letter 7.

4 Manson discussed hepatic abscesses in his *Tropical Diseases* (1898a), 343-78. See, especially, 362-363.

Letter 12
02/071

Secunderabad

10th July 1895

Dear Dr Manson,

During the last fortnight I have not been able to find a single fresh case of malaria though I have been hunting all round the station for them. I find by statistics that this is the least feverish time of year; it is cloudy, windy, rainy, with temperature about 75° or 80°. There are a few cases of rather severe continued fever. One of my May spring tertians has had a relapse – the same parasites again, quite different from quartan or summer tertian. In this relapse the parasites were very few & all, except one, the youngest & smallest amoeboid forms (never ringed); yet I *spotted* them almost at once; so that when I don't find parasites I am now confident that I don't overlook them. Moreover I don't believe Crombie's statement that an intermission is pathognomonic of malaria,[1] because several of the continued fevers show often one intermission at the end; & I have two curious cases in which the temperature is normal every morning & rises to 100 or 101 every evening, & yet there is not a sign of pigment or parasites in the blood while quinine has no effect whatever & there is an intensely sore spot to left of umbilicus in each case, also pultaceous[2] stools. Crescents have gone from Abdul Kadir's & the prisoner, Ramasami's blood; the latter had never more than a few crescents & was not a good case to work with; but I took over my mosquitoes & was disappointed to find no crescents to receive them. I have looked in all sorts of cases for crescents without result. In spite of offering rewards to hospital assistants of the civil & other hospitals I can't get a case. I thought I should find cases in the civil hospital the other day to a certainty, but was disappointed. I don't know what's up with the place. Yet there are tanks & marshes everywhere & only a scanty rainfall. The huts of my regiment are practically just over a great tank with muddy, drying margins – yet out of 800 odd men, no malaria. I will tell you why – because the mosquitoes don't thrive this windy weather. I will bet on your suggestion that malaria is in the first place a disease of mosquitoes – hence the idea of it being carried by winds etc. It is the *mosquitoes* & not the *germs* which are carried by the wind. They probably deposit the germs in the drinking water. This is the reason why I am beginning to work with drinking water instead of with an artificial marsh as you suggest. If the germs were so numerous in the air as to infect one person they ought to infect *many*; this will not explain isolated cases satisfactorily. It appears much more likely that only those persons are infected who have drunk water by chance out of a chatty or water pot in which an infected mosquito has laid her eggs – the infected mosquito may of course have been blown from a marsh, where the disease is rife among the mosquitoes, or may have recently bitten a malaria case. During windy weather mosquitoes don't thrive. I have received your letter of 21st June; & many thanks for it; I am very glad that you think the first finds from Abdul Kadir encouraging & much annoyed that I haven't been able to confirm them with another case & above all, that I can't send you a series of specimens. I was often on the point of attempting such a series with Abdul Kadir; but I had determined before-hand not to make specimens but push on & obtain as much certainty as possible about the *first step*. I had only a fortnight to do this in & expected every day that the crescents would disappear suddenly. Next case will enable me to send you specimens; also dried infected mosquitoes, I hope. *The* point of importance brought out from Abdul Kadir's case was that *all* the crescents are transformed in the mosquito – don't you think so? It is a fact I am convinced. The crescents & spheres are so different that it is impossible to make a mistake. About the absence of digestion of the parasite it may be said simply that this will require time & that therefore we can't expect them to be digested at once. The blood doesn't become viscid for 1/2 an hour about.

It may also be argued that since the crescent - sphere - flagella transformation takes place in all blood drawn from the body, why shouldn't it also take place in blood drawn by mosquito? I can only answer that it takes place there to a much greater extent; all the crescents become spheres, even after quinine; numbers of flagellate bodies may be seen; 70% of parasites become spent pigment.

If I am luckier than lately I may be able to send you a series of specimens by next mail, in time for the B.M. Association meeting. Am going crescent hunting furiously tomorrow again. It is *very* annoying that I can't get a case.

Why did not I find more *free* flagella? Either they dash away into the tissues at once, or, I am beginning to think, cease to move almost as soon as they free themselves from the cyst. They have to scurry out of the cyst for fear of the phagocytes; but after that may develop without movement in the contents of the stomach – again what do you think? Oh for another case! I make this conjecture because there ought to be numbers of free active flagella in mosquitoes' blood, whereas I saw only two or three; while on the other hand they may be seen to cease moving in a few minutes. In mosquitoes 18, 21 & 24 there ought to have been swarms of free flagella apparent, *if they had continued wriggling.*[3] I think that this point requires study before attacking the question of the tissues; I shall work with much thinner films than, for fear of bursting the spheres, I did before. Don't you think that the flagella ought first to be found free in the stomach? Staining etc must be tried. As soon as this is done, I shall go on & follow your advice exactly about the tissues.

Many thanks for your intention to bring my first attempts before the Association; it will be just the thing; but I wish I had specimens to send you. It may be useful however just to mention the results obtained & also touch on the experimental case of fever. I may have a similar case by next mail.

Many thanks again for your letter; it was a great pleasure to get it. Also for the tip about amoeba coli. I shall certainly try the guinea worms etc when I get an opportunity. I have one case of beriberi contracted at Cuttack. Tomorrow morning I am going to see some horses said to have intermittent fever. Am thinking of sending an account of the mosquitoes to South Indian branch of B.M. Ass. in order to work them up a little.[4] Nobody is doing anything in the microscope line. The Patiala investigation has collapsed entirely owing to opposition of Lieut. Governor of Punjab.[5] Owen does not want the British Medical to take it up; so there is nothing further to be done. It is a pity. Will write to you about it later & hope to send you some letters I have received; they are amusing. With kind regards, I remain

Yours truly

R. Ross.

1 Alexander Crombie, 'Presidential address in medicine and pathology', *Indian Medical Gazette* (Jan. 1895), 8-14, discusses the relationship between malarial and other kinds of fevers, using intermittence and remittence as central criteria in their differentiation.

2 semi-fluid; pap-like.

3 See Letter 4.

4 Ross read a paper on his researches in December 1895 which was subsequently published in the *Indian Lancet* in 1896; *Memoirs*, 156.

5 Sir Dennis Fitzpatrick - see Letter 4, note 2 and Letter 25.

Letter 13
02/005

28th June 1895

My dear Ross,

Your last letter[1] was supremely interesting and, if the experiment you describe turns out to be something more than a mere coincidence, you may be congratulated on having clenched the whole matter of the rôle of the mosquito as alternative host of the malaria parasite. It is most interesting and, moreover, of the highest practical and scientific importance. Prove it by one or two more experiments and the Indian Government will give you anything you like in the shape of opportunity for further work. If they won't they ought to and if they don't I shall take care that it is made pretty hot for them here.

In my last I think I told you that I had to open a debate on the subject of malaria at the meeting of the B. M. Association at the end of July. Try to have me in possession of all your facts & some slides if possible up to date and I shall make a carefully prepared statement of how things stand and bring the matter out so to speak officially. I think it would be a mistake to make any definite announcement yet or before we were quite certain. This much we might say even now viz. that the crescent evolutes in the mosquito; but that is not enough; it is an interesting fact and a necessary fact for our theory but it does not prove it. Your experiment on malariating a man with mosquito water does prove it if repeated experiment gives similar results.

My idea about the beast in the mosquito is as I think I told you that it is transmitted in a sort of hereditary way from mother mosquito to sons and daughters as a cell parasite; that it gets to man in mosquito dust - the debris of dead mosquitoes in which the germ has been encysted; that these germs on entering the human mouth, air passages, or swallowed in the saliva or what not, or as in your experiment in water, penetrate the human mucous membrane as they do the mosquito's stomach and so get into his circulation. An experiment I should like to see tried would be to evaporate some water in which malariated mosquitoes had died - say in some small glass bottles, to evaporate it thoroughly, so that the sediment will not decompose, but to evaporate it in the sun so as not to scorch it and also so as to resemble what occurs in nature; to have this transmitted to England; to add there a little water to the dried sediment and then to drink it. I am willing to try.[2] A positive result to such an experiment would be irrefutable. Another experiment worth trying would be to pulverise this same sediment or the bodies of desiccated malariated mosquitoes and then inhale the dust.

A suggestion I would make about these experiments is that the mosquito water, or mosquito dust, should be taken or inhaled first thing in the morning and on an empty stomach so that there would be no danger of its having its included germs destroyed by the stomach juices.

Pay some attention to the mosquito grubs in malariated mosquito water; it may be that they take in the germ in the water they swallow.

Another hint I would give you. Send specimens of the mosquito for identification of species. Possibly different species of mosquito modify the malaria germ; that the differing degrees of virulence depend on the difference of species of mosquito that has served as alternative host to the parasite.

Collect as many malariate mosquitoes as you can bottling them in some preservative - as glycerine and water and labelling the bottles with date and time from hour of blood ingestion.

If your experiments have turned out successful I would advise you to apply to the government for leave to devote yourself to the matter and for assistance and some sort of a laboratory although I don't think the latter is very necessary - in fact it is a man's work to keep it laboratory-like and that is not its purpose.

Simplicity is the best guarantee of success. As little machinery as you can get along with. Let the other fellows, the men who are going to come after you, worry with these things and elaborate in detail the big principles which you indicate and establish. Go for principles - not details too much.

I have not had a malaria case for a month. I hear of some mosquitoes at the docks and if I got my case I should have a try for the malariation of the insect and the consumption of his infusion myself.

Meanwhile I am still observing from time to time my guinea worm embryos which are still alive - seven weeks - in my cyclops. They are slowly evoluting. Many have now cast their skins once, some I think twice, and have dropped their tails. I have a good mind if the development goes on to try, when it is completed, to persuade myself that it is justificable to swallow one or two. What do you think is the duty of the father of a family in such as case. Would he be justified?

My lectures are getting on and I am well through my session. I have also been made lecturer to Charing Cross Hospital[3] on the same subject and will do my course there in the winter - probably in January and February.

Wishing you every success in your most important work I remain yours very truly

Patrick Manson

I have seen the proofs of the Hunterian Lecture. I corrected them, but have not had any copies yet: I shall send you some as soon as they arrive.

1 Letter 6.

2 Cf. Letter 11, where Manson cautions Ross from performing such an experiment on himself.

3 See Letter 6, note 3.

Letter 14
02/072

Secunderabad
17th July 1895

Dear Dr Manson,

Your very pleasant letter of 28th June reached me only yesterday. It is very encouraging to me to get your letters; but you *must not* feel called upon to waste your time in replying to mine unless you have absolutely nothing better to do. It is a great pleasure to me to write to you on work in which I take so much interest; but if I find myself encroaching on your time I shall stop!!! I know how busy you are, you see. I enjoy sitting down once a week to scribble to you; & you must excuse me doing so, even when I have nothing particular to say as, alas! has been the case lately; remember that I am an exile with no one to talk to about malaria germs! but you must not waste time over replying unless you think it necessary.

First about my results during the week. It has been an interesting one, but not a single crescent or case to work with on mosquitoes. I am nearly wild, & have been able to do nothing for nearly six weeks now. I have been all round the hospitals again & have touts out everywhere &, with great difficulty have obtained three bazaar people - no crescents. The bazaar people won't come to me even though I offer what is enormous payment to them. I offer 2 & 3 rupees for a single finger prick & much more if I find crescents - they think it is witchcraft. Even my own gardener woman refused to allow me to prick her finger more than once. However I think luck is about to change. I must depend clearly on the sepoys of the native regiments who are not so superstitious; and during the week I have had five beautiful cases containing fever forms. One a relapse of spring tertian - only a few parasites. Two small amoeboid unpigmented ring-forms, either quotidian or tertian. One containing the same together with pigmented leucocytes; & the last my first case of quotidian - a beautiful case - several nearly mature forms, with the exact characteristics given by Marchiafava,[1] & also a swarm of young amoebae, sometimes two in a corpuscle (conjugating - Mannaberg).[2] These four summer-autumn fevers ought to yield crescents next week - I think the last will. I am studying them very carefully. I think that the Italian classification[3] must undoubtedly be accepted. Our typical 'old gold'[4] corpuscle seen, but no sporulating form as yet. These four are all fresh infections. Also, do you know, I believe that I have come upon a new variety altogether; but have not observed it sufficiently yet to let you know about it; the corpuscles seemed to be infected with 1, 2, or 3 very minute forms like this 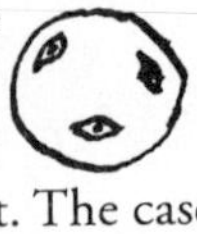 which oscillated within them & on turning sideways became like this 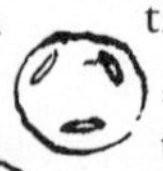, without the central dot. The case is a child & I found three bodies with some similar but much larger ones 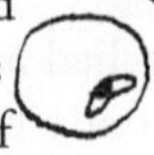 in four specimens. Perhaps after all they are some kind of vacuole - but they move & turn around! - we will see.[5]

I also examined five horses with fever - chart not intermittent - no parasites seen.

The fourth *experimental case* has had no result (now 15 days). But the malarialised mosquitoes contained only a few parasites each & were kept too long dead I think. Thus only one out of 4 cases contracted fever; and though that fever *looked* like a malarial one (summer tertian - not clear) I could find no parasite. Yet the incubation period was quite correct and when we come to think of all the chances of failure in such experiments we must by *no means* expect success in more than a small percentage of cases, at least at first. We have to find how long to keep the malarialised mosquitoes, because it is not at all unlikely that there is a definite point of time when they or their eggs or excreta must be given in order to produce fever - don't you think so? The malaria germs must be mature on the one hand & on the other if the dead mosquito be kept too long they may be devoured by other putrefactive organisms. In all my cases I did as you suggest - gave the mosquito water first thing in the morning. I think it more advisable to begin by experimenting with drinking water, because, here at all events, the exceedingly small number of cases out of a force of 800 men suggests a very localised cause. The men willing to be experimented on are moreover very few. Don't for heaven's sake mention at the B. M. Association that Lutchman is a dhooley-bearer - did I tell you so? - he is a Government servant. To give a Government servant fever would be a crime! (Also, I will add here, to give a lecturer on tropical diseases at two London hospitals guinea-worm would be a worse one).[6]

Now for your kind offer to bring the matter out officially before the Association - you see I have no specimens to send you & it would now be too late even if I had. I have already however put you in possession of 'all my facts up to date.' These facts prove, as you say with such precision, that 'the crescent evolutes in the mosquito'; it is 'an interesting fact & a necessary fact for our theory, but it does not prove it.' That is exactly how I would put it; but I think we may fairly add that the evolution goes on to a greater degree in the mosquito than in finger-blood specimens; and also that 1 out of 4 malariating experiments gave some sort of fever after 11 days, the correct incubation period; the chances against such being an accident being considerable. Still, all this is *very far* from a certainty.

I fear you will have been much disappointed in the absence of progress during the last few weeks; but wait till I get on the track of those crescents again! Myself & family of mosquitoes (which I keep in stock) are raging for them. But I have now seen and worked on all the varieties of malaria & have dissected many ordinary mosquitoes. Wait till my quotidian shows crescents!

You must not think of trying the cyclops. What I suggest is this. Bribe the man at the bar in the House of Commons to put the cyclopses in the drinks of the M. P.s. It would draw attention to science, put a stop to much useless talking by keeping the M. P.s off their legs, and not injure anyone of consequence.

With kind regards
Yours truly
R. Ross.

The Patiala business is quite dead. I am not sending any notice about the mosquito work to the South Indian B. M. Association.

I have heard no more of your malaria charts which I sent to government.

1 Marchiafava and Bignami (1894), 39-49.
2 Mannaberg (1894), 289-292.
3 Marchiafava and Bignami (1894), 5, where Marchiafava and Bignami classify malarial fevers into the mild winter and spring ones, including quartan and tertian, and the severe summer and autumn ones, consisting of the quotidian and malignant tertian.
4 Presumably a reference to the colour of the corpuscle.
5 See Letter 30, although the observation was of no consequence, *Memoirs*, 165.
6 See Letter 13.

Letter 15
02/073

Secunderabad
18th July 1895

Dear Dr Manson,

At last!

Just as I said in my letter yesterday, Abdul Wahāb, the man with ring-forms & pigmented leucocytes only, showed crescents this morning - 1 in 4 fields. At work again. Eight hours today.

I said I was going to watch free flagella. With my usual luck I found a beauty in my very first specimen & watched it for three solid hours exactly, without taking my eye off him. So much for my absurd theory of the flagella becoming quiescent. What he did you will think interesting.

He riggled [sic] around for 20 minutes like a trypanosoma, so that I could hardly follow him. Then he brought up against a phagocyte & remained so long that I thought the phagocyte had got a hold of him. Not a bit; he was not killed or sucked in; but kept poking him in the ribs in different parts of the body. I was astonished; & so, apparently, was the phagocyte. He kept at this for about 1/4 hour & then went away across two fields & went straight at another phagocyte! He pushed into this in several places with one end for a long time; & the phagocyte seemed to rear up & try to get round him, but could not. At last the phagocyte seemed to give up & flattened itself against an air-bubble, the flagellum still poking away at him. After 50 minutes the beast seemed to be getting tired, when a very curious thing happened; a third phagocyte came at him with mouth open right & straight across the field, but had no sooner got near him when the flagellum left his fallen foe & attacked the new one, holding on & shaking like a snake on a dog. In one minute the third phagocyte turned sharp round & ran off howling!!! - I assure you. I won't swear I heard him howling, but I *saw* him howling. He went right across a whole field, the flagellum holding on to his tail like this 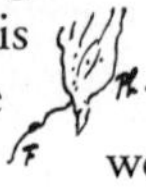 . This continued for five minutes, the poor phagocyte literally *legging it*, after which the flagellum left him & went away. By this time the beast had become much more visible & had a large swelling in the middle  . I watched him steadily, & his movements gradually became slower. He was certainly able to attach himself to the cover-glass (as shown by touching it with a pen) by *either* end & even perhaps by the swelling. At last this swelling moved to one end [DRAWING][1] nearly of the beast &

became very large and distinct, until after three hours the creature evidently died - at any rate, curled up & ceased to move. Isn't this interesting? I think it shows, first that the phagocytes have no more power over free flagella than over trypanosomes; secondly the beast was evidently attacking the phagocytes, probably *mistaking them for some other kind of cell* - so I judge by its leaving the phagocytes after a time.[2]

After this I put the mosquitoes on. Results of Abdul Kadir completely confirmed - & more. The first mosquito was killed at twenty minutes. My usual luck again - *all the parasites were flagellate & there were scores of free flagella.* I say *all* the parasites - all except about 5% which were spheres.

In the second mosquito at 40 minutes I saw four flagellates; the rest were spheres & spent pigment. In neither mosquito was there a single crescent, though in the first control specimen 50% of the parasites remained crescents after three hours. I killed no more mosquitoes, being tired out, but kept 8 for malarialising experiments. After this it is not much use bothering about going over the "first step" again - but I shall make you some sets of specimens & try to stain the flagella; Mannaberg does it.[3] The spectacle of the first mosquito was really wonderful. I shall dream of it. Good night. So was the fight between the flagellum & the three phagocytes. I shall write a novel on it in the style of the Three Musketeers.

24th July. Five days of severe work spent mostly opposite to one of those brick-walls you advised me of; but with one result. Two more of the summer fevers have got crescents, as I expected; & four fresh cases have come in; also one spring tertian and one *quartan*; the last being a case I had judged formerly to be summer tertian on strength of only two parasites seen. It differs apparently from the European quartan in that the infected corpuscles are smaller than the others & the "babies" show a tendency to the ring form. Numbers of perfect rosette forms found yesterday. The man saluted, said he was quite well & fit for duty. 'Wait a minute, my friend' I said 'you will have a bad attack of fever presently.' 'Ah, no' he said 'I am quite well.' I told him to wait; in a hour his teeth were going like castanets. They now take me for a prophet. I put the mosquitoes on to the two other crescent cases.

You may now rest assured that the "first step" is completely proved. I have tried four cases with identical results. In the third case there were very few parasites; but again I found them *all* flagellate at 25 minutes; in the fourth case same results as before. It is quite clear that within 20m or $^{1}/_{2}$ hour all the parasites become spheres & numbers become flagellate. In control specimens this happens to, often, only a small percentage of crescents. I think moreover that I am now able to state with much reason, that the mosquito's stomach is the *best place possible* for the evolution of the crescent - don't you think so? The last cases show much more extensive flagellation than did Abdul Kadir, who had been given a good deal of quinine.

Two more men were given mosquito water this morning; five & six infected mosquitoes kept for six days in each bottle & the water exposed to the sun yesterday for some hours. I am afraid to try with a number of men at once, for fear the induced fever may be severe.

The *brick wall* is the behaviour of the free flagella. I have not been able to follow one more. Though found free in the mosquito they seemed to disappear rapidly, probably owing to the yellowness of the serum. However I know now that they *can* live for three hours. The work is very severe, especially when I have to examine some ten ordinary specimens a day first, besides many other duties. Today I must rest.

Another small brick wall is making dried specimens. You must never expect, I fear, to see in dried blood what I see in liquid. First in liquid mosquito blood the parasites can be seen with the utmost distinctness even in fairly deep layers. Thus the whole contents of a mosquito need not be pressed out much; so that we can find usually one or two spheres in every field. But we *must* use thin films in dried blood; & in making them by the usual smear process, the parasites seem to disappear almost entirely. When found they are nothing like as clear as in liquid blood. Out of some dozens of attempts I have obtained only two tolerable specimens. Perhaps I am not skilled enough; but the failures have been very disappointing moreover the parasites are not nearly as numerous in these cases as in Abdul Kadir. The best result I think is obtained simply by drawing the insect's abdomen, with the blood oozing from it, across the cover glass, which is then mounted without staining or any medium, as Laveran recommends.[4] Yesterday I examined a mosquito which gave 2 parasites a field; on smearing away the cover-glass & drying I could barely find one or two in the whole specimen. But I will try again & hope to send you some fairly good specimens by next mail.

With kind regards
Yours truly
R. Ross.

Plenty of flagellate organisms seen in all the mosquitoes. Your lecture not come yet; nor any news about the charts. Will send you bottled mosquitoes. Am going to try bugs & fleas.

1 Drawing missing due to a hole in the letter.
2 Ross, *Memoirs*, 167, notes that the flagellum had probably 'mistaken' the leucocytes for female *Plasmodia*, an interpretation which Ross could not have made before the discovery of sexual reproduction of *Plasmodia* by MacCallum in 1897. See Letter 105.
3 Mannaberg (1894), 273.
4 Laveran (1893), 28.

Letter 16
02/006

21 Queen Anne Street, Cavendish Square,
10th July 1895

My dear Ross,
Your post card of 19th June just arrived. I sympathise with you in your difficulties. The period of hitch is always followed by the spell of progress and I have little doubt that by this time you are again in full swing on a new lead. I am very sorry about the Patiala business being burked by the Government.[1] You will not get listened to at head quarters until your work has come out. I am preparing a manifesto for the B. M. A. meeting, now only some three weeks off, and I think that after this comes out you will be boomed perhaps more than you wish. Meanwhile I am intending to interview Hart and perhaps the Lancet people, at all events the former, so that he may be put up to the ropes and be prepared with a stiff leader as soon as the paper is read. I think you should push on with your work as fast as possible now, as after the thing has become public there are sure to be many workers on the same lines; not in Europe, for the season will be getting too late for the merry mosquito, but in India and South America and the West Indies. I do not know of any one as yet working on these lines but it is only a question of a few months I think before it is taken up by dozens now you have given them the lead.

I have also some chance of making influence in your favour at the India office. I know Sir Charles Crosthwaite[2] and I am sure he would lend a hand if he is approached; I also know Sir A Macdonnell[3] who I understand is a power in the state. I do not know him well but I have seen him as a patient and expect to see him again soon. Him too I shall try to influence. Meanwhile work as hard as you can and try to move the peg up one step higher.

Preparations of mosquito blood showing the flagellated organism in quantity would be a most convincing argument. I think you would do well to send some of them; also mosquitoes preserved at different stages.

Your mother sent me the cutting from the Indian paper 'Pioneer'[4] and I saw the same or a similar notice in the Friend of India.[5] Why did the Govt refuse the Patiala man? I should like to get out very much but I cannot afford to leave my work and the Royal Society have declined to give me the grant I asked for.[6] I shd like to come though.

You say in your letter of 10th June, referring to your examinations of Hutchman's [sic] blood, "that though I saw many *ring-forms* and pseudo-parasites I never saw one which I was convinced was a parasite". Were not these "ring-forms" parasites? Surely they were. I have often seen them at the commencement of a fever spell and never had any doubt that they were. They disappear in a very short time. I hope this man did get crescents eventually but if these ring forms were what I understand by ring forms I am convinced he had parasites in his blood. Those cases in which you do not see the parasite are cases of summer-autumn fever in which the young forms are present in the blood for a short time only and this time can be easily missed. Try such a case at the beginning of the fever crises; you are sure to meet parasites then. It is merely a question of the proper time.

You saw Thin's article in the Lancet of last week.[7] A long rigmarole about staining. It will do harm and frighten people off the business. Reading it one would suppose that nothing but the very finest lenses and an apothecary's shop full of stains and chemicals and an elaborate training will suffice to find the malaria bug. It is a great mistake to frighten people off in this way.

I recognise your classification of the fields of the microscope.[8] I classified them into three zones in describing them to my class; yours is much more complete.

I have never seen the phagocyte burst the parasite as you describe. They are much more languid in their operations here.

Your programme is a good one. If you succeed in infecting with mosquito water once or twice again you may be sure you are on the right track and that you are justified in claiming the fact, that the mosquito is an active agent in propagating malaria, as proved. I cant say what these bodies you find in the mosquito are. Very possibly as you suggest coccidia. Might they be malarial? I should look out in five or six-day-old malariated mosquitos for bodies like the crescent;

for some body which is more or less encysted and prepared for a lying in wait period. I should also look out for some intracellular form like the sporulating stage in the human body. You may find the latter in some particular organ analogous to the spleen or bonemarrow. Look inside the eggs. Look inside the mosquito larvae. The latter may take it in in the water their mothers die in perhaps and probably by the mouth.

It is blazing hot here still, almost tropical and very oppressive and no rain. I am off to shoot grouse about the 9th or 10th of next month and I assure you I need it.

With kindest regards and all good luck I remain
Yours very sincerely
Patrick Manson

1 See Letter 4, note 2.
2 Sir Charles Crosthwaite, (1835-1915), permanent Under-Secretary of State at the India Office at that time. See **Biographical Appendix**, and Arnold Kaminsky, *The India Office, 1880-1910* (London: Mansell, 1986).
3 Sir Antony Patrick MacDonnell, (1844-1925), 1890, Chief Commissioner of the Central Provinces; 1895, Lieutenant-Governor of North Western Provinces and Oudh.
4 Untraced.
5 Untraced.
6 Manson had applied for a Royal Society grant to pay his expenses to go to Demerara to study the mosquito theory himself; see Letter 8, note 6.
7 George Thin, 'The parasite of malaria and malarial fevers', *Lancet* (6 July 1895), 12-19. Thin's long and technical article probably offended Manson by its concentration on Continental malarial work; see Letter 25 and **Biographical Appendix**.
8 Letter 8.

Letter 17
02/074

Secunderabad

30th July 1895

Dear Dr Manson,

Your very kind letter of the 10th. First of all about the ring-forms in Lutchman's blood - I have always forgotten to write to you about the matter. I remember perfectly that I saw C1 & C4;[1] but at the time I examined the case I had not obtained any summer autumn fevers. I remembered also that one form similar to C1 was due to a speck on the glass, as proved by pressure on the cover-slip, & I thought that all these forms were vacuoles because I remember having seen similar appearances often before. I *did* see them before, but they were parasites not vacuoles. I saw them in this very station when I arrived in June 1893 *after the spring fever season*. As the soldiers are usually sent to duty three days after the fever abates, *I missed the crescents*. Hence chiefly my former want of success in finding the parasites here. I have actually long been familiar with C4 under the name of "eye - form" vacuoles; one was certainly in Lutchman's blood - I remember it very distinctly in the first specimen I took of him when the fever was beginning; & now by repeated observation I am certain that the form is parasitic. Still I could certainly never find crescents in his blood; so won't claim him as a complete success, but will certainly confess myself a fool for being so pig-headed about my vacuoles. It is very annoying to be such an ass by nature. About what you say concerning ring forms appearing at the beginning of the fever - it is borne out exactly in my observations. In a fresh case yesterday beginning at 8 a.m. there were numbers at 8.30 (temp. 105° F), but *all* were gone at 12.0!

Again about the eye-forms C4 - there were numbers in the case I told you about as belonging possibly to a new variety. Unfortunately the case is a child 2 years old & the mother fights me about pricking its heathenish little black toe - but I have found numbers in 5 specimens now. Yet they differ from the usual C4; some, it is true, are exactly similar, but most of them are far smaller - so small often 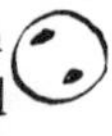 that they can only just be seen; & they do not show amoeboid movement, but *turn* frequently in the corpuscles & are certainly some form of life. Oddly enough the child's fever has passed off, yet these bodies, of different sizes but similar shapes, are still to be found; and they are found in the best fields where vacuoles *are* not. No crescents however - curious.

A very useful way for finding crescents & pigment, suggested by your marginal clot & the mosquito's stomach in which pigment is found almost instantly. Put a large drop of blood on a slide without spreading it out & stir it with a needle & breathe on it for two minutes until it is half dry; then put on the cover-glass. The corpuscles are found to be in a viscid yellow mass in which the black pigment of the crescents etc. is seen in a moment. We may thus examine a large quantity of blood in a very small area. This method enabled me to find crescents at once where I had failed after a long study of two ordinary specimens. Useful for diagnosis.[2]

On 26th I put 3 mosquitoes on to my quartan. Numbers of intraglobular forms, beautiful rosettes, but no flagellate form seen. (morning before fever)

Same day one *flea* on Abdul Wahâb. Only four parasites found in the whole insect, which however had drunk freely. Two of the parasites (at 40 minutes) were dead spheres & two spent pigment. Crescents were plentiful in mosquitoes (1 in a field) the same day. Bugs tried - refused to bite.

Working along the whole line at the transformation of flagella. Watched another for half an hour, after which I lost him. Again of this form  ; wriggling chiefly at the ends as if it were a *body* with two arms.

Malarialised mosquitoes examined after 2, 3 & 4 days - abdomen & thorax simply teazed out & crushed to see what is to be seen. In all except one, the coccidia-like bodies, of which more tomorrow. In one at 2 days, irregular masses of size & shape of dead leucocytes without amoeboid movement, in insect's stomach. Each contained one oval distinct vacuole- looking body, which however stained deeper than the rest 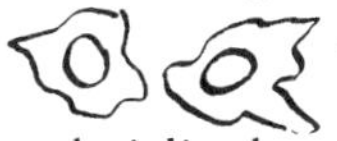 . All the vacuoles (nuclei) of same size nearly.

Today in malarialised mosquito of five days, teazed out (eggs developed), numerous oval bodies about 20µ in longest diameter, with a peculiar indented margin, nearly round, containing about 15 circular spores 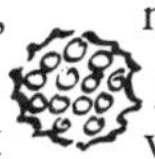 perhaps more. I send you the specimen in glycerin & water, stained by irrigation & then dried (specimen 8). A number of these bodies were in one part found embedded in some tissue. Stained irrigation turned them all blue in a moment - so blue that the spores were lost sight of.

7.30 p.m. At incessant work since 6 a.m. More tomorrow.

31st July. Absolutely no time to finish this letter - cases swarming in - three ring forms & one mixed, mostly spring tertian, this morning. Rat's blood full of surra.[3] A mosquito fed on *healthy blood* killed at two days this morning & searched for coccidia-like bodies. None found. Shall examine three more tomorrow at three days; but I believe that I have seen these bodies in healthy mosquitoes. I shall send you a few specimens next week including some coccidia-like forms. Owing to paucity of crescents in all my cases up to date, specimens referring to evolution of crescent are very poor. There is enough work for three men to do in my regiment alone; & I am unfortunately saddled with another man's work. By next week I hope to have a clearer view of the coccidia & also of the above bodies full of spores. Your intentions respecting my first work are indeed encouraging! I hope the theory will turn out right; at all events I have no doubts now about the first step. The Patiala affair was opposed by government for a reason which I am not allowed to mention, but which in my opinion is bosh. The fact is that the Indian government & especially the medical services are utterly ignorant of the importance of this kind of work. I have long been thinking of a project - to send you a careful criticism of faulty points in the construction, regulations & management of the service. At present I have no time - but it *ought to be done at all costs*. The B. M. J. ought to bring out a series of leaders on the subject. Unless this is done there will be a scandal. The medical services are becoming truly in a deplorable state.

With kind regards
Yours truly
R. Ross.

1 A reference to Manson's Chart, Figure 3.

2 Ross, *Memoirs*, 168, notes that this is the beginning of his 'thick-film' method, on which he published three papers in 1903, e.g. 'An improved method for the microscopical diagnosis of intermittent fever', *Lancet* (10 Jan. 1903), 86.

3 Surra is a disease of horses caused by a trypanosome; *Trypanosoma lewisi* was originally described in rats in 1878 and similar parasites were first noticed in horses in 1880. For a discussion, see Lise Wilkinson and Anne Hardy, *Prevention and Cure: The London School of Hygiene and Tropical Medicine, a 20th Century Quest for Global Public Health* (London: Kegan Paul, 1998), ch. 2.

Letter 18
02/075

Secunderabad
5th August 1895

Dear Dr Manson,

I am sending you 8 specimens numbered in red ink they are

1. Finger blood opened after 1 hour & dried & stained - crescents & spheres.
2. A mosquito at 5 minutes.
3. Another mosquito of the same batch as 2, at 35 minutes.
4. A mosquito at 30 minutes.
5. The same as 4 stained.

These are all poor specimens selected out of some dozens attempts solely because they showed the greatest number of parasites. I can't send you good specimens until one of my cases shows a large number of crescents; as soon as this happens I will send you a series or two. 2 & 4 are made by dragging the mosquito over the cover-glass, 3 & 5 by smearing in the usual way. As I told you before these give you no idea of what is seen in liquid mosquito blood. I shall try to think out a method which will give better results.

6. Is a malarialised mosquito at 2 days containing the psorosperm.[1] Like bodies in large numbers (coccidia-like bodies).

7. Is one (malarialised) at 5 days containing the same, a little larger I think.

All these from 1 to 7 are mounted dry.

8. Is *not* the sporulating bodies I mentioned in my last; that specimen having changed in some way & become useless. It is a very interesting specimen however of a dissected mosquito mounted in glycerine & water & containing crowds of the psorosperms in the broken end of the intestine, apparently the lower end. If you look with a low power you will find not far from the *insect's tail* a part of intestine broken off, with crowds of psorosperms tumbling out 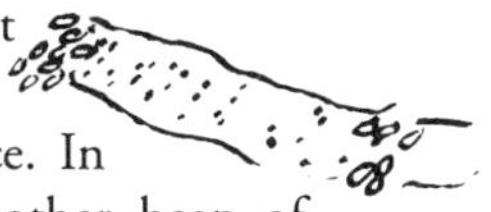

They occupy the intestine for some distance. In another place there is another heap of psorosperms either in another piece of intestine or in a *gregarine*[2] 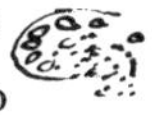 . The mosquito's tail-piece comes between these two heaps. I want to know whether these bodies are psorosperms or not. If so where are the parent gregarines or coccidia? The psorosperms are about 10μ long, shuttle-shaped & showing something like sickle-shaped bodies along the sides. You should open 6 & 7 & let in glycerine I think. They do not stain with stain-irrigation or otherwise readily (meth. blue). They will be seen easily with strong dry lenses. 8 is mounted in glycerine & water & I *do hope* that it will not be spoilt. It is a malarialised mosquito at 3 days (from Abdul Wahább). I have found these bodies however (in small quantities hitherto) in insects fed on healthy blood; though a lot of my specimens were ruined by my finding a man whom I thought healthy to contain a crescent or two (by my new method); I saw a spent-pigment mass in one of his mosquitoes at *2 days* & diagnosed malaria instantly though he had had no fever for two months! Crescents found by my method.

Don't you think that these bodies must be looked to very carefully? I have spent the whole week over them. It seems to me that they must still be watched even though they do turn out to be psorosperms. Leuckart & Blanchard[3] say that the sickle shaped bodies when freed from the psorosperm become amoeboid (as for instance the intracorpuscular forms). The bodies appear to be very common among mosquitoes here. I remember finding however a much larger form about 20μ in length with a little rosette near one end 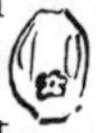 . I think it was in a mosquito which had not bitten; but I have not seen it again. Clearly by your theory it may be present in non-malarialised mosquitoes & yet be connected with the malaria parasite. The bodies appear to me to belong to the sporozoa, and to be of a size which we may well imagine the flagella to grow into in a day or two. But you must not be surprised if I go on many a wild-goose-chase. They certainly appear "encysted & prepared for a lying in wait period."

Finding parasites in every case now, but no time to *work* at them. Have not a moment's leisure from 6.30 a.m. to 8 p.m! It is now 7 p.m. & barring half an hour for breakfast I have been at it since 6.30. Luckily feeling fit & full of energy. It takes 3 hours to hunt through a mosquito; but for my statistics I would throw over examining fresh cases of malaria any more for the present.

6th August. The two men to whom I gave mosquito water a fortnight ago have apparently failed; no fever nor parasites in the blood. These are the 5th & 6th experiments. It seems as if Lutchman's fever was accidental, but if so it was a strange coincidence because he had never had fever before & because the ring-forms had not set in at the time. Shall try a number of experiments as soon as I get a good crescent case: Abdul Wahább has *dried up*.

Have now examined carefully 5 mosquitoes fed on healthy blood, at 2, 3 & 4 days (all same batch); no psorosperms. Still, I think that they are to be found in healthy mosquitoes (not malarialised). Am going to hunt in mosquito grubs & unfed mosquitoes presently. The body in specimen 8 which I thought might be a gregarine is certainly only a piece of broken off intestine. Perhaps the parent sporozoa live in the grubs. I am now becoming more familiar with the anatomy & the changes in the fed mosquito & can work more quickly than when I began.

7th August. Two more mosquitoes of the same batch at 5 days (not malarialised). No psorosperms. Also a baby grub; no psorosperms. The spore bearing bodies I wrote about seem to come out of the mature eggs & are probably some normal cell; have seen them again.

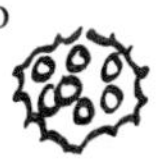

Waiting for your Hunterian lecture to press your charts & my microscope. Cases coming in daily; nearly 50 now, I believe, since I came here. Reuter's telegram about Hart's attack on I. M. service.[4] If you can get India Office to send a hint about malaria investigations it would certainly be useful. The people here not likely to move. Owen has no objection to a hint from the India Office but thinks the B. M. Journal could do no good otherwise. The India Office might ask politely *why* the Punjab government refused to allow the Patiala investigation. Specimens despatched registered & prepaid. Nearly dead with work; but intend to live on a little longer! Will send you a list of malarialising experiments. With kind regards,

Yours truly

R. Ross.

1 For definition see **Glossary**.

2 For definition see **Glossary**.

3 Rudolf Leuckart, *The Parasites of Man and the Diseases which Proceed from them*, trans. by William E. Hoyle (London: Young J. Pentland, 1886), 211-214; Blanchard (1889-90), I, 33-4.

4 Ernest Hart's address at the opening of the Section of Public Health at the British Medical Association Annual Meeting in London, 'Public health legislation and the needs of India', *BMJ* (3 Aug. 1895), 287-291.

Letter 19
02/007

21 Queen Anne
Street, Cavendish Square
26th July,
1895

My dear Ross,
Many thanks for yours of 26th June and of 10th July. The lack of suitable cases is very disappointing. I labour under a similar famine. Not one case of malarial fever for a very long time and on Wednesday next have to demonstrate the parasite to the B. M. Association and with nothing but stained slides to fall back on. My paper is ready but it is too long for the quarter of an hour they allow so I must curtail the first part of it devoting the best part of the quarter of an hour to your work. I saw Hart about the Patiala business and he is quite ready to take up the cudgels for you - but as you say Owen[1] does not want this. I shall try to keep him from being too energetic. I am writing today to Cleghorn,[2] who is an old friend of mine, and I shall tell him all about the malaria-mosquito business and ask him to befriend you in the matter so far as lies in his power and I fancy he has a good deal to say in such matters. I am also writing to Leslie[3] who is at Simla.

I have been very much occupied of late otherwise I would have hunted up the pebrine literature for you; there is a long paper in the Journal of Experimental Medicine, Paris,[4] on the subject of blood protozoa but I forget just at present the number. If I get time I shall go to the Col. Of Surg. one afternoon before I leave for my holiday and look into the matter.

Drinking water may be a source of malaria but not the only one - by source I mean medium. Dried water sediment or even soil on which a mosquito has died if raised in the shape of dust might very well contain the desiccated and perhaps encysted spore. I believe it does. Hence the danger of turning up the soil. The soil full of encysted spores which had been formed in the bodies of mosquitoes now defunct, spores which being encysted may retain their vitality for a very long time.

I saw a man some days ago about my guinea worm preparations - a man who is an exquisite mounter of the more delicate forms of infusorial life and I spoke to him about the difficulties of mounting flagellated bodies. He said the best plan with the mosquito would be to fix the blood and beast in quarter per cent osmic acid for quarter of an hour; wash very thoroughly in distilled water and then put up in 4 per cent formaline. He says the mosquito will keep very well in this and he promised to try to mount the flagellated body for me if I got him the mosquitoes. So if you can spare a few remember me. Also, do not forget to send me dried mosquito dust and dried sediment of mosquito water. I shall try it on myself or some one. A positive result after such an experiment would be absolutely conclusive.

I kept my cyclops for 70 days at the end of which time I found the form represented in Davidson's book[5] with the tripartite tail

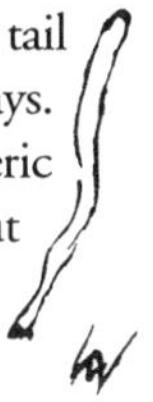

Fedschenko[6] found the metamorphosis completed in 36 days. It takes longer here, doubtless owing to the lower atmospheric temperature. I can't say why you did not see more flagella but I imagine that the flagella rush away from the sphere very rapidly - in fact as soon as they get free. It is manifestly in their interest to do so to avoid the phagocyte. Besides those you mention another objection to the mosquito theory might be founded on the viability of the phagocyte in mosquito; Objectors might say that if the mosquito does not kill the phagocyte what right have we to think it would kill the malaria parasite. But the argument does not quite apply. The phagocyte is in operation *inside* the *circulating* blood; the malaria parasite does not come into operation until *outside* the circulating blood - it develops under conditions which are not favourable to life as a rule - only favourable to parasitic life: Why should it only develop under such conditions if it were not that it had got into suitable conditions. The life of the phagocyte is a mere survival - the life of the malaria germ in the mosquito is a development; they are not parallel.

I suppose these bodies you draw are coccidia, but they are worth study. I have an idea that you will find the larval mosquito at its very earliest development the best medium for studying the mosquito-malaria disease. I conjecture it becomes infected either through the egg or while in the water from the maternal parasites. If this is so the transparent tissues of the grub will be much easier to work at than the scaly mess of the adult mosquito. I used to find these scales and the fragmented ova a horrible nuisance.

There is not much doing in medical circles here just now. I had a look at Osler's article (in manuscript - not printed yet) on malaria for Clifford Allbutt's System[7] the other day. There was nothing new in it and the article was not a good one. You will rouse them however I am sure and there will be a fresh spurt in malariology as soon as your work comes out. The Frenchies and Italians will pooh pooh it at first, then adopt it, and then claim it as their own. See if they don't. But push on with it and don't let them forestall you. They won't have time this autumn and they will not have a chance to work seriously at the matter till next June or so. You have got a year ahead of them and in that time you should have solved the problem in its principles at all events. Leave the details for them to work out which they will do well and with much wrangling. I can see a big field of work springing out of yours; the influence of different species of mosquito on the parasite; does the difference in spring and autumn fevers depend on the difference in species of the mosquito medium? - the symptoms of malarial fever in the mosquito; the determination of efficient species of mosquito; and so on. I believe a splendid work for a man to spend his life over would be the influence of the mosquito as a pathological agent. I don't think the filaria and the malaria bugs end him. He or rather she is a carnivorous animal and like all carnivores acts as intermediate or definitive host to the parasites of the animals or tissues of animals it devours - the blood in this case.

Yours very faithfully
Patrick Manson

1 See Letter 12.

2 Surgeon-General James Cleghorn, (1841-1920), Director-General of the Indian Medical Service at the time. See **Biographical Appendix**.

3 John Tasman Waddell Leslie, (1861-1911), Secretary to Cleghorn. See **Biographical Appendix**.

4 Probably a reference to A. Laveran, 'Des trypanosomes parasites du sang', *Arch. de Méd. Expér. et d'Anat. Path, Paris*, 4 (1892), 257-269.

5 P. Manson 'Diseases of the skin in tropical climates' in A. Davidson (ed.), *Hygiene and Diseases of Warm Climates* (Edinburgh and London: Young J. Pentland, 1893), 928-95, on p 956.

6 Aleksiei Pavlovich Fedchenko, [On the structure and reproduction of Filaria medinensis L.] *Izvest. Imp. Obsh. Liub. Estes. (Mosk.)*, 8 (1869-70), 71-82; translated in *American Journal of Medicine*, 20 (1971), 511-23. Manson always spelled it Fedschenko.

7 W. Osler, 'Malarial fever' in Thomas Clifford Allbutt (ed.), *A System of Medicine*, 8 vols (London: Macmillan and Co, Limited, 1896-1899), vol. ii, 721-742.

Letter 20
02/076

Secunderabad
12 August 1895

Dear Dr Manson,

Very many thanks for your letter of 26th July. Your letters are most encouraging & keep me up to my work; and I can't thank you enough for all your kindness. I am looking forward much to the B. M. Ass. meeting which will be reported soon I hope; and it is indeed an honour to me to have my work reported upon by you in this manner! However I hope to show better results soon. I have today got to the bottom of the psorosperms - this *is* what they are. After writing to you I tackled a number of unfed mosquitoes finding psorosperms in many. I told you that they were in the intestine; but I find by a plate of insects' digestive apparatus in Blanchard[1] that what I thought were the intestines are the Malpighian tubes, five of which in the mosquito are inserted into the *pylorus*. They are long blind tubes consisting of tessellated cells, full of black granules & easily seen as white threads by the naked eye, as of course you know; and they are present both in larva & pupa. I have now found a way of drawing out the whole apparatus with the ovaries or testicles away from the body cavity; so that I can make beautiful specimens, some of which I will send you. Well, I found the psorosperms in numbers of unfed mosquitoes mostly at the closed ends of the Malpighian tubes where, if they are very numerous, they render the tube friable. I then began to study *grubs*, but found no psorosperms. This morning I took to the pupae, just before hatching into mosquitoes. In the stomach of the first were a number of gregarines of this shape 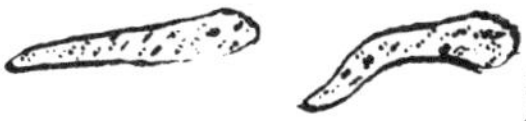 , about 100 to 150μ long, moving rapidly just like slugs, thick end forward. They ceased to move in five minutes. They are full of dark brown granules, but I couldn't see the nucleus. Next I looked at the end of the Malpighian tubes - full of large oval bodies about 70μ long, evidently *encysted gregarines*. On pressure these and a number of encysting gregarines poured out of the ruptured tubes.

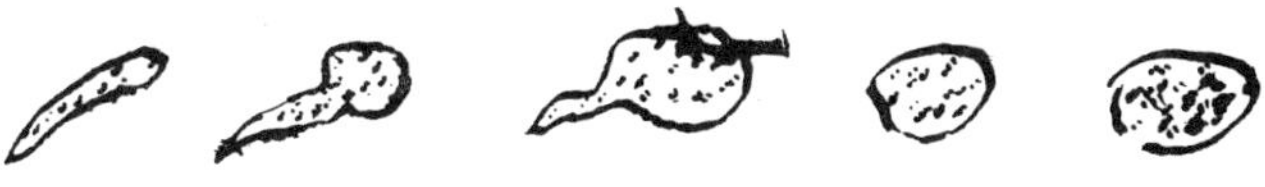

I saw no conjugation forms; the gregarines appear to be single. It was now clear by the *position* of these bodies at the end of the tubes that they were the parents of the psorosperms; but the next pupa put this beyond a doubt by *showing psorosperms inside the encysted gregarines* -

so here is the whole chain at once.

Now what do you think? Is it still possible that these bodies are another form of the malarial parasite? Please let me have your opinion. So far as I have gone the gregarines live in the pupae, the psorosperms in the mosquitoes. They seem to be hard encysted little bodies capable of enduring much rough usage, & may be discharged either in the faeces or when the insect dies & breaks up. Now the next stage is that of the falciform bodies, which, so far as I can gather from Leuckart & Blanchard, become *amoeboid.* Is it possible that this amoeboid form is the *intra corpuscular malaria parasite*?

I think, by your original article,[2] that you have had this idea. It is clear in the first place that if the mosquito is the alternative host, the malaria parasite must be capable of living in it without man necessarily as an intermediary; we cannot conceive that the insect does no more than carry the parasite from an infected man to drinking water or mud; malaria must be a general endemic disease among mosquitoes; the germ must only take an excursion into men for change of scene & refreshment, so to speak. If this is the case then, we must expect the parasite to be a common one among mosquitoes and capable of being propagated from mother to children ad infinitum; but also capable of rushing off into human beings, probably in its immature form. Such I read your theory to be; and such would probably be the case if the malaria parasite is the amoeboid form of the mosquito's gregarine. These gregarines are evidently a very common disease among mosquitoes in this station; and so far as I can see, all the facts which I observe respecting the occurrence of malarial fever here can be explained *best* on the supposition that the poison is conveyed by mosquitoes into *isolated pots of drinking water* in the houses of the men. My reason for this is the following. The whole regiment lives in barracks or rather huts about 1/2 mile from a large tank over which the wind blows towards us; the whole regiment drinks water from one large well. Now if the air or well-water were infected, we should expect nearly all susceptible people in the regiment to get the fever almost simultaneously, as happens in the case of cholera-poisoned wells. But what is the truth? The cases keep dropping in, one or two a day only, out of 700 men. Surely this suggests a most limited & isolated source for the poison; such in fact as the infection of a chatty or two of drinking water in the men's huts by ripe, infected mosquitoes. The mosquitoes themselves of course may come from the tank; and it is thus that lakes & marshes have got the reputation of being malarious; but, so far as I can see, the poison, however general it may be in a district, must be absorbed from very localised, & not general, sources, in order to explain the scanty & successive, and not general & simultaneous, occurrence of cases of fever.

On the whole then, I think these gregarines fall in wonderfully well with your ideas of the alternative form. Even if they are not the malaria parasite, I can't help thinking they will be found to have some human pathological import, because, as you say, men & mosquitoes fall exactly into the usual parasitological circle. The question is what do the free flagella develop into? Why not straight into young gregarines? I have not observed gregarines in malarialised mosquitoes, but I may easily have mistaken them for normal cells; because I would not have recognised them today, if I had not seen them crawling about, which they ceased to do in a few minutes. Then again, the gregarines I have seen must have entered the young grubs, because they were fully developed in the pupa. Do you think that it is possible for them to enter the mature insect by way of human blood, & develop into psorosperms before its death? Why not? I will look very closely. I must also try to find gregarines in the grubs, & must see how the psorosperms leave the mosquito, whether by the intestine or only after death. I am certain too that I once saw a much larger kind of psorosperm, I believe in an unfed mosquito (don't remember).

You can imagine my excitement over all this - though it may turn out to be a wrong scent. My work is tremendous - I have *twenty* malaria cases in hospital - can't possibly work at them properly. Still a few negative cases which worry me a great deal. One case with extraordinary large *amoeboid red corpuscles* & no parasites. One of pernicious access, nearly died. Not a single *good* crescent case; the crescents appear to vanish & leave a slight daily rise of fever to 100° or so - can't make it out - quinine perhaps. Think I shall send a short list of cases to B. M. J.[3] in order to correct Crombie's statements. My spring tertians relapse, contrary to Mannaberg's statements[4] made possibly under stimulus of the idea that crescents cause recurrence. I am *feeling* some undiscovered malaria parasite; but have seen no more cases like the child I told you of with numbers of small C4s, though I have seen one or two small C4s in ordinary fevers. Talk of malaria investigations. I am in the thick of it here. Three men working would not be too many. But I think that the Indian government ought to be made to recognise the necessity of doing these things; and accordingly thank you very much for writing to Cleghorn & Leslie & speaking to Hart. Hart's utterances on the I. M. Service[5] has set them all raving with rage; but I hope he won't say too much about the Patiala business, as they may be down on Owen. If you could say a word to Sir C. Crosthwaite[6] & Sir A. Macdonnell[7] on the subject in general it would doubtless help a great deal.

13 August. Gregarines found in two more pupae & in a number of larvae, down to small ones, but not down to the smallest size yet. Encysting gregarines in one old larva. They occur also in the intestine. Nuclei often clearly made out. By oil immersion the granules are seen in continual motion and a sort of bubble forms at the creature's big end. 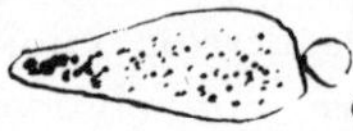. Granules at tail bigger than the rest. Clear double contour. Length measured by micrometer = 200μ for about the largest size & 100μ or less for the smallest. The youngest grubs contain the smallest gregarines, which are mostly of this shape , with a curled up tail in segments (apparently of course) &  perhaps contained in cells of stomach. I missed these in larvae before, for reasons given above. I think now that I remember your mentioning the mosquito's gregarine.

14th. Have been demonstrating malaria parasite to an A. M. D. man[8] all day & must close to catch post. Extremely sorry not to send you more specimens yet. No crescents. With kind regards

Yours truly

R. Ross.

1 Blanchard (1889-1890), vol. ii, 532.

2 Patrick Manson, 'A clinical lecture on the parasite of malaria and its demonstration', *Lancet* (6 Jan. 1894), 6-9.

3 Ross never got around to this.

4 Mannaberg (1894), 345.

5 Hart, (1894; 1895). See Letter 18, note 4.

6 Letter 16, note 2.

7 Letter 16, note 3.

8 Unidentified member of Army Medical Department.

Letter 21
02/077

Secunderabad
20th August [1895]

Dear Dr Manson,
Before reporting progress I will answer two questions which I know you will have been asking. First why don't I send you good specimens of the "first step"? Because I have seen scarcely a crescent for a long time now. They are present in the summer - autumn fevers but only in small numbers. I might go hunting for them again but it would cost me more time than I can afford, as you will admit I think. A case is sure to drop in soon. Secondly why don't I try malarialising experiments on a large scale? Because I am too much afraid of success; & don't want to get the reputation of trying these experiments on a large scale, or the authorities will be down on me. One fatal case (not experimental) today. I shan't try malarialising experiments again until I am ready for them. For the same reason I don't send you mosquitoes yet.

Having worked on the connection between the gregarines & psorosperms, the next thing to do was to find how the latter leave the insect & how far they mature within it. Though gregarines are to be found in almost every grub, I have often failed in finding psorosperms in mature mosquitoes. Hence, if I had not overlooked them, I concluded they must pass out during life. I examined a number of unfed mosquitoes which had died naturally - no psorosperms; then a number of fed mosquitoes at 2, 3, 4 & 5 days - only a few psorosperms occasionally. On the other hand they were often plentiful in newly hatched mosquitoes; in one I found a single *gregarine*; in two others cysts full of psorosperms. Hence it is probable that they pass out about the 2nd day after hatching; but how I cannot make out; I cannot find any in stomach, intestines or about the anus.

At the same time I examined water at the bottom of bottle in which mosquitoes were kept - no psorosperms to be found. I looked at eggs which had been laid - same result. On considering large number of gregarines in grubs & pupae & often small number of psorosperms in even newly hatched mosquitoes I began to think that they were got rid of during pupa stage. I looked accordingly at the *cast off skin* of *pupa - numbers of psorosperms*. This fact is always confirmed by examinations up to date; so that this is at least one way in which the psorosperms pass out; though I can't imagine how they get from the blind end of the Malpighian tubes to the skin. They are most numerous generally in the head-piece of the pupa-pelt & are seen as numerous hard little bodies with a collection of granules at one part 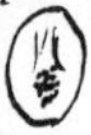 or 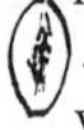. I have seen no development yet in specimens kept in water sealed for two days. In the M. tubes there seems to be often another form without the granules 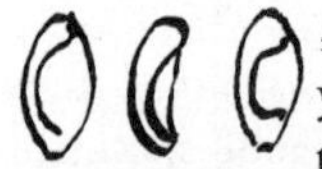, & sometimes curiously curled, ? empty shells. The youngest psorosperms (inside the parent cysts) seem to be rounder & full of granules 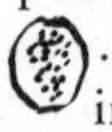. It may be that the psorosperms are evacuated by the bowel into the pelt in the efforts of the insect to change its skin. I find none in the pelts of the grubs hitherto. Anyway it is pretty clear that the large majority of these spores pass out between the end of the pupa stage & before the mosquito is two days old; the oldest mosquitoes have the fewest. Well now, you see, if there are malaria germs by any chance I have been doing the worst thing possible in giving the matured insects in malarialising experiments; & if I had sent you such mosquitoes you would have possibly seen nothing in them & failed in your experiments. And it is necessary to investigate still a little further. I want to know exactly how the psorosperms escape & whether they develop at all in water. Surely they must be passed out by the bowel; & possibly not only dropped in the water by the escaping imago, but scattered over the country in its flight afterwards. Do the Malpighian tubes open into the rectum by any chance? I am also going to try drying the psorosperms & wetting them again to see what happens; & as soon as I have cleared the way a little I shall try to malarialise with them. Give me a little more time & I will send you a number of mosquitoes too. I fear however that you will be able to make nothing out of mosquitoes sent to England: because a few hours after death they either dry up & crackle to pieces, or else decompose (even in glycerine I think). What a pity that you cannot come out here!

I have also had a shot at trying to trace the gregarines in the grubs down to their youngest forms; but am not far enough advanced to report, though I think that the smallest gregarines are encysted in some kind of cell, & start life from a round nucleus-like body but may be mistaken.

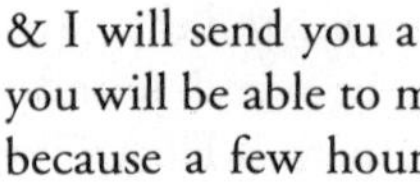

21st August. The B. M. J. of 3rd[1] to hand, with a mention of your speech at the association. I see Thin opposed you - how it would have interested me, you can imagine. Am very anxious to hear more. Hart's speech was tremendous & thoroughly needed; but the only way to get anything done will be to go at the heads of the department in all the

Presidencies by *name*, ask what they are doing, etc., or else they won't move. Not a man doing microscopic malaria diagnosis in the whole presidency yet, so far as I know; the science not taught at Madras medical schools (of course every hospital assistant ought to be able to find the parasite); microscopes not supplied; no official circulars on the subject; no reply yet about your charts; simple hoggish obduracy. You must prick them up by name; ask what they are doing not to stir in this malaria matter; ask why every doctor in the country is not using the microscope in malaria. Wish *I* had the power to do so. The fact is by some fatuity the worst men rise to the top of the service here, that is the so-called smart men, the regulation-wallers, never the scientific men. Why was not V. Carter made Surgeon-General?

Amusing. I wrote a little paper in the light scientific vein for the Pioneer on the mosquito theory,[2] broaching it, the other day. The editor now sends me for review Harvey's report on the causation of malaria for the proposed Sanitary Drainage Bill.[3] In this report 4 out of 12 doctors whose opinions were asked on the subject, deny Laveran's organism! (*my* fault in some measure possibly). Think I shall review the report cautiously, chiefly insisting on need of investigation; & shall ask permission to send on the papers to you, as the question at issue, that of plunging into large surface drainage schemes, is a very important one.

A point of interest - *none* of the recruits 50 in number have had fever during the last 4 months, though nearly 100 cases have occurred in regiment. Yet they live in close vicinity, but in a stone built house & are fed by means of a well-conducted mess; whereas the Sepoys live in mud-huts surrounded by water-pots full of mosquitoes. Also I think some of the companies get more fever than others; which since the companies live in distinct blocks, will be a useful fact to make out.

As soon as I get crescents again I shall resume attempts to follow the flagella & shall work at the cellular structures of the mosquito with which I am getting more familiar; in fact, whether the gregarine theory be right or wrong, I am much better prepared for the work than I was.

With kind regards believe me
Yours truly
R. Ross.

1 'Report of the section of Pathology and Bacteriology', *BMJ* (3 Aug. 1895), 312.

2 'Malaria and the mosquito', *Pioneer* (3 Aug. 1895), 3. **RA** 05/002.

3 Surgeon-General Robert Harvey, (1842-1901), see **Biographical Appendix**. As the law stood, local bodies could be formed to carry out drainage works of 'collective agricultural interest'; legislation was being considered to allow the formation of local bodies to carry out drainage works exclusively for sanitary purposes. A. J. Hughes 'Some points relating to sanitary polity in India', *Transactions of the First Indian Medical Congress, 24th to 29th December 1894* (Calcutta: Caledonian Steam Printing Works, 1895), 227-230. See also W. J. Simpson, 'The need of a sanitary service for India', *Ibid.*, 222-227.

Letter 22
02/078

Secunderabad
31st August 1895

Dear Dr Manson,

I was obliged to miss the last post owing to being suddenly engaged in a medico-legal case.[1] It lasted from morning to night for three days; a hundred rupees a day, but forced me to waste some malarialised mosquitoes I wished to examine.

I have worked the gregarines pretty fully except the gap between the psorosperms (? pseudonavicella) & the youngest gregarines. The smallest gregarines are certainly to be found curled up in cells (perivisceral) of about 20μ in diameter, & I am not sure that they don't arise from peculiar spherical bodies with a fringe of cilia ; but I have still to work more in this direction. I think that I have found 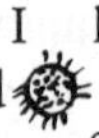 another smaller species of gregarine, without the big head; but of this after more study. In one batch of mosquito grubs obtained from a distance I could find no gregarines at all - so that they are not always present. As I told you the gregarines encyst in the pupa stage; & the psorosperms are mature & discharged *by the bowel* at the end of the pupa stage & the first days of the imago stage. I have now frequently seen psorosperms in stomach, intestine & about the anus. It appears that the gregarine cysts break up in position (that is in the ends of the Malpighian tubes), so that the psorosperms are passed out entirely free & are found free in large numbers in the Malpighian tubes themselves. The cast-off skins of the pupae often contain numbers of psorosperms, as I said, but still numbers are carried away by the flying insect & evidently scattered abroad through its bowel as it flies. Thus I caught a mosquito which was trying to bite me; a stream of psorosperms was issuing from its anus & could be traced up the intestine, the stomach & the M. tubes. I have kept psoropserms in water for a fortnight now, but have not observed any change. The psorosperms themselves show certain differences which I will work at. They are seldom to be found I think in old insects either fed or unfed; & seem to be almost always got rid of before death. In order to find psorosperms in pupa-pelts it is necessary to separate the pupae from the larvae, because the latter have the habit of sucking the cast off skins, evidently for the numbers of infusoria & amoebae, etc, which they contain; in this process the psorosperms are shaken out & sink to the bottom of the vessel being *heavier than water*, or are *swallowed by the larvae*. If however the pupa is put in a bottle by itself the skin is generally found full of psorosperms, & so is the digestive apparatus of the living insect which has emerged.

I think these are *facts*, as I have worked long and hard at the various points. The upshot is that the psorosperms must be discharged into two *different worlds* as it were; some are left in the water in which the grub lived & others are scattered - where? Now I will reason in the way you have taught me to. Suppose that the psorosperms were meant *only* to infect mosquito grubs, or perhaps some kind of fish or water-insect, would not the gregarines *make haste* to complete their development in time to allow of all the psorosperms being discharged into the water in which the grub lived; or would they not *retard* their development in order to allow the discharge to take place when the *eggs are laid*? But as a fact most of them are got rid of just at a time when the insect is *furthest* from water & is busy *hovering round men*. It is indeed almost certain that *while the insect is biting* it is discharging psorosperms upon the human skin; which may be directly conveyed to the mouth by the man scratching himself & then accidently sucking his finger. How does this look? Or the psorosperms may be simply scattered over a sleeper's mouth.

I must say that this *psorosperm* theory is looking very promising especially this latest development of it, into which I have been driven by hard facts. Nature would I apprehend scarcely waste the psorosperms by causing them to be evacuated just at the moment when the insect is furthest from the water - that is supposing they are meant only for grubs or water animals. In short, I believe that the psorosperms are *meant* for *men*, as well as for reinfecting the grubs, of course; hence their being discharged into *two worlds*. But what disease can they possibly cause; not dysentery I suppose; malaria seems the only supposition. Well, I have got three tubes containing psorosperms, & I hope to give each of these tubes to a man tomorrow; but I must begin with small doses of psorosperms - so you must not be disappointed if I fail at first.

1st Sept. Sunday. The contents of three tubes given to three healthy young men at 8.45 this morning. Each tube contained psorosperms from three insects (direct from the Malpighian tubes). One contained a pupa-pelt. All given in water by mouth. If the experiments fail I will try spraying the psorosperms into the lungs.

I consider that these experiments are justifiable for the following reasons.

1. They afford a certain test - I must be able to produce malaria.
2. The importance of the theory is immense.
3. We have a specific in quinine.
4. Malaria rarely affects natives badly and generally causes only one or two days fever (with tendency to relapse if quinine is not given). In over 100 cases, I have had only 1 death, a child, & 1 or 2 severe cases, in all of which quinine was not given energetically at once, the patients having delayed coming to hospital.

The nature of the experiment was fully explained in the presence of witnesses to all the men who submitted to it.

I have a sort of feeling that it will be successful, and, as you will readily understand, a kind of religious excitement over it. God knows what will be the result. If the experiment fails I shall have to take a holiday, because the work & excitement are telling upon me; but I shall soon begin work again on other lines. I feel convinced it is the mosquito.

2nd September. You will perceive that I am becoming superstitious - in other words overworked. Must give it up for a little, as the *fixed idea* (that of psorosperms) is bad for one. Today & yesterday I have been trying to make you specimens from a man with a few crescents. I mentioned a batch of mosquitoes that have no gregarines - very odd, they refuse entirely to bite. I hope however to send you by this or next mail about 12 gregarine specimens, 10 or so malarialised mosquitoes in glycerine, some grubs, pupae & young mosquitoes containing gregarines & psorosperms & a set or two of mosquito specimens from the crescent case. The only way to make these I find, when the crescents are rare, is to lump the blood together, dry, fix slightly with heat, apply aqueous solution of methylene blue to stain parasites & wash out haemoglobin. This gives the parasites close together and pretty distinct; & will show clearly, I think, the evolution of the crescent into the sphere, though spent pigment is apt to be lost sight of. If the blood be spread out thinly the parasites are clear enough, but extremely rare. No dry stained specimen will give you any idea of the liquid mosquito blood, in which the spheres stand out with the definition of spheres of glass; you will see what I mean by watching crescent evolution in partially dried viscid blood. Do you care to try in your next case? I must warn you that in such blood *crescents often look just like spent pigment*, since their pigment only often is visible (this you have observed perhaps). But it is high time that I sent you specimens of the first step, & I must do what I can with what cases come in. Have tried fixing the parasites in liquid blood by osmic acid (Laveran)[2] but evolution & phagocytosis seem to go on unchecked. Will try the way you tell me for flagellate bodies; but I must have numerous crescents surely for this. I wish to goodness that I had made specimens of Abdul Kadir's blood while I had the opportunity. The gregarine specimens are mounted in glycerine or Farrant's solution,[3] in which the tissues become a little discoloured & the psorosperms tend to curl up . When voided in water the latter are perfectly full & clear with 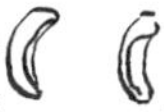 granular ball at centre or near one end - they are much 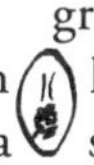 less visible in glycerine. I send two pupa pelts also; and a specimen of faeces voided by a just-hatched mosquito caught by me coming out of the pupa - it passed three droplets each of which contained some hundreds of psorosperms, which would naturally have fallen into the water. The same happens I am sure *while the mosquito is sucking the blood* - I will tell you later. I have never examined the evacuations before, as you told me to. If the present feeding experiments fail, I intend to give the men daily doses of psorosperms for some days to make sure that the psorosperms have no effect.

3rd. Holiday today (only the sick of 3 regiments, one court marshall & a medical board). Lawrie[4] disbelieves in the parasite. I saw your letter about him & will write & offer to convert him. He & Hehir are a curious couple & I will tell you later my amusing relations with them. *Your charts have been refused by the P. M. O. Indian Army on the score of* ***Expense****.* I will send you the correspondence. The fact is that these men are simply too lazy to do anything; that, I assure you is the secret of it; the excuse of expense is only a cloak to cover their laziness. I think that the correspondence should be shown to Hart & if you like to the Bills Committee;[5] & the B. M. J. should go at these men by *name*. It is the only way. They now feel themselves perfectly secure & irresponsible. They cry "expense"; but why does government support about a dozen secretaries to surgeons general? the appointment is quite unnecessary.

Moreover there are scores of sinecures all over India; if these were abolished & the men set to doing real work it would be a gain surely. The fact is that the B. M. J. should strike now while the iron is hot after Hart's speech, & strike hard. In this station there are about a dozen doctors, not one of whom possesses an oil immersion or works at malaria. Is this to go on for ever? Yet Laveran's discovery is essential to treatment. I have just been adding up my results for four months. I have recorded 110 cases (ague or simple continued fever). But of these I have found the parasite in 65 or 59%, having missed it in numbers of other cases simply owing to pressure of work, I expect. Two children with swarming summer-autumn forms had bronchitis & colds in the head; one died. Other cases might easily have been mistaken for S. C. Fever.[6] But for this malaria my regiment would have been quite healthy. Malaria causes about $^1/_3$ of the admissions in the country (I have quite discarded my old theories you see).[7] Now is not the apathy of the heads of the department quite monstrous? It amounts to a national scandal. Why don't they supply proper microscopes & make their men work at the subject? Why don't they teach it in medical schools? In districts where fever is prevalent why don't they have the fever investigated by the microscope? Really if nothing is done soon there will be a scandal. The fact is that our surgeons general don't seem to recognise their position or their duties in respect to new scientific discoveries. It is the same with amoeba coli - Hart ought to come out in a very decided & particular manner about all this & should ask pointedly what surgeon general so-&-so is doing, & threaten to put the matter into the Bills Committee. That would wake them up at once. Moreover qualified men should be sent round the country to teach *Laveranity* apostles. Oil immersions ought to be supplied at once.

But what is all this to psorosperms? Enough - "that way madness lies."[8] I have sworn not to think of them for some days. I forgot to tell you one thing. I have not had a single fresh case of fever since 22nd August. Before all the men's houses there are numbers of pots of stale water - usually full of mosquitoes - for putting out fires. About the middle of August regimental orders were issued to change the water in these every few days, & the men were recommended to keep their drinking water covered. I wonder if the fever is really going to stop altogether here! It may be only laughing at me. For many years this has been a most unhealthy part of the town & August & September the most unhealthy months. We shall see.

I have examined the stomach, intestine, kidneys & ovaries of three malarialised mosquitoes pretty carefully, but have seen nothing which I can swear are parasites. They were killed at 3 & 4 days. If the psorosperms fail I must of course work entirely in this direction. But except the psorosperms I have seen nothing yet which looks sufficiently hard & encysted to withstand *out-of-door* life. The hitch in the psorosperm theory comes in when we enquire what the flagella develop into. Is it possible too that a single animal can undergo so many metamorphoses? I am looking forward anxiously to your opinion of it all.

With kind regards
Yours truly
R. Ross.

1 *Memoirs,* 174, quotes the passage but does not give further details.

2 Laveran (1893), 17.

3 Farrant's solution, used in mounting specimens, consisted of gum arabic, glycerine and a solution of arsenious acid.

4 Edward Lawrie (1846-1915), then head of the Medical Services of the Nyzam of Hyderabad. See **Biographical Appendix**; Patrick Manson, 'Malarial parasites in the blood', *BMJ* (10 Aug. 1895), 394; and R. Ross, 'Surg. Lt. Col. Lawrie and the parasite of malaria', *Indian Lancet* (1 Oct. 1896), 311-312, **RA** 06/010.

5 The Parliamentary Bills Committee of the BMA was established in 1863/4 "to watch the progress of all bills introduced into Parliament, affecting the medical profession", Hart was the chairman between 1872 and 1897. See Peter Bartrip, *Themselves Writ Large. The British Medical Association 1832-1966.* (London: BMJ Publishing Group, 1996), 124-129.

6 Simple Continued Fever.

7 In R. Ross, 'Some objections to haematozoic theories of malaria', *Medical Reporter* 2 (1893), 65-71, Ross had argued that most fevers in India were gastrointestinal in origin.

8 *King Lear*, Act III, sc. iv.

Letter 23
02/008

Littlewood Park
Alford.
N.B.
22nd Aug, 1895

My dear Ross,

Many thanks for your letters – the last dated 30th July. Those - what you very aptly described as "my eye forms" are funny things. They remind one of the eye in Egyptian inscriptions. I have often seen them but never gave enough attention to their interpretation. I wish you wd give an *eye* to them & find out their real significance. I hope to find your slides awaiting me when I return home on the 2nd. I may go to Rome for a week or two, but so short a time is of very little use. My principal mission would be to bring back some mosquito eggs & grubs with me. I have permission to keep a "house" in the orchid house Roy. Bot. Soc. Gardens & mean to try to keep a stock going during winter so as to avail myself of any good case that may turn up.

Those coccidia-like bodies you draw I can't recall seeing - unless they are the opercula of the mosquito eggs - but I suppose they are too small for that. They are well worth careful study. Dont conclude that anything you may see in mosquito which has *not* fed on malarialised blood - but which has fed on healthy blood - is not malarial. I believe mosquitoes get malaria independently of man - perhaps in the egg from the parent - perhaps in the water passing from dead parent to water feeding larva. The trouble will be on finding a suspicious body to prove it malarial. I would suggest systematic examination of mosquitoes from non malarial district. These proving satisfactory - that is having no malaria bodies - feeding humans on such mosquitoes looking for negative results & then feeding humans on malarialised coccidia bearing mosquitoes looking for a positive result. I wish I were in your boots - hated warts & all.

Here I have been on holiday since the 9th shooting grouse & black game and walking over awful hills 10 hours a day. It does me a power of good. I want it as I have undertaken to write a Cassell's series manual on tropical diseases[1] this winter besides other things. I dont know when the B.M.J. will publish my paper on your work - I suppose soon. The accounts given of it, as usual, are inaccurate. Thin tried to throw cold water on it,[2] but the feeling of the meeting was distinctly in its favour – not that that makes any difference to the facts. The merry microbe goes its own way regardless of what people think and say about it.

I look forward to your slides with great interest. Wishing you all good luck and a happy issue out of all perplexities.

I remain
Yours very faithfully
Patrick Manson

I fancy the Italians are on mosquitoes now. Clifford Allbutt has asked me to add a section to Osler's chapter on malaria on the subject before October. So hurry up and try to give me the latest.[3]

1 Patrick Manson, *Tropical Diseases: A Manual of the Diseases of Warm Climates* (London: Cassell, 1898).

2 See Letter 21, note 1.

3 See Letter 19, note 7. Manson added an appendix to the publication 'Malarial fever', vol. viii, 941-950.

Letter 24a[1]

INDIAN TELEGRAPHS
11.9 [1895]

TO
Dr Manson
21 Queen Anne Street
Cavendish Square
London
Post Registered Bombay

FROM
Ross

Suddenly ordered Bangalore cholera investigation two of three cases had slight fever after psorosperms probably malarial but no parasites found.

1 Letter in the possession of Dr Gordon Manson-Bahr.

Letter 24
02/079

Bangalore
18th Sept 1895

Dear Dr Manson,
I have just half an hour to write before the post starts. I wired last mail to Bombay to you, being suddenly transferred here on 8th Sept to work at a cholera outbreak & to report on & reorganise all the sanitary conditions of this big city. You can imagine my work - from 6.20 a.m. to 10 p.m. The psorosperms must be dropped for the present. Very many thanks for your letter from Scotland; I note contents carefully. Now forward. On 1st Sept. I gave psorosperms to 3 young men. I gave about 1500 to each kept in a few minims of water for a day or two. They were separated by the needle from the Malpighian tubes etc. the scales of the insect not being given. To one man I gave a pupa-pelt & Govinda had as well the stomach of a malarialised mosquito which died at 24 hours; the stomach contained some old malarial blood.

Govinda: age 17 - male. Says no fever for eight years. Fat & very healthy. Blood not examined (evidently useless) 1500 psorosperms (about), on 1st Sept. 8 a.m.

5th Sept. 1.45 p.m. Complains of headache. Tongue clean. Pains in loins. Says began to feel ill half an hour ago. Says feels chilly, looks a little ill. Specimen, no parasites.

Temperatures $\frac{98.4}{13.45}$ $\frac{99.2}{14}$ Feels cold. $\frac{99.6}{14.30}$.

Specimen one (β) not amoeboid ? parasite.

$\frac{99.8}{15.0}$ $\frac{100.2}{15.30}$ $\frac{100.4}{16.0}$ $\frac{100.5}{16.30}$

Bad headache. $\frac{100.5}{17.30}$ $\frac{99.3}{19.30}$ $\frac{99.3}{21.0}$ $\frac{99.0}{22}$ $\frac{99.0}{23}$

Repeated specimens one doubtful double ring - no undoubted parasites.

6th Sept. $\frac{98.8}{6}$ $\frac{98.6}{8}$ $\frac{98.4}{10}$ $\frac{98.8}{12}$ Slight chilliness. Headache continues. Bowels not open. Pains in bones. Repeated specimens - no parasites

$\frac{99.7}{14}$ $\frac{99.7}{16}$ $\frac{97.7}{18}$ Slight sweat.

$\frac{98}{20}$ $\frac{97.6}{22}$ Repeated specimens - negative.

7th Sept. $\frac{97.0}{6}$ Still headache. Tongue white.

$\frac{98.5}{10}$ $\frac{98.5}{13}$ $\frac{98.6}{18}$ $\frac{97}{20}$ Repeated specimens negative.

8th. Temp. normal Feels quite well today. Not seen after today

Benketnaraina.[1] Healthy young man age 19. Says no fever for three years. Blood not examined. 1500 psorosperms on 1st.

7th Sept. Says headache began last night. Tongue clean. Not looking well. Says is chilly.

Temperatures $\frac{98.6}{8}$ $\frac{98.8}{14}$ $\frac{98.2}{19}$

undoubtedly slight fever. Chilly & headache. Only two specimens. No parasites. No time to examine further.

8th. $\frac{98.1}{6.0}$ Temp. normal. Feels better. 1 Spec. no parasites. Not seen after today.

I have had no reports of these cases nor of the third man. The two cases were like Lutchman's & I think that the psorosperms bring on some reaction, *probably malarial.* The cases strike me as malarial, due to *insufficient* doses. Will try 3000 psorosperms next time.

Have sent you all my specimens by this mail. Alas! only two malarialised mosquitoes - blood jumbled up to get parasites near together. Ought to have sent to you good specimens long ago. A fresh cholera case & must be off at once. Will try to write next mail. Excuse scribble. Starting bacteriological work here for detection of cholera in water. Have plenary powers to reform all sanitary details. With very kind regards. Yours truly

R. Ross.

1 The patient's name and those mentioned earlier are likely to be correct although Ross had probably not seen them written and, like many place names, spelt them phonetically.

Letter 25
02/009

21 Queen Anne Street,
Cavendish Square,
9th Sept., 1895

My dear Ross,

I have to thank you for your last three letters - the last dated 20th Aug. and only just received. They are full of interest and I look forward to receiving them as a sort of intellectual meal of weekly recurrence. I have been in Scotland shooting and hence non-reply to the last two or three. The gregarina culicidis is interesting; but I look upon it as a good lesson merely and not as the final outcome of your work. The plasmodium is a sporozoon, true, but not a gregarine; it belongs to a special order of sporozoa I believe and not quite in line with the gregarines, coccidia, sarcosporidia, microsporidia and so forth the already recognised genera. So that I would not be led too much, in investigating it, by analogy. The change of host and its position in the blood impress on it necessities which those others do not feel. The life of the plasmodium is complete in the blood of man and there is no evidence in this life of gregarine spore formation, or of coccidial pseudonavicella and so forth; and if it is complete in man and from the fact that it multiplies in the mosquito may it not also be complete in the mosquito and why therefore should we look in the latter for any important differences between the parasite in man and the parasite in the mosquito; in both hosts the necessities of the parasite are the same and it is more than probable that these necessities will be met in the same or a very similar way. Still it is necessary to clear the ground of gregarina culicidis and you do right to get clear conceptions in this point before going further.

I think you would find out a good deal about the life of this gregarine if you grew it in pure cultures. To do this I would suggest starting with mosquito eggs; these I would remove from the water in which they were originally laid and place them in distilled or rather boiled water in which no adult mosquito had died or had access. Then you could see when and how the gregarine got into the larvae and could experiment with them at will. I have no doubt the parasite comes from the insect, gets into the water, and is thus swallowed by the larva and through it passed on to the insect. It is curious finding the psorosperms about the cast skins of the pupa. You say you dont understand how or in what channel the parasite leaves the mosquito. But in the preparations you sent me I could see in the malpighian tube crowds of pseudonavicellae and in one preparation there were similar bodies in great profusion in the blood in the stomach. Does not this point to the alimentary canal as the channel by which the outer world is reached. I suppose the infant pupa uses its cast shell as a sort of diaper - dirty little beast. Those boat shaped bodies are exactly like pseudonavicellae (collapsed owing to medium of mounting) the younger granular bodies inside the psorosperm cysts an earlier stage of these pseudonavicellae. The story of the beasts life then would be - pseudonavicella passed into the water in which the larvae are swimming; a degree of development herein and then swallowed by larvae; in stomach developed into gregarines which creep up malpighian tubes, enter epithelial cells and on maturity become psorosperm cysts and in which after a time spores and pseudonavicellae are formed and so on ad infinitum. Probably the cycle is completed several times in the larvae and pupae and what the latter contain continue developing in the perfect insect which is the medium of carrying the infection from one pool of water to another.

I should make careful drawings and keep careful records of your observations on this gregarine because some one going over your work by and by will be sure to stumble on it and say you are on a wrong track, and that you have allowed yourself to be misled.

I had a whole forenoon over your slides for which accept my very best thanks. I could make out the crescents in the mosquito very well and I thought they were much more numerous than in the finger blood. I could also see the pigmented spheres in the older mosquito blood spent spheres or perhaps flagellated bodies. They were quite distinct enough to convert me.

I like your dodge of finding crescents and shall try it in the first case I get. It ought to answer with other pigmented forms as well and should prove a great gain in diagnosis. If it comes out all right I shall send the part of your letter referring to this to the B M J adding that I have tried it and find it good. You see what a fuss they are making over staining the beasts. Thin did harm by his paper frightening the modest microscopist and Daniels of Demerara[1] is inclined to follow suit. You ought to write to some of the papers and tell them to give up the staining cry. It is keeping back things very much. I have no end of letters about it.

You are right about the young gregarines being enclosed in some kind of cell. The gregarines are cell parasites in most instances at some time of their lives. You ought to find the *young gregarine* in the cells of the malpighian tubes.

You say you cant find the psorosperms in the intestine or about the anus. Have a look at the little specks of gamboge[2] coloured faeces you will find studding the inside of the bottles you keep your mosquitoes in. I fancy you will find them there. It may be however that they don't escape until the mosquito dies and breaks up in the water only in this case you should find them later than the second day after hatching of the insect which you seem to think is the period of their stay in the mosquito. Try the faeces.

Next to the establishment of the fact that the mosquito's stomach is the most favourable place for the evolution of the flagellated body, the most important observation you have made is the discovery that the free flagella can live three hours at least as independent organisms and that they attack cell structures. The free flagellum is not a feature of gregarines or coccidia so far as we know at present and in this is another argument against supposing that your gregarine is malarial. Still it may be so. There is surely a stage in the life of the coccidia in which they multiply in the definitive host; for how comes it that they are so numerous in the coccidia tumours in the rabbit's liver. It cannot be that all the coccidia ingested by the rabbit on the falciform bodies becoming amoeboid they all follow the same route and bring up in only two or three points in the liver. Some multiplication must take place in the liver - some multiplication by repeated division of the amoeboid body - before they finally bury themselves in the epithelial cells of the bile ducts. Still, flagellated spores have never been observed so far as I know in any of the sporozoa except that of malaria. This fact justifies I think placing it in a genus by itself - it and the other haemogregarinae.

Peg away; you are doing most valuable work and I firmly believe, that a light will dawn on you soon such as will astonish you and the rest of mankind and be a complete reward for all your efforts.

By way of hint let me suggest your examining the grubs of a malarialised mosquito. They are sufficiently transparent for you to see the hearts and blood vessels. It may be that in the oat-shape blood corpuscles you may find something similar to the human beast. They need oxygen in man and they may need it in mosquito.

I could write for a month about these things but must have consideration for your time and patience.

I had a letter from Cleghorn[3] a week ago. He now knows you are working at malaria and if he can help you I think he will do so. He tells me that being in Madras you are not under his immediate supervision but his sympathies are with your work. He also tells me that there is to be a stirring of the dry bones in the service soon and I hope when the waters are agitated you will be able to step in.

My friend Muir Mackenzie,[4] who has just gone out to Poonah, spoke about these malarial researches to Sir Edward Buck.[5] Mackenzie writes that Buck thinks "it unlikely that the difficulty has lain in the seconding of Ross, particularly since I told him that your latest information was that the obstacle had come from the Punjab government. He will talk to the Lieut Governor, Sir Dennis Fitzpatrick,[6] and to Cleghorn if he is in Simla, and advises me to write to the Punjab Government [sic] who is a personal friend of mine". Mackenzie also says he will try to influence Lauder[7] who has something to say with the Nizam. Buck he says was strongly of opinion that the Nizam could be approached. If you think of this write Muir Mackenzie using my name and ask him to help you. I am sure he would do it and he takes a lot of interest in matters malarial.

I dont know when or if the B. M. J. is to print my paper. I suppose they will. You were amused at Thin's criticism and so were the people who heard him. He is somewhat in the opposition shop to me, as I suppose you guess, and is not likely to speak favourably of anything I am engaged on. Perhaps a little small in this respect. I suppose you saw the article on Crombie[8] and guess where the facts come from. Crombie is absurd and does not understand what he is speaking about.

By the way I forgot to mention that Thin has gone to Catania,[9] I presume malaria hunting, and very likely he will come home with something against mosquito. I am well primed now with your work and shall be quite ready for him. The beggar in an article in the Lancet,[10] although I was the first to show him the malaria bug, made no mention of my work on the subject; not that I care a twopence about this, only I am sorry he should be so small spirited for he is in a way a clever man and a good worker in his own particular line.

I must close now with apologies for this long letter and many thanks for yours and for the slides you sent me.

Yours very sincerely

Patrick Manson

I had some blood slides from Thornhill of Ceylon[11] the other day. He cannot find the filaria and sent me those to see if he had by any chance overlooked them. In about ten slides I found the filaria in three. I cant understand how he managed not to see them. I suppose he was looking with a twelfth immersion or making some such absurd mistake.

What on earth has Lawrie[12] been up to with his white corpuscle nuclei! I suppose he has burst himself over his staining. These are thy prophets O Israel.

1 Charles Wilberforce Daniels, (1862-1927), Colonial Medical Service, seconded to British Guiana; see **Biographical Appendix**; for Thin, see Letter 16, note 7.

2 *Chambers Dictionary* (Edinburgh: Chambers Harrap, 1993): 'a yellow gum resin, obtained from any number of Asian trees, chiefly Garcinia morella, used as a pigment and in medicine.'

3 Not traced.

4 Sir John William Pitt Muir-Mackenzie, (1854-1916), was Under Secretary to the Government of India in the Revenue and Agricultural Departments and subsequently Director of Agriculture and Chief Secretary to the Government of Bombay and Commissioner in Sind. Member of the Indian Irrigation Commission.

5 Sir Edward Charles Buck, (1838-1916), Secretary to the Government of India, 1882-1897.

6 Sir Dennis Fitzpatrick, (1837-1920), Lieutenant-Governor of the Punjab 1892-1897.

7 Unidentified.

8 'Medical research in India', *BMJ* (24 August 1895), 488-489.

9 City and province in Sicily.

10 See Letter 16, note 7.

11 Hayman Thornhill, Senior Medical Officer, North-Western and Sabaragamuwa Provinces, Ceylon.

12 'Condition of the blood in malaria', *Times* (6 August 1895), 3. Lawrie reported that there was no parasite in the blood in malaria, but through a staining error, the nuclei of the white cells in the blood had been mistaken for parasites connected with the red blood corpuscle.

Letter 26
02/080

Bangalore
4th October 1895

Dear Dr Manson,

Since my last scrawl to you I have not had a moment to write to you, but now do so to thank you for your very interesting letter of 9th Sept. just received. You need be under no fear for my "time and patience". I carry about your letters in my pocket until I know 'em by heart, and they deserve it. Your objections to the gregarine are very weighty, and perhaps conclusive. I am of course not sure as to the result of my experiments of the 1st Sept. but two of the men certainly got something like malarial fever of a very slight kind; my only conclusion is that the psorosperms cause some kind of reaction, query what kind? Further experiment however may still prove me to be mistaken. Now about some points of your objections. I have partly forgotten what I have written to you in the hurry of my last letters to you. Did I tell you about the specimens of psorosperms in the stomach of young grubs which I sent you? I put some young grubs belonging to a batch which were not infected by gregarines into water containing psorosperms. As you will see in the specimens many of the psorosperms were empty; but though the grubs had been eating psorosperms for several days (I have forgotten how many alas!) they did *not* contain young gregarines, at least I could not find any after pretty careful search. The experiment requires repetition with greater care; but I am not at all sure that the psorosperms can directly infect the grubs, as I thought at first and as you think. Then again I doubt whether the gregarine "cycle is completed several times in the larvae & pupae", because I have never found mature encysted gregarines & psorosperms in the larvae; they would of course be most apparent objects in them. No, the psorosperms are ejected only at the end of the pupa stage & beginning of the imago stage. Why the latter, if they are meant only to infect other grubs. The young mature mosquito leaves the water and hunts *men*; as I told you, a mosquito which was biting at me & was killed on my hand (males also *try* to bite one; it was a male) was ejecting psorosperms. Perhaps as you say this is only on the chance of infecting fresh pots of water; but it requires careful looking into. Then is the whole history between the psorosperm and the young gregarine fully known yet? I can't find any very complete description in Leuckart or Blanchard;[1] it seems all hazy. It would indeed be very curious if the same parasite were capable of going through two separate life cycles; but doesn't something like this occur in the distoma[2] - the [nurses?] (circaria, are not they - I know nothing about them, because I always forget what I only read & haven't a book with me)? I admit all the difficulties, especially about the flagella, and don't presume even to put forward a gregarine theory; but it is curious that (I believe I haven't told you) I could find gregarines only in the mosquitoes at Begumpett (my regiments quarters) the most feverish locality in Secunderabad. Just before leaving Sec'bad for this place I examined five or six batches of grubs from other parts - no gregarines at all! Then again after I suppressed the gregarine bearing mosquitoes at Begumpett on 22nd August, there appears to have been scarcely any more fever in the regiment. I left on the 9th Sept. & am awaiting a list of cases since then from the Med. Officer who relieved me. Will let you know result. Nor can I find gregarines in the few mosquitoes which I have examined here. Certainly your view that the parasite within the mosquito is likely to have much the same appearance & history is much the more probable one. You may depend on my looking carefully when I can set to work again. Another point however which I must watch out is *what comes out of the psorosperms.* I recognise clearly the difference between the full & the empty psorosperm.

8th Sept. The difficulty, if the mal. parasite in the mosquito is like what it is in man, will lie in distinguishing it from the nuclei of cells; I have seen so many things like malaria parasites in the mosquito & the grub; but I have a lot to learn about their anatomy. Many thanks for all your kindness about the Patiala business. I may now whisper that the real reason why it broke down was a *cash* reason. The Surgeon General, however, ought to insist on a special appointment for the work being made. The cry of want of funds is utter nonsense. The fact is that all the funds are wasted in the pay of sinecures. It is monstrous that any Surgeon General should have a highly paid secretary when money can't be afforded for doing necessary work - put it that way - that will rouse them. The office of secretary to surgeons general is not only useless, but vexatious & simply an impediment to business, besides being often I fear a source of the most corrupt jobbing. Leslie wrote to me for my malarial experiences. I have found in 112 fever cases

21 spring tertians
38 summer autumns
2 quartans
3 mixed
5 doubtful

69 Total parasites found

Of course in numbers of cases of only one attack of fever (in hospital) I had really no time to look properly. There were only four or five cases in which I found nothing after fairly careful search. Should I send a note to the B. M. J. of my experiences? I will certainly write to the Ind. Med. Journal about staining when I have a moment to spare. I enclose two cuttings from the Pioneer of articles by me.[3] That against Lawrie I found it absolutely necessary to write because everyone was beginning to follow his lead. Just before leaving Sec'bad I wrote to him offering to demonstrate the parasite & he sent a silly reply but a guarded one. He deserves what he has got. As for Hehir & his cholera microbe,[4] when I had a case of cholera I wrote to ask him to come & demonstrate his haematozoön - no reply. Next case I wired - answer, he was too busy. Then I wrote strongly saying I thought it incumbent on him to do so - no reply at all. He has gone home sick. I must send you your charts with reply from government. As I haven't received your Hunterian Lecture I am going to send your charts to Ind. Med. Gazette to advertise.[5]

9th. And now in the midst of all this work to be suddenly snatched away & put to the duty of reforming the sanitary arrangements of a city of 100,000 inhabitants, & one of the finest, if not the finest station in India! But I have no more time to write on this interesting point - my life being a continual rush. Would the B. M. J. like to copy from the enclosed paragraph in the Pioneer.[6] Needless to say I am the "medical expert" referred to, but don't mention that. The city has long been in a vile state which has not been remedied by the municipality, although the Residency (Civil) Surgeon, Surgeon Colonel Dobson,[7] my friend, a very able man, has used every endeavour to stir it up, an endeavour which owing to want of real power (a want of power common in the medical department in India generally) has been fruitless. At last owing to the presence of the successive strong Residents, Mr Lee Warner[8] & Mr Mackworth Young,[9] a special medical man has been sent for correct matters. As my reports go up to government, you may be sure I am going to make something indeed out of this for Sanitation in India. To tell you *privately* I have been credited, *perhaps by a slip of the pen*, with almost unlimited power; & I have seized upon the order (or mistake) & immediately *commanded* the municipality to make *three* great reforms. Dobson is at my back, & I doubt much if, though the new Resident should wish to rescind the order, he *could* now do so. There will be a tremendous stir presently. I may want the B. M. J. at my back, as it will be a precedent for all India. I have acted with such celerity that the astonished President of the municipality, who has been muddling matters terribly, has conceded my provisional demands and has allowed me actually to *carry my reforms half through* before he or the resident or anyone understands the tyrannical nature of my actions. The reforms are so obviously beneficial that, now they are already on foot, no one will dare to oppose them; they are, good latrines, municipal conservancy & registration of water-carts (the last a thin-end-of-the-wedge measure). One final victory took place this morning; it is a regular coup d'étât. More by next mail as I am sure you will be much interested. If it does not lead to improved sanitation in a score of big towns like this it won't be our fault. I shall try to send you my printed reports, but at present it would not be allowable. Mr Hart's words are bearing fruit though he has certainly made one or two painful mistakes (who has not?).[10] With kind regards

Believe me
Yours truly
R. Ross.
Excuse this terribly thin paper & dreadful writing.

1 Leuckart (1886); Blanchard (1889-1890).
2 For a concise discussion of the life-cycle of the parasitic worms of the genus *'Distoma'*, see Henry Power and Leonard W. Sedgwick, *The New Sydenham Society's Lexicon of Medicine and the Allied Sciences*, 5 vols, (London: New Sydenham Society, 1882). The Distoma do have a complicated cycle within two separate hosts.
3 A handwritten copy of Ross's article against Lawrie's view that there was no malaria parasite, survives in the Ross Archives (**RA** 05/003). This was published in *Pioneer* (28 Sept. 1895).
4 See Letter 10, note 5.
5 This did not appear in late 95 or early 96.
6 Untraced.
7 Andrew Francis Dobson, (1848-1921), then Brigade Surgeon Lieutenant-Colonel, IMS Madras and Residency Surgeon i.e. medical officer to the Resident, the civil staff and the Bowring Civil Hospital.
8 (Sir) William Lee-Warner, (1846-1914), Indian Civil Service, Resident at Bangalore.
9 (Sir) William Mackworth Young, (1840-1924), Indian Civil Service, Resident at Bangalore 1895-1897, succeeding Lee-Warner.
10 See Letters 2, note 4 and 18, note 4.

Letter 27
02/010

21 Queen Anne Street, Cavendish Square,
11th October, 1895.

My dear Ross,
Your telegram[1] and your letter of 15th Sept.[2] were duly received but the specimens despatched by that mail are not yet to hand. I suppose they have gone round by Gib.[3] and will turn up in a day or two. I am truly sorry you are off malaria and on to Cholera. I trust that by this time you are back to your first love who urgently claims your

attention. Laveran is inclined to take up the mosquito hypothesis and I have no doubt that by next summer the French and Italians will be working at it. So for goodness sake hurry up and save the laurels for old England. It is in your power. There was an important gathering at the Academie de Medecine[4] the other day discussing malaria prophylaxis in connection with the Madagascar business and Laveran was strong on the mosquito, so that I am sure that the fat is now in the fire and it is going to burn quickly. You have the advantage and can come in an easy first with a little luck.

The psorosperms are very interesting not to say promising but dont give up working on the old lines. Dont quit the thread. Follow up the flagellum. Experiment by feeding but observe directly. I have spent a lot of time over the specimens you sent me. About the psorosperm I have an idea it is too big an organism in the mosquito to be related to that of man. Of course this is mere fancy. But were it smaller I should be more hopeful. The psorosperms are also too distinctly capsulated to tally with the soft minute spores of the malaria bug. Still the changed conditions may be enough to account for all this. Certainly the habits of the two beasts run very well together and certainly the habits of the mosquito gregarine are just what we would expect of the malaria parasite - the double provision for life in one bunch of mosquito and also for the spread of the parasite from puddle to puddle by another bunch. Why not give a rattling big dose of mosquitos, grubs, pupae and all together selecting malaria fed beasts - insects for the experiment. If you got a positive result you could then be assured that it was the mosquito and by a series of experiments with insects and larvae of known ages you could afterwards determine the exact ages, conditions and so forth.

Another line of observation I would strongly recommend is to fix and section malarialised mosquitos. I am trying that here on some insects I got from Old Calabar. I shall let you know the result. The beasts have been preserved in glycerine and the blood in them is hard as nails. I fear therefore that they may be useless. I think insects fixed in osmic acid and afterwards preserved in formaline as I wrote you some time ago would do better. If you can get a batch of these - as many as you like - duly marked with date of catching and death I would take a lot of trouble with them and see if I could trace the flagellum in stained specimens.

Also try to malarialise mosquitos with ordinary tertian blood. Select the hot & sweating stage of the fever for feeding the mosquitos. That is the time when the flagellated form abounds most in tertian blood. This I had a remarkable demonstration of the other day. They had a case of malaria at University College. They could not find the parasite so Dr Ringer[5] asked me to come round and look for it. All that was wanted was a proper film; the man was full of beasts. It was a pure case of tertian and I was anxious to find out if the flagellated body in the simple tertian was really an ordinary intracorpuscular body which for some reason missed sporing. I went round at the end of his next attack. I found one or two minute unpigmented forms and a large number of very large pigmented circular free forms. Keeping one of these under observation after quarter of an hour or so it projected flagella; another the same; and I have no doubt that all or many of them would have done the same. It is evident therefore that the flagellated form of the simple tertian comes into the blood - or rather has completed its development so far as the human host is concerned at the time of fever, and that it is then ready to proceed with development in its extra corporeal medium the mosquito. Is it not curious as well as suggestive that this is just the time when the mosquito has the best chance - the patient is prostrated and cannot defend himself - very probably asleep; he has thrown his clothes off to cool himself and is well exposed to the mosquito; and his skin is bathed with perspiration, damp and attractive. Truly this looks very like an adaptation, and it looks as if the febrogenic property of the malaria parasite was not an accident but like everything else in connection with the beast an incident designed to subserve its interests. Similarly the crescent parasite in its persistence in the blood seems to point to adaptation; the fevers it gives rise to are not always associated with sweating or the extreme prostration of a smart ague; and so the thing is permanently (for the time being) in the blood that it may have a good long chance of its mosquito absorption - a good long chance so as to compensate for the superior attractiveness of the human host sweating and prostrate in the tertian ague.

The flagellated body in the simple tertian is very different in appearance from the flagellated body derived from the crescent; as a sphere it is larger and the flagella are much finer so far as I can make out not bulbous at the ends or in their continuity.

I have got some mosquito larvae from Gib. and some eggs from Italy which I am trying to rear in the hope that if I get insects they will bite the first malaria case I can lay my hands on. But I may not trust to that and if you could possibly send me some material I will do my best to make sections of mosquitos and in that way supplement and happily confirm your work in India.

I have had some correspondence with Cleghorn[6] lately and have posted him on what you are doing. You will find a friend in him I think. Lawrie, Hehir and Co it seems are well known at headquarters and their scientific value properly assessed there.

Yours very sincerely
Patrick Manson

1 Letter 24a.
2 Actually 18th, Letter 24.
3 Gibraltar.
4 Reported in the *Indian Medical Gazette* (Dec. 1895), 496-7.
5 Sydney Ringer FRS, (1835-1910), Professor of Clinical Medicine, University College.
6 Correspondence not located.

Letter 28
02/081

West End Hotel [Bangalore][1]
26th Nov. 1895

Dear Dr Manson,
I am just scribbling a line to tell you of the state of things & how I have not been able to touch malaria work owing to this Bangalore Sanitary business. We are carrying everything successfully here, you will be pleased to hear; & I am drawing toward the end of my report which I hope will put the place in a way to be fairly healthy. As the report touches everything, I have been so busy as not even to have a moment for anything but meals & two hours golf daily. I went down to Madras however to meet my wife who has arrived with the children from England,[2] & I took the opportunity of showing them all the malaria parasites & now they are at it keenly, especially a man called Sturmer[3] who writes me that he has found the parasite in 5 out of 9 cases already. I showed them a triple quartan & a summer - autumn, the latter occurring in a case of elephantiasis which a man showed me in order to catch me, thinking that he had elephantoid fever. The laugh was turned against him. I hope that you got the specimens all right & have been able to make something of the mosquitoes bottled in glycerine, but doubt whether they were of any use. I received a number of bottles the other day from London but without a letter. I

wonder if you sent them for me to return full of mosquitoes.[4] Anyway I shall do so as soon as my report is finished. I have not found a good crescent case yet, in the few cases I have had time to examine. My labour has been frightful - working from 6. 30 a.m. to 11.30 & 12 at night & I am dead beat but have a week's work or more still to put in. I got a letter from you a month ago, by the way, for which many thanks. You may be sure that I would not have left malaria for cholera of my own free will; but it was a case of hukam[5] or command. Everyone will be on malaria shortly. I have not been able to find any psorosperms here or in Madras. It is annoying not to be able to get on with the work; what if the Italians do come in first! I am sending a short paper on parasites in Secunderabad, especially with reference to ease of finding them etc. to the B. M. J. Doubtful whether it is worth publishing.[6] I enclose a letter from Sturmer[7] to me which will show you how keen he is; but his observations on flagella are a bit startling - I can't make out what he saw. None of them in Madras were able to find the animal till I went down there. I forgot to mention arrival of your Hunterian Oration for which many thanks. I saw Cleghorn in Madras & spoke about malaria. Everything is now merely a question of want of time with me; there are only 24 hours in a day. I reported about mosquito investigations to government in response to a circular which Cleghorn sent round.[8] Have seen no notice in the B. M. J. of your speech on the subject at the B. M. Association, & everyone is asking for it. Will write again when I start real work. Kind regards from myself & my wife to you & Mrs Manson.

Yours truly
R. Ross.

1 Ross was living in a tent in the hotel's compound; *Memoirs*, 180.

2 Ross by then had two daughters, Dorothy (1891-1947) and Sylvia (1893-1925).

3 Arthur James Sturmer, (1851-1930), Surgeon Lieutenant-Colonel, IMS, one of the district medical officers in Madras.

4 Manson had sent them; see Letter 29.

5 OED: Hookum (hukm, or hookm) [Hindi] A command, order, or instruction from a person in authority.

6 R. Ross, 'Observations on malaria parasites', *BMJ* (1 Feb. 1896), 260-1.

7 **RA** 02/304 Sturmer describes some malaria parasite and a strange unpigmented body, Mary E. Gibson, *The Ross Archives Catalogue* (London: London School of Hygiene and Tropical Medicine, 1983).

8 Not located.

Letter 29
02/360

21, Queen Anne Street,
Cavendish Square
21st October, 1895

My dear Ross,

The long looked for consignment of mosquito slides arrived in good order and condition - with the exception of the malaria mosquito blood - last week, and I have had two long studies of the very interesting and important revelation of facts they represent. Yesterday I spent nearly all day over them and made a number of drawings - such as they are - of the various forms of the gregarine they contain. They bear out all you have said about this beast and one can read the life history of the little brute in your slides as in a book. How do you manage to get the alimentary canal out so perfectly without injury to malpighian tubes and other delicate structures. It is a strange instinct that sends the gregarine up the tubes to encyst and sporulate. How complete the adaptation of the beast is to the cannibalistic habits of the mosquito grub. I tell you that the sight of the alimentary canal of the mosquito grub stuffed with fragments of the parental body is a sight and one might argue from it that after all the Congo negro and the South Seas islanders were not so far wrong when they killed and devoured aged parents and fellow men generally. Next Sunday I shall have another round with these gentlemen and endeavour to complete my set of drawings. The only link I cannot find is the passage of the ingested psorosperm to young gregarine. The latter I can trace up to very minute proportions but I cannot find him emerging from psorosperms. Can you? I presume he becomes an intra-cellular parasite at this stage but I cant find him in mosquito. I presume he gets into the cells of the stomach wall for a time as is the manner of gregarines. This is a point well worth settling.

But, as I said in my last, I do not think this particular gregarine has anything to do with malaria. In the first place it is much too big when mature and is a free parasite during the greater part of its life, the only intracellular period being that which transpires after the psorosperm stage and before free gregarine stage and this even is questionable. Whereas the malaria parasite in humans is free only for a very brief period - at the time of sporulation in the intra-human stage and at the time of flagellation at the extra-human stage I fancy. The latter I believe will run on the same lines as the former - slightly altered but very nearly the same. You must go back to flagellum again and try to follow it up. But the gregarine lesson is not lost for it shows how cunningly nature provides for the spread of mosquito disease. I believe the malaria haemogregarine or haemamoeba - whatever you like to call it - completes its life in man and just in the same way and probably very much after the same fashion completes its life in the mosquito and that in both hosts the forms of the parasite will resemble each other in size and structure & habit.

I got some mosquitos - non-malariated - from Old Calabar the other day and tried to find out something from them. I found that having been preserved in glycerine the blood in the stomach had become so hard that I could not soften it and could not make anything out of the beasts at all at all. So I determined to get them sectioned and I send you by this post two slides to show you the result. I am sure you will be delighted with it for it opens up a method by which one could easily follow up the malaria parasite in the insect and at the same time preserve a permanent record of the most graphic character of the whole business. You can see from the slides how well a crescent or a flagellated form would show up.

I also send you out a box of small bottles with some formaline in the hope that you may be willing and able to fill the bottles with malariated mosquitoes which if you send home I can have sectioned stained and studied. I am very anxious to be able to demonstrate in a convincing manner to sneering sceptics that the crescent does really undergo change in the mosquito and I would fain hope that by studying sections of the mosquito stomach in series we may be able to trace the progress of the flagella after they have broken away. I think we could do so easily by following this method which I feel sure will appeal to you.

I am so vexed I did not have the chance of getting such sections of the mosquito when I was working at filarial metamorphosis. You can see the muscles of the thorax how plainly they stand out and how easy it would have been to study the encysted and metamorphosing filaria in them. I was born too soon I sometimes feel. I wonder if you could get filariated mosquitoes for me. If you could it would be a great boon for me. I have in contemplation the preparation of three Gulstonian lectures and am at my wit's end for a subject. It would seem that my mind won't work on two lines at a time - that so to speak my heart is where my treasure is; that is to say I am thinking of malaria all the time just now and cant get my attention diverted to any other subject until this one is worked out as far as it can be. Thus full of the subject I contemplate taking your work as my theme for the lectures and to illustrate the process of reasoning would like to bring up the story of the life of the filaria in the mosquito and if I could only illustrate it by such slides as I feel I could now prepare from filariated and malariated mosquitos I think it would make the lectures not quite uninteresting. Do you think you could get me a series of filariated mosquitos. It would be easy enough if you can get a case of filaria disease in a complacent native. Years ago I sent home lots of filariated mosquitos but like a fool I kept none for myself and here I am in the lurch when I most need the material I chucked about among people who did not appreciate it.

If you can do all this for me I shall be under a big load of debt. I hardly expect you to take so much trouble; I would not ask you did I not know you are willing to help on a good cause.

Perhaps if you can't get a filaria man you might get some one about Madras where the filaria is so common to get the necessary filariated mosquitos for me. The malaria ones you alone can do as you know exactly what is wanted. The filaria mosquitos should be simply immersed in the 5% formaline in batches after fixing in $^{1}/_{2}$% osmic acid - first, soon after they are fed one set, next at 12 hours, next at 24 hours, then a batch at a days interval up to the time of laying eggs. If I get these say half a dozen more or fewer of each I am all right and shall be easy in my mind about my lectures. The malaria of course you will understand will have to be formalinised - either with or without previous immersion in osmic acid half per cent - at much shorter intervals; say immediately after feeding and then for every five or ten minutes for the first hour or so and then at such longer intervals as in your judgement you think most likely to give good results. From such insects I hope for much.

My lectures are in March and I would therefore have to be hard at work all February or earlier if possible. You would therefore require to have the box or some specimens despatched so as to reach me by that time. Any expense you may be put to on my account please send me a note of. Perhaps you could contrive to send me a few mosquitos in the course of a mail or two after this. It is a very great pity you did not get a big stock from Abdul your first crescent patient. That was an opportunity that may not recur very soon again.

I have got the reprints of my Hunterian lecture but the publisher, owing to the blunder of the secretary of the society, has not included either the charts or the coloured plate. The charts are published in the speech as it appears in the transactions of the society[1] but they have left it out where I most wanted it. I shall send you some copies probably by this mail.

By the way the formaline should be diluted with water - 40 parts formaline to 60 parts water is the strength I send; of this one part to 20 of water - that is 5% of the commercial = almost 3% pure. Fix first in $^{1}/_{2}$% osmic acid - then preserve in the formaline 5% sol.

If you have plenty of mosquitos you might try some in glycerine but unless you have plenty I would not risk this as I am not quite sure if it would not shrivel the parasites too much.

If I receive some of these valuable insects in the course of a mail or two, after reply to this is possible, I shall ever bless you and you will have the consciousness of having done your best to get me into a more comfortable frame of mind than I am in at present.

Lawrie's manifesto has not appeared yet. He will get it hot if he has the hardihood to publish his absurd views. The Lancet as well as the B. M. J. has been asking me about it.

Yours very sincerely

Patrick Manson

The two slides of malariated mosquito blood in this latter consignment show nothing - I fear they have gone wrong.

1 Manson, (1894-1895).

Letter 30
02/082

West End Hotel
Bangalore
3rd Dec. 1895

Dear Dr Manson,

Three days ago I received your letter of 21st October, *three weeks late.* It had been wrongly forwarded to Madras & kept at the club there. This explains the arrival of the bottles, formaline & specimens for which many thanks. You will have thought it very [un]grateful of me not to have sent your specimens or replied to your letter before! In fact I am very distressed about it; and you may imagine that my disgust reached its climax when, happening to open my box of microscope nick-nacks I found the dozen malarialised mosquitoes in glycerine which I thought I had sent you months ago with the other specimens! Well it can't be helped. I sent off your letter at once to Maitland[1] & have just heard from him that he will procure filariated mosquitoes. I have also told the people here that whether they want my report quickly or not they must wait & give me time to get some specimens together. So I have spent the morning hunting for crescents without finding. My golf boy has about 2 in a specimen. Will go out again after breakfast.

4th Dec. Have found a good case of crescents & having been trying to get mosquitoes on; they would not bite; try again tomorrow. Sending 12 old malarialised mosquitoes in glycerine today. No time to write more. Am inclined to claim discovery of a new species of malaria parasite namely the eye-forms. Found two cases one dysentery & fever, the other fever with numbers of these. They are certainly living creatures & are *motile* to a small extent but not amoeboid. Are they young crescents? Hope the B. M. J. will bring out your speech about mosquitoes & the crescents. Smith[2] at Madras wants an article for South Indian Branch. Think I had better send him one. Writing next mail I hope. With kind regards

Yours truly
R. Ross.

1 John Maitland, (1852-1907), IMS, Madras. See **Biographical Appendix**.

2 Presumably Ross means Surgeon-Major John Smyth, IMS Madras (1857-1927), Editor of *Transactions of the South Indian Branch of the British Medical Association*. See **Biographical Appendix**.

Letter 31
02/083

West End Hotel
Bangalore
12th Dec. 1895

Dear Dr Manson,

I am afraid I have to disappoint you again about the specimens. The day after I wrote I tried the mosquitoes again, but, probably owing to low temperatures, 65-70°, they refused again to bite. As they were a young batch I determined to keep them for two days (until they should become hungry) & then try again. I did so; all the crescents except one or two in a specimen disappeared in the meantime. It is most annoying as I have spent the middle of five days over it, and, what is more it is out of the question my making another attempt until my report is written. The Govt. of India, the Resident & the municipality are all waiting for it before introducing the sanitary reforms which the place requires; & in fact it is impossible for me to spend any more time except on writing the report which is already three weeks over due. I calculate that it will take another fortnight or even three weeks, after which I shall have all the middle of the day for tackling specimens & will do my best to send you some good ones. I expect to find plenty of crescent cases by hunting for them, as there are men down from Chitral & Burma.

I had better leave off now & set to work; but hope you will excuse not receiving specimens. It is quite impossible for me to undertake the work until the report is finished. I am naturally worried that it is not sent in already, as the report will be or ought to be one of the biggest things attempted in a sanitary way in India, because I have an invitation to say what I please about the present insanitary state of affairs in the town (which may be taken as an example for the whole of India) & to suggest & carry out almost anything which is advisable. Ernest Hart's tirade has wakened them up.[1] But don't think that I do not clearly see that the mosquito affair is much bigger. Will write as soon as I start work. With kind regards -

Yours truly

R. Ross.

1 Above, Letter 2, note 4; Letter 18, note 4.

Letter 32
02/011

21 Queen Anne Street,
Cavendish Square
23rd December 1895

My dear Ross,

I was just on the point of replying to your letter of 26th Nov when that of 3rd Dec was handed me. I thought some of my letters had gone astray and also that some of your mosquitoes had wandered from the right path. Now I understand what happened. I shall welcome the twelve apostles – I mean the twelve mosquitoes in glycerine for I hope to make them apostles in a malarial sense - preachers of the gospel of Laveran and of the cause you and I have at heart. I have at last succeeded in getting a filariated mosquito. Many years ago - 17 or 18 I sent to Cobbold[1] a lot of filariated mosquitoes.

I knew that Cobbold's collections had gone to the Col. of Surgeons and so got permission to look over them for my mosquitoes. I could not find them although I found my own letters about this and other helminthological subjects. I knew that Cobbold had given some of my mosquitoes to Stephen Mackenzie[2] so I went to him and asked if he had any left. He did not know but said he would look. He looked and found a small bottle with one solitary mosquito floating in the glycerine I had sent it home in. So I got the beast, had him sectioned and stained and behold in its abdomen there were my Amoy filariae and in its thoracic muscles there they were too most beautiful to behold. Of course being in horizontal section some of the filariae appear only as little circles, others in more oblique section show as long ovals, but some that lie more in the plane of the section are quite characteristic and cannot be mistaken. In some sections the sheath that they have discarded can be seen distinctly. But in the muscles of the thorax there they show up the best. The trend of the muscle fibres tends to keep them straight out and in more than one section the line of the filaria corresponds very closely with the line of the section. They lie straight out separating the fibres for all the world like a travelling trichina. Evidently the particular mosquito I got had been captured and bottled only a few hours after it had fed so that the permanent location taken up by the filaria in the thorax is not apparent. I am anxious to ascertain this and look for light from the mosquitoes you have been good enough to get Maitland to promise to send to me.

I cannot spare a sectioned mosquito otherwise I would send you a slide; but by and by when I have got them drawn I may find it in my heart to part with one. Dont think me selfish.

About your eye-parasite. I have often seen it but unfortunately I have not kept notes of the cases nor of the circumstances in which I saw it. I put it down to injury of the blood corpuscles. In my own mind I accounted for it by supposing that it arose from injury of the corpuscle by a minute speck of dust on the slide, the speck wounding the compressed disc and starting a rent at the same time the haemoglobin uncovered so to speak by the rent agglomerating round the offending particle of dirt. Fool I was not to look more critically. Only last week I saw it in a case of Indian fever. Before publishing anything about it be very careful about your position. Get a case in which they are numerous and try to stain the things and try to stain them so as to show nucleus or nucleolus. Unless you succeed in this people will say vacuole.

I am looking forward to great things from your glycerine mosquitos. I shall section them first; treat the haemoglobin with weak acetic so as to dissolve it out and then stain for the parasite. I believe I shall see the flagellated body in full form and I believe I shall see flagella on their way to the walls of the mosquitos stomach. Shall I be able to trace them further? ? ? ? If I cant you must take it up in fresh insects and if you fail with the microscope you must try what experiment will do.

I have an idea that the fever state induced by the parasite is a condition invoked by the parasite in its own interest. I think that the prostration caused by the fever favours the chances of the mosquito getting a good meal and so absorbing the parasite and moreover that the sweating of the sweating stage provides a moist skin which is very attractive to the insect. We know that in ordinary tertians and quartans the flagellated organisms are most abundant in fact are almost confined to the febrile stage of the disease. What do you think? The chances of the flagellated organism of the crescent fevers are so much multiplied by the persistency of the crescent in the blood during all stages of the fever that there does not seem to be so much necessity in its case of making the skin specially attractive to the mosquito and accordingly sweating is not so marked a feature in this form of malarial infection. Nature is very dodgy and I believe that the fever caused by the parasite is a dodge in the interest of the parasite. Nothing walks with aimless feet.

As I told you in my last that I have asked the B. M. J. not to publish my paper on this business seeing that I was to take it up as the subject for my Goulstonian lecture.[3] They put it off so long that I thought it would be a mistake now the subject has advanced a bit to print what is becoming more or less stale. Dont you think I was right[?]

As soon as I get sections of your mosquitos I shall write in full. Meanwhile work away in the assurance that you are casting bread on the waters and that it will come back to you with full interest ere many days are past. I shall not fail to give you full credit for what you have already done and if I can give you a leg up in any way you may rely on me.

Publish in the Indian papers if you think it would be of use but send to the English papers as well and dont forget to send to the Royal Society. If your work leads to a successful issue you have the ball at your foot.

Wishing you and yours a merry Christmas I remain,
Yours very sincerely
Patrick Manson

P.S. I forgot to say that I had a call from Hehir. He is a queer fellow. An enthusiast and ambitious certainly. Knows a little about much but is not precise in his knowledge. I cant tell what he really does know about malaria. He is Lawrie's "*plasmodist*" he says - the Dr P. that famous pathologist demolishes.[4] He says Lawrie knows nothing about the microscope and he is right in this respect at all events. I am not sure about Hehir's own knowledge however for I cannot conceive that if Lawrie - who in a sense is no fool - could not be converted to plasmodism by Hehir's preparations he could not have seen the parasite - that is Hehir could not have shown it and he did not show it because he did not know it. I dont know what to make out of Hehir. He is funny. This of course is confidential in the highest degree. Lawrie is ignored here. He has made such an ass of himself that the papers for the credit of the country shut their eyes to his fiascoing. But I see the Americans have got a hold of his report or whatever it may be and are making great fun of it. They say - The Medical Record - New York[5] - I think it is - that if the science of malaria is no further advanced in India that Lawrie's report seems to represent they are sorry for India and the medical profession there. I hope you will soon give Uncle Sam one on the eye for this.

I send this to Secunderabad - on the chance that you have returned there. Please let me know your one and certain address.

I cant work out Sturmer's body I believe it to be filaria something of that sort.[6] Your visit to Madras will do good. It will stimulate Madras as against Calcutta and counteract Crombie's repressing discouraging attitude. I saw a paper by one of his men in Nov. I. M. G.[7] He found nothing in first batch of 50 cases - 30 or so in his second batch of seventy. Moral: He is only beginning to know how to look for the parasite. The more he works - the more he will find.

1 T. Spencer Cobbold, (1828-1886), the leading British helminthologist. See **Biographical Appendix**.

2 Stephen Mackenzie, (1844-1909), Physician to the London Hospital.

3 Patrick Manson, 'The Goulstonian Lectures on the life history of the malaria germ outside the human body', *BMJ* (14 March 1896), 641-646; (21 March 1896), 712-717; (28 March 1896), 774-779.

4 For Lawrie's doubts about the plasmodium see 'Condition of the blood in malaria', *Times* (6 August 1895), 3, and 'The malaria parasite' *Lancet* (9 Nov. 1895), 186.

5 The *Medical Record* printed Lawrie's report that there was no malarial

parasite (Nov 23 1895) 756, but does not appear to have had any immediate discussion on the subject, but see Letter 36, note 4.

6 See Letter 28, note 7.

7 F. P. Maynard, 'Notes on the examination of malarial blood', *Indian Medical Gazette* (November 1895), 412-420.

Letter 33
02/084

West End Hotel
Bangalore
29th January 1896

Dear Dr Manson,

At last I have finished my report on the sanitation of this place, after three months incessant work which has reduced my brain to a pulp.[1] But I am still so busy that I have time to write only a line or two. Many thanks for the copies of the oration and the charts. I am sending these to our Indian medical papers. Would you care to have the oration or parts of it reproduced? – I think it would be distinctly useful. I am also sending you copies of my paper on the crescent-mosquito business,[2] most of which was written in Secunderabad, the conclusion (on the gregarine) being put in very hurriedly. I took the liberty of quoting some parts of your letters which I thought apropos. I have done the same in connection wih a paper on the parasite generally which I sent the other day to the Indian Medical Gazette[3] – I quoted your remarks on the flagellate bodies of the intermittent fevers & your inductions from the same, as they seem to me to be very valuable, and believe you will not mind because the theory must be pushed forward. I have been corresponding with Maynard[4] who is very eager, but has just been sent away on the Persian Boundary Commission. You see our duties are apt to carry us off on all sorts of errands at any moment. Many thanks for your last letters which I read, as ever, with great interest & care. Also for the sections of mosquitoes which I have not examined yet with sufficient care – I fear that the method won't help much with the malarial parasite for a simple mathematical reason, namely that unless the blood is *swarming* with parasites you won't find more than one or two in the whole section – however I may be mistaken & it is worth trying. At Christmas Sturmer[5] came here for a week on purpose to hunt for germs & I spared him a couple of hours every day & showed him ring forms, crescents &

flagellate bodies. We made a determined attempt to put on the mosquitoes, but on three occasions they failed to bite. A few days ago however I tried again with Carr White,[6] Staff Surgeon here. The case had pretty numerous crescents & the mosquitoes bit fairly well but not so voraciously as to fill themselves all at the same time. Hence I cannot vouch for the accuracy of the times at which the mosquitoes were killed, the blood of which I send you (ten specimens). They are all dry smears not mounted in anything, nor stained. I hope that you will be able to find something in them – I have not had time even to look at them. I also send some mosquitoes dipped straight into formaline & some others (discoloured) dipped first into 1% osmic acid. This strength was necessary in order to kill the parasites before the transformation in the insects' stomach; though I doubt whether even this was able to do so. Hence you must not be surprised if you find only spent pigment. It was no use attempting a regular series; I think it is too cold here now for the animals to bite simultaneously. I enclose a paper written by Carr White[7] which he is sending to the Indian Medical Gazette; you will see it confirms my statements exactly, and he is a smart man. He found six flagellates in one mosquito — we were not very lucky. There is absolutely no doubt about the "first step" & you may set your mind at rest about it, I am sure; but I don't believe that any dried specimen will ever demonstrate the change with anything like the distinctness of a liquid specimen. I will however try again for you – it is absolutely necessary to get swarms of parasites, though. We had only two or three days at the case, after which the crescents became too few to work with.

I must now leave off & think out my *speech* for tomorrow. I have imposed a scavengering cess tax on the public here, who are howling in the press, & we expect a row at the municipal meeting tomorrow. I am going to give it them.

30th Gave it them with great success – tax passed & my services applied for for six months from date. Hope to write again very shortly.

With kind regards,

Yours truly

R. Ross

I enclose a letter from Messrs Thacker, Spink & Co[8] about selling your malaria chart & temperature charts. Can you get your publisher to send say 20 copies, as soon as possible?

1 R. Ross, *Report on Cholera, General Sanitation and the Sanitary Department and Regulations in the C. & M. Station of Bangalore* (1896). **RA** 04/001; 04/081.
2 R. Ross, 'Some observations on the crescent-sphere-flagella metamorphosis of the malaria parasite within the mosquito', *S. Ind. Branch of the B. M. A.*, (17 Dec. 1895), 334-350.
3 Ronald Ross, 'Some practical points respecting the malaria parasite', *Indian Medical Gazette* (February 1896), 42-49; (March 1896), 86-88.
4 Frederic Pinsent Maynard, IMS Bengal, (1864-1921). See also, Letter 32, note 7, and **Biographical Appendix.**
5 Letter 28, note 3.
6 Percy Carr White, IMS, (b. 1865), succeeded Ross in the Staff Surgeoncy at Bangalore.
7 P. Carr White, 'A short note on the change the malarial parasite undergoes in the mosquito', *Indian Medical Gazette* (April 1896), 121.
8 Publishers of the *Indian Medical Gazette.*

Letter 34
02/012

21 Queen Anne Street,
Cavendish Square
29th January, 1896

My dear Ross,

I have been hoping to send you an account of the results of my examination of those twelve glycerine mosquitoes which in your letter of 3rd December you said you had sent off to me. But the infernal things have never turned up and I am in despair about concluding my Gulstonian lectures fearing that the bottle has miscarried or come to grief somehow. I got filaria slides from Simla, which were despatched on the 28th of December, a week ago so, that if yours had come forward at the same rate they ought to have been here nearly a month ago. It is a great pity for I feel sure I would have got some valuable results from the plan of sectioning I have found so effective in filariated mosquito. Would you ask at your post office and if you have one or two malariated insects handy on receipt of this they might yet be in time if sent off at once and via Brindisi. The first lecture is on the 10th of March; the last not till the 17th I think. They are likely to be published soon after delivery and I shall try to send you an advance proof before.

The B. M. J. sent me your paper on the parasites of Secunderabad[1] and asked me to comment on it. This I have done. It will be published soon I fancy as there is rather a boom on in malaria lately in consequence of the death of Prince Henry of Battenberg.[2] I am worried every day by the papers for information and articles. Be therefore ready to strike now that the iron is getting to welding point. I give your experiments and results as fully as the time at my disposal will permit in the Gulstonian and do what I can to advance your interests and the interests of the plasmodium. I think you might publish categorically all your observations on plasmodium in mosquito either here or in the Indian Medical Gazette timing the publication so as to chime in with my lectures. If the government will move then you are sure to be the man and I do think that any reasonable application for leisure to pursue the work, money and opportunity will be given you.

But you must follow up your flagella. Depend upon it that is the next step. It means work; but success is everything. The sectioning of the malariated mosquito is the method I feel sure is best and I also think that the formaline preparations will turn out the best for the purpose. I have an idea that they will show best in mosquitoes treated with weak acetic acid so as to dissolve out the haemoglobin and then stained with logwood – vide Mannaberg's logwood process.[3]

I hope you are through with your cholera report and are once more on the plasmodium. I miss your letters and feel disappointed when a mail comes in without one.

Yours very truly
Patrick Manson

1 Ross (1896a).

2 Prince Henry of Battenberg had died from an attack of a 'malarious form of African Fever' whilst visiting the Gold Coast, reported in *Lancet* (25 Jan. 1896), 245, 305-6.

3 Mannaberg (1894), 256. The active ingredient from logwood is a red haematoxylin dye.

Letter 35
02/086

West End Hotel
Bangalore
27th Feb. 1896

Dear Dr Manson,
Just returned from a rush to Poona & Bombay in search of some sanitary details. Was shown my article in B.M.J. of 1st Feb[1] with your very flattering remarks, and also your lecture. Have only a few minutes before post goes to thank you. Preached Laveranity at Poona & Bombay, making one convert in the former (found parasites in 4 out of six cases, one examination each), a young chap called Kilkelly, I. M. S.[2] saw the Parsee doctor, Surveyor[3] whom you know in Bombay, & showed him a spring tertian & also saw some relapsing fever "spirilla". Do you know I believe it is an *animal parasite*? Some possible connection with Surra (?) - hardly perhaps, but does not look like bacterium.[4] The Bombay men don't care a rush for the malarial parasite; they wouldn't take the trouble to look at my spring tertian. Madras men are waking up well. See also Ind. Med. Gaz. of Feb 1896[5] - Crombie, Rogers & myself on malaria. Next month Carr White's confirmation of the mosquito business will be out I hope. Rogers has been messing with dried specimens. I don't believe Crombie is *good* at finding the animal; hence his sluggish advocacy of it; he quotes Maynard's 25% results. Rogers[6] however believes nearly all fever cases in India are malarial. I enclose another of Lawrie's follies - quoted from Times of India, Bombay,[7] about 17th Feb. His conduct in getting unknown persons to wire to the lay press in this manner & in not issuing a single signed article on the subject in the medical press is most highly reprehensible I think & unprofessional. He ought to be severely wigged for it, because he influences the muffs. Many thanks for yours of 29th Jan. I shall enquire why the bottle of mosquitoes did not reach you before - this post-office is disgraceful. Hope you got my other specimens. I have still been immensely busy over sanitation. We hope to carry matters with a higher hand than Mr Hart dreamed of, I think; if not we shall make it a test case to fight over. I shall be able to set to steady mosquito work very shortly now & shall begin by giving a few more doses of psorosperms & then "follow the flagella". Shall also try the *bites* of malariated mosquitoes.

Must leave off. With kind regards

Yours truly
R. Ross.
I only want one thing - *time*. Scurrying all day long.

1 Ross (1896a). The 'flattering remarks' appeared in an unsigned leader, 'The microscopic diagnosis of malaria', *BMJ* (1 Feb. 1896), 293.
2 Patrick Percy Kilkelly, (1869-c.1948), IMS, Bombay.
3 Probably either N. P. Surveyor or N. F. Surveyor, both of whom subsequently published on malaria.
4 For surra, Letter 17, note 3. Relapsing fever is caused by spirochaetal organisms of the genus *Borrelia*.
5 A. Crombie, 'Treatment of malarial fever', *Indian Medical Gazette* (February 1896), 41-42; Ross (1896b); Leonard Rogers, 'The etiology of malarial fever with special reference to the ground-water level, and the parasite', *Indian Medical Gazette* (February 1896), 49-55.
6 Leonard Rogers, (1868-1962), then Surgeon-Lieutenant IMS Bengal. See **Biographical Appendix**.
7 Lawrie had reported that as well as there being no parasite in the blood of malaria, malarious fever was not primarily a disease of the blood at all but a disease of the spleen and liver. Laveran's bodies were not parasites but developments of embryonic forms of blood cells, like those found in the liver and spleen of frogs. **RA** 02/085.

Letter 36
02/013

21 Queen Anne Street,
Cavendish Square,
4th March, 1896

My dear Ross,
Very many thanks for the consignment of mosquitos and blood slides of mosquito blood. The latter show the spherical bodies very well indeed but I cannot as yet manage to bring out any flagellated form. The mosquitos so far have not turned out well - the stomach contents especially in the osmic acid ones are too dark and opaque. But I shall go on trying different methods and may sooner or later succeed. My present impression is that the glycerine preserved insect is better than the osmic acid or the formaline beasts but about this

I shall let you know later on.

There was a discussion on malaria some time ago in the Medico-Chirurgical Society.[1] A very helter skelter sort of business. Thin was down on the mosquito theory. Naturally I was for it. Thin said what we want is facts - not hypothesis. And so on. I said we had the facts and wanted a hypothesis to string them on; at the same time we would be very glad of a few more facts. Thin sees no good in any one who has not a continental name and does not believe that any good thing can come out of Nazareth.

In my lectures I make a point of suggesting to the Indian government to encourage you and to give you opportunity and I do hope they will act on the hint. I fancy they will. I shall also try to get the B. M. J. to urge the same thing. They really seem inclined to move just now. I have not seen your paper yet in the Indian Medical Gazette but intend going this afternoon to the library in the hope of seeing it there.

I shall also see Danielssens[2] people this afternoon about malaria charts for Thackers people. Carr White's paper is of value as confirmatory.[3] What has Lawrie done in the matter? He is a rum fellow. None of his publications have seen the light in England yet. The Yanks still continue to make fun of him and of the service he belongs to in consequence of his silly statements.[4]

I am glad your cholera - sanitation labours are near a close - at all events that the acute stage is over and that you may have some time for higher things. If you get the mosquito business just one step further you are a made man. As the voices said to Sir Galahad so say I to you "O just and faithful knight of God, Ride on the prize is near".[5] For God read plasmodium.

I had a very bad case of Ashanti fever the other day - three or four pigmented plasmodia in every field and albumen in the urine - perhaps some haemoglobin. The parasite is the small malignant lightly pigmented form occupying about a third of the corpuscle when the pigment becomes central. I am waiting now to see if crescents come in. Send me a note of progress occasionally.

Yours very sincerely
Patrick Manson

1 'A discussion on the parasite of malaria', *Proceedings of the Royal Medical and Chirurgical Society*, Ser. 3, viii (1896), 118-151. Thin and Marshall's paper was published: R.J. Marshall and G Thin, 'The parasite of Malaria as observed in the malarial fevers of the south of Spain', *Medico-Chirurgical Society Transactions*, 79 (1896), 101-141.

The paper by Thin and Marshall, read on 11 February 1896, dealt with malaria in the south of Spain. Most of it was taken up with clinical histories, with microscopical analysis, but in the concluding pages, the authors argued that the distribution of malaria in Spain suggested that the malaria parasite 'hugs the soil', and that it was probably acquired through the air. They dismissed the possibility of mosquito transmission by the fact that mosquitoes were not found there in sufficient numbers, and that biting flies were more numerous. The resulting discussion lasted over two meetings, 11 and 25 February, with Manson defending the mosquito hypothesis, though deferring details to his Goulstonian Lectures, which he was shortly to deliver. Dr Galloway discussed Grassi's view that the flagellum is a degenerative body, and while not coming up with any conclusion of his own, criticised Thin for paying too much attention to French and Italian workers, to the exclusion of British and American ones.

2 Danielssen and Co, Lithographers – publishers of Manson's malaria charts. See Letter 33.

3 Letter 33, note 7.

4 An editorial, 'On the value of blood examinations as a test for malaria', in the *Medical Record* 49 (8 Feb. 1896), 200, concluded that Lawrie was 'prejudiced, ignorant, and incompetent'. A subsequent letter argued, in support of Lawrie, that the malarial parasite to the untrained eye was very hard to find, but that Lawrie's proof based only on negative evidence showed 'a tendency to be easily led astray that is, to say the least, mournful and embarrassing.' *Ibid.* (22 Feb. 1896), 280-281.

5 Alfred Lord Tennyson, *Sir Galahad*, II. 79-80.

Letter 37
02/087

West End Hotel
Bangalore
25th March 1896

Dear Dr Manson,

It is now two months since I finished my report, and in spite of your letter in which you said you miss my effusions, one month since I wrote to you (and over). But directly I came back from Poona I found the town in the middle of a severe outbreak of small-pox, measles & influenza, which together with the task of reforming all the sanitation has kept me in an "acute stage" of work which seems to be unending. Moreover on 1st April I take over the whole conservancy of 85000 people & start four filth depots & the reconstruction of 10,000 latrines. I am almost in despair about malaria work, but am insisting on getting assistants, who will relieve me, I hope. The report was highly complimented by the Resident.[1] I am sending copies all round - one to you I hope. I have secured full powers for the sanitary department of the town; which has never yet been given in India, and will serve as a model, I trust, for the rest of the country. But you can't imagine the labour all this costs; and the whole time my conscience pricks me for neglecting the parasite. Well, I *have* done a little lately.

First about your last letter. I am disappointed about the consignment of slides & mosquitoes. It was extraordinary that the insects sent in January (I think) did not reach you. Unfortunately I did not register the parcel & all the post office people are thieves out here. How did the *slides* look? Were they all spheres, or were there numerous crescents. I shall never be able to send you good specimens until I find a case swarming with crescents; and it will then cost me a week's work. In the meantime I must make more demonstrations of the whole first step to people here. Carr White & I went crescent hunting all over the station again - none; but we expect a crowd of cases from Burma in a few weeks. Hence I have been forced to fall back on psorosperms; with the following results.

I don't think the psorosperms are capable of directly infecting the grubs, because (a) I find grubs with numbers of unchanged psorosperms in the *rectum*, and (b) grubs kept in water full of psorosperms & containing psorosperms in their stomachs may be entirely free of gregarines. Next psorosperms seem to infect the striped mosquito most. Thirdly the sediment of the water in which such mosquitoes are kept swarms with psorosperms, which however decrease in numbers day by day even when there are no grubs in water. Lastly in about a fortnight or more the psorosperms change somewhat. The mass of granules becomes surrounded with an amoeboid (?) fluid & begin to oscillate. I have noticed nothing else. Rotiferae don't eat psorosperms. There is evidently some step wanting, I think. Where do the crowds of psorosperms at the bottom of a bottle go to? What happens to them? I often find empty shells & psorosperms which look as if degenerated. Perhaps the above amoeboid fluid is a degeneration.

On the 2nd March Carr White & I made another feeding experiment. You remember the three men to whom I gave psorosperms just before I left Secunderabad, one of whom had slight fever & the other of whom looked ill. We gave about I cub. inch of sediment containing say 3000 psorosperms to two healthy men aged 25 & 16.

Both remained quite well until the 19th inst. when Chowriappen (25) came to me in the evening with fever (Temp. 101.8). He said he was seized suddenly with shivering at 9 a.m. followed by fever; but as I was out all day he did not see me before. Very annoying. However, examined blood for $1^{1}/_{2}$ hours - no parasite whatever. Temp. 102.0 at 7 p.m. He said he had got slightly wet in a small shower of rain on the 17th. I told him to come to me early next day.

On 20th inst. *man absent* & I had engagements which could not be broken, all day. He came again however at 7.30 p.m. Said fever went away at night & recommenced with rigor at 9 a.m. Temperature at 7.30 (certified by Carr White) 102.0 - Pains in head & bones. Blood carefully examined - no parasite whatever.

Next morning (21st) temp. 97.9 at 7.30 a.m. - 98.8 at 12.0 (no fresh fever) - 99.0 at 3 p.m. No more fever. Blood examined repeatedly - no parasites. No crescents as yet (25th).

The vile luck of the case was that I did not examine in the mornings either on 19th or on 20th when I might have noticed the intermission & second rigor, if not have found rings.

Bye-the bye I have *entirely forgotten* to tell you up to date that I myself took some psorosperms in October & again in December - no result at all. I took about 1500 & 2000 on the two occasions but then I have never had fever though I have been in malarious places. Three days after the second dose I thought I felt ill, but it was probably liver. Well, I have given psorosperms now to six persons, of whom two certainly got fever & one was undoubtedly not well. There was also my first case, Lutchman, who drank water which probably contained these parasites; so that I think you will agree with me that a case or two more of this kind will deserve to rouse our closest attention. In this last case the fever was beyond all doubt & if the man's statements were true (and he is an honest looking fellow) should be malarial.

I have been thinking a great deal lately about the subject & am inclined to hold that the reaction should, ceteris paribus, be in proportion to the amount of the dose. Hence I am unwilling to give a very large dose of the psorosperms for fear of producing dangerous results. Such a course would certainly set the question quite at rest one way or another; but is it justifiable? Isn't it better to proceed as I am doing by giving larger and larger doses? I am now getting some fresh grubs for renewed experiments, which I shall in future conduct, as in the last case, before professional witnesses. I shall also send you living psorosperms in water in a mail or two. Then again, in spite of all objections to the gregarine theory, these bodies seem to me to be just the bodies capable of producing such disease as malaria. They are hard-shelled little things, capable of any amount of resistance when placed amongst the numerous forms of life found in stagnant water. Lastly I cannot find any other protozoal parasite (though plenty of fungi, etc) in the grubs; and I can't help thinking that something mysterious goes on between the psorosperm & the young gregarine. In the specimens I sent you, you say that you could not find young gregarines in grubs which contained psorosperms - nor can I *ever* do so - there is a phase wanting. Why, if every psorosperm which gets into a grub becomes a gregarine, the grub would not live at all.

I sent you a copy of my paper on the crescent-sphere metamorphosis, which has lately been reprinted in the I. M. Gazette.[2] It was very hastily written & I fear that you will think I took rather a liberty in quoting your letters. But they were very much to the point & I did not anticipate that they would be printed. My paper on the m. parasite in the I. M. G.[3] is also hasty, & I don't like it at all. However, life is short and can't be spent in getting things absolutely correct.

26th. Chowriappen complains of headache every day at about noon. Temp. at 11.30, 98.4 which is slightly above normal for a native. Perhaps he will get fever again. Examined blood very carefully again. Corpuscles absolutely without a mark. No crescents in two stirred-blood specimens.

Examined a batch of grubs - not a single gregarine or psorosperm. In another small batch which was full of psorosperms a fortnight ago, scarcely one is to be found now though the batch contains nothing bigger than rotiferae which, as I have frequently observed, won't swallow them.

I read Thin's paper.[4] There is absolutely nothing new in it & his remarks are of the usual stupidly trite kind when a theory is propounded. Nobody says, I presume, that the mosquito theory is *established* as yet; but he is quite wrong when he says that we have got no facts to go upon. Your remarks were very good & so were Galloway's.[5] When & where are the lectures coming out? Would you like to have the Hunterian oration reprinted in whole or in part in some of our Indian medical journals? Carr White's paper on the "first step" will be out in the April number of the I. M. Gazette.[6]

Now about my affairs here. At the end of May, I am going to act for six months for the Residency Surgeon and it is not unlikely that I may get the appointment as a permanency if he gives it up. This I shall like as it is one of the best appointments and perhaps the best station in the country. One can keep ones children here almost as well as in England. As I shall be head of the Public Health Dept. of the municipality I shall have my own little laboratory & assistants I hope. On the other hand if I don't get the Residency Surgeoncy I shall be entirely free in November & only wish that Govt. would use me for malaria work. Anyway I shall apply to leave here in Oct. & Nov. & travel in this Presidency in order to study the different species in different stations.

With kind regards
Yours very truly
R. Ross.

1 William Mackworth Young, (1840-1924), Resident at Mysore, 1895-1897.
2 Ross (1895).
3 Ross (1896b).
4 See Letter 36, note 1.
5 See Letter 36, note 1.
6 Carr White (1896).

Letter 38
02/014

21 Queen Anne Street,
Cavendish Square,
18th March 1896

My dear Ross,
I sent you last mail the proofs of my two first Gulstonian lectures. The proof of the last I have not yet received in such a form as to be able to send it to you but it will follow I hope in a short time. I have seen your paper in the Ind Med Gaz of Feb[1] and have to thank you for your paper in the trans of the South Indian B. M. Branch.[2] The latter is by far the best from a literary point of view and is bound to do a great deal of good in propagating the faith. I have been working as I could find time and health - for I have been very seedy lately - at the mosquitos but cant find much. The crescents were too few in the case but I shall work through the lot and try to get some light. I think the glycerine specimens were better than the osmic acid and formaline ones. These things did their work too well and have left so much haemoglobin that it is difficult to make out the parasites even in very thin sections. What do you think of trying glycerine and

water the dilution being so adjusted as not to shrivel the parasites. This and then sectioning after they have become hard enough.

I am looking forward with interest to the continuation of your paper in the Ind Med Gaz.[3] That about the different zones on the blood slide is good. Each has its lesson and each requires to be studied. I have lately had two cases of malaria - one from Ashanti the other from Kurrachi. Both were very instructive. The African parasite was the small malignant type. It produced crescents after a week which slowly disappeared in the course of 10 days or so. I am anxious to get some good cases this summer to try the English mosquito on. I have a cage all ready for breeding purposes but want the temperature, the patient, and the mosquitos - in fact everything except the will.

I write now specially to tell you that I had a letter last mail from Hankin[4] - Agra - telling me that he was likely to have a man told off to him to work on the mosquito theory. I hope you are the man. If not you must not allow any one else to forestall you in this work. In my last lecture I detail your work and - patting the government on the back - mildly hint that men like yourself should have every opportunity given them to carry on such investigations. I hope they will take the hint and push you. But if they dont for goodness sake dont let anyone else take the silver spoon out of your mouth. Hammer away as hard as you can and get ahead of everyone else. Dont trouble with detail too much. Seek general principles. Above all run the flagellum in to its appropriate cell. Had I the chance I would work day and night at this. If you want money apply to the Brit. Med. Ass for a grant. I think they would give it.

Get Thayer and Hewetson's book on the Malarial fevers of Baltimore[5] in the Johns Hopkins[6] Hospital reports; Also get Labbé's article on the Haematozaires du sang des Vertebres in tome 2, 3rd series of the Archives de zoologie experimentale et generale.[7] I send you the former but cant run to the latter but I think you would not regret buying it. They dont sell the article separately - so that you have to take the volume - it is about 40 francs but for you well worth the money. I cant get any special book on the mosquito but you told me there was one published in Madras[8] which I daresay you can lay hands on.

These other men who have been writing on the malaria parasite in India are a long way behind you and have a lot to learn yet. They dont seem to apprehend the life history of the beast properly and seem to miss the parasite in its intracorporeal forms in the irregular fevers.

Lister tells me that sudden exflagellation is a common occurrence in some of the mycetozoa so that Grassi's objection on this score does not hold water.

Excuse haste. I write principally to tell you about the appointment impending in connection with Hankin's laboratory at Agra. Keep it private however. I suppose Cleghorn is pulling the strings.

Yours very sincerely
Patrick Manson

1 Ross (1896b).
2 Ross (1895).
3 Ross (1896b).
4 E. Hanbury Hankin, (1865 -1939), appointed in 1892 as first organiser and director of the bacteriological laboratory in Agra investigating cholera and typhoid. See **Biographical Appendix**.
5 William Sydney Thayer and John Hewetson, *The Malarial Fevers of Baltimore: An Analysis of 616 Cases of Malarial Fever with Special Reference to the Relations Existing Between Different Types of Haematozoa and Different Types of Fever* (Baltimore: Johns Hopkins Press, 1895). For Thayer see **Biographical Appendix**.
6 Manson wrote **John** Hopkins, see Letter 105, note 1.
7 A. Labbé, 'Recherches zoologiques et biologiques sur les parasites endoglobulaires du sang des vertébrés', *Archives de Zoologie Expérimentale et Générale*, 3rd series, 2 (1894), 55-258.
8 Unidentified, though see Letter 49, note 3.

Letter 39
02/015

21 Queen Anne Street,
Cavendish Square,
20th March, 1896.

My dear Ross,
Just a line to say EUREKA. That is to say that your mosquitoes have turned out so far first rate. I have only done one of them yet but this one showed after proper preparation dozens of the pigmented sphere and a suspicion of flagella in one or two of these so that I have little doubt as we work our way through the lot that we will find one or more of them with flagellated organisms and perhaps we may be able

to follow this up into my hypothetical cell. The method I have adopted is to soak the insect for 24 hours in strong (not glacial) acetic acid, then for a short time in alcohol and then celloidin, section and stain with alum haematoxylin. The acetic acid removes all the haemoglobin and leaves the section beautifully clear the ghosts of blood corpuscles showing, the leucocytes staining well and the parasite staining a lightish brown and the pigment showing up characteristically. This is the method I think you should start in to work with. I have not tried the osmic acid insects in this way yet but I fear that set of insects will not be so good. Last night I received a consignment of crescent fed mosquitos from Demerara.[1] When I can I shall have them sectioned too and compare with the Bangalore batch.

On the whole I think things look very hopeful again. My first attempts with the mosquito sections made me somewhat depressed but I am quite on the other tack again. I shall send you a slide or two probably by next mail. And if you can let me have as many crescentic mosquitos as you like fixed in the formalin at various times I shall be for ever grateful. I would like some fixed immediately after feeding so as to show crescents and the gradual evolution at the very earliest stages for the benefit of the sceptics.

Excuse me bothering you thus again.

Yours very sincerely

Patrick Manson

I have been using your diagnostic microscope a great deal lately & find it very convenient.

1 Undoubtedly from C. W. Daniels, for whom see **Biographical Appendix**.

Letter 40
02/088

Bangalore
8th April 1896

Dear Dr Manson,

I have received your two letters of 18th & 20th March, for which many thanks, and have been much concerned to hear that you have not been well. I fear that you have been feeling anxious about the theory not getting on & alas disappointed at the specimens &

mosquitoes which I sent you, though, I am glad you have succeeded at last in finding the spheres in the sections. You must not be anxious about the theory, much less about the acceptance of the parasite. I feel pretty sure that I shall be able to produce fever again very shortly. It *can't* be a mere coincidence that three men should have got fever shortly after drinking mosquito-water. I don't say it was the psorosperms or anything else; but undoubtedly three men *have* acquired fever after the experiment. Another case or two will clench it. I have not been able to do any more experiments unfortunately. A servant broke my bottle of glycerine bearing grubs & I can't get any more. Since the last successful case moreover, volunteers won't come forward; but I hope to be on the job in a day or two perhaps, if I can find some fresh psorosperms. You must think that I am very backward & slow over so important a matter, but I can only assure you that I have scarcely time to eat & sleep & have a hundred anxieties over the sanitary work, the extent of which you have probably no idea of (& could have no idea unless you were doing it). All the papers in the Presidency are continually talking about it, most of them hostile (these people love filth) so that I have to show the utmost energy & care. On receiving your letter, however, *re* the appointment under Hankin of a man to study the theory, I have written post haste to him & Leslie[1] to find out exactly. Of course I can't throw over this work at least for two or three months, & if I throw it over at all, it will only be at a cost of a good appointment & the best climate in India, which are serious matters to a man with a family. However, I would do this for the theory; but will not wonder if another man is appointed. I know the ways of the India Govt. & think that they are likely to put anyone in. When I hear from the Surgeon General[2] however, I may be able to arrange matters. If an arrangement could be effected whereby *half* my time could be devoted to the parasite (and such an arrangement can be made) I could do a great deal. I will try. More by next mail. The Gulstonian lectures are *splendid*.[3]

Yours very sincerely
R. Ross.

1 Letters untraced.

2 i.e. Cleghorn.

3 Manson (1896a).

Letter 41
02/089

Bangalore
29th April 1896

Dear Dr Manson,
Just a hurried line to tell you that I am afraid it is impossible to work on the theory. I am in despair about it. Since last writing I have had a sweepers' strike, have had to form my Health Committee & do a thousand things the worry & anxiety of which gave me symptoms of cerebral exhaustion so that I had to rush off to Ootacamund for five days' rest. My work lasts me from six a.m. to 5 p.m. every day Sundays included & it is *impossible* to investigate. I have found however several batches of mosquito grubs with psorosperms & if they are numerous enough will try to give them to six men I have got in a day or two which I hope will clench the psorosperm business one way or another. I have also been to several hospitals in search of crescents – not a case. But it is hopeless to talk of working at the theory properly under such circumstances. I am in despair about it. It makes me depressed. I even spoke to the Resident about giving up my present work, but he would not hear of it – it is impossible as you will see when you get a copy of my report. But I have an idea – that is to hire an intelligent young hospital assistant and train him to work at the theory under me. It will cost about 30 rupees a month and I shall try to get the South Indian Branch of the B.M.A. to help me. Do you think that you could get the B.M.Ass. to give me a little money to the above amount for the purpose of providing me with an assistant? Well, anyway I think I shall look out for a man in a day or two & shall write to John Smyth[1] of Madras to help me. I wrote to Cleghorn on receipt of your last letter & also to Hankin.[2] The first said that no special appointment to study the mosquito malaria theory had been sanctioned; the second said that he had unintentionally misled you & that he proposed only to get the next man who came to study with him, to tackle the theory - that was all - there was no fixed appointment contemplated.

Well, I am very down in spite of my five days' leave. Temperature even in Bangalore 90° to 95°, and I have just come off an *eleven* hours spell of work with one hour for breakfast. How many will do that in England? Now (5 p.m.) I am going to sleep. Better luck soon.

Yours very sincerely
R. Ross.

1 Letter 30, note 2.
2 Letter 38, note 4.

Letter 42
02/016

21 Queen Anne Street
Cavendish Square
London W.
April 18th, 1896

My dear Ross,
Your letter of the 25th of March reached me in due course. I congratulate you on the completion of your sanitary labours, or rather of your report, but regret very much that these have taken you away from what I look upon as your proper work - the investigation of the mosquito stage of malaria. - I read with great interest all your papers in the Indian Medical Gazette,[1] that were last published. One was first rate; you always write best when you let yourself go and don't trouble to pick and polish. Those eye parasites are interesting, and I hope you will make something out of them. I have already told you that I, too, had seen them, but like a fool, I passed them over as vacuoles, or effects of injury from dust to the corpuscle. Since you have written so positively on the subject, I want to take back all I have said about that, and whenever I come across the things, I shall look at them with renewed interest and try to make something of them. Do you do the same and work up a case or two, stain them and send the paper home. Carr White's confirmation of your mosquito work will be of value.[2] I have had many of your last batch sectioned, but except in one or two instances, and even in these, somewhat doubtfully, have failed to make out the flagella. I have had some lately, from British Guiana, but in them the parasites were even scantier than in yours and showed nothing further. Lately I had a magnificent case of crescent infection which showed the high value of the microscope in diagnosis. The man was admitted with phthisis and had the usual evening rise of temperature; the house physician, who is now an expert in malarial diagnosis, suspected something more than this. He examined the blood and found crescents by the hundreds. Quinine administered and rapid improvement; the phthisis, of course, remained. I have been making a good many experiments in this man's blood, principally with the view of accelerating microscopic diagnosis and the preparation of good films

for staining and I think I have succeeded. In elaborating methods of real value I dispense altogether with cover-glass preparations; they are difficult to prepare with even films; they are easily broken; and they cannot be labelled unless with a lot of trouble. This is my plan: say I want to prepare fifty films, I can do it in five minutes and much better films than you can get on cover-glasses; clean fifty *slips* and lay them side by side on a table near the patient. Cut three or four oblongs of tissue paper, (an inch and a half long by five eights of an inch broad); prick the patient's finger; get a good drop of blood; lay one surface (near one end) of the tissue paper on the blood; then apply the charged surface to a slip; wait till the blood runs out a little and pull the tissue paper along the surface of the slip; and so on for your fifty slides, recharging the tissue paper every four or five slips as it appears to be exhausted; allow the blood to dry; label and store. When you wish to stain, fix the blood by dropping a little alcohol on each slide; Dry stain with half minute of borax methylene blue; dry mount with zylol balsam. The result, perfect preparations. Another plan I practise has for its object the examination of a large quantity of blood rapidly. Practise it thus: clean the slip; prick the finger; get a good drop of blood; dab the slip on the blood; spread the blood out in a fairly thick film and allow to dry; fix with alcohol and then wash out the haemoglobin by a very weak solution of acetic acid, (two drops to the watch-glassful of water); wash in water; dry; stain with methylene blue. Crescents show up perhaps fifty in a field and other forms of the parasite are recognisable to the practised eye. I sometimes dispense with the acetic acid, but in that case, before fixing with alcohol, pass the charged slip once or twice through water, pouring a little alcohol on immediately afterwards, so as to fix at once; Dry and stain. Result:- for crescents good, only they are apt to be slightly deformed. Try these plans and let me know your opinion. Today, examining some blood which had been sent from Demerara for filaria purposes, and which was thick and opaque, by using this method I succeeded in recognising crescents very easily. I noticed on the label of the slide that the patient from whom the blood came had been suffering from malarial cachexia. I am very much interested in your psorosperm experiments; go on with them but I beg of you not to leave hold of the flagellum. I suppose that the psorosperm on getting into water may pass through one or two elementary phases, before they are ready to infect the mosquito grub. Don't experiment on yourself, as a married man and one whose life is of value to medical science, you have no business to take risks of this nature. I hope you received my Goulstonian lectures[3] and that they represent your views. I had a letter from the editor[4] of the Indian Lancet, I think, asking permission to publish the Hunterian oration, I said "publish". What is Lawrie doing now? Is his pipe out yet? It ought to be. I wonder if he has the pluck and candour to take back what he has said. Sometime ago, I had a letter and also a report from Surgeon Captain Bruce[5] who is now in Zululand investigating the Tsetse Fly Disease. His results are most interesting and most important. He finds that the Fly Disease is caused by a trypanosome, exactly like that of Surra but, unlike the Surra of India, it affects horned cattle and dogs as well as solipeds. I wonder if the Indian and African parasites are identical. I have asked a man here, connected with the British Institute of Preventive Medicine,[6] to inject trypanosome-containing rats' blood into horses to see if the horses will get Surra or any analogous complaint. Be sure to keep me posted with the progress of your work and let me know if there is any chance of your getting into Hankin's Laboratory.

With kind regards,

Believe me,

Yours very truly

Patrick Manson

1 Ross (reprint of 1895; 1896b),
2 Letter 37, note 6.
3 Manson (1896a). See Letter 40.
4 Laurence Fernandez; Manson's lectures were not republished in an Indian Journal.
5 David Bruce, (1855-1931), See **Biographical Appendix**.
6 Renamed Jenner Institute in 1898, and Lister Institute in 1903.

Letter 43
02/090

Bangalore
27th May 1896

Dear Dr Manson,
None of the experimental cases has come in yet & all look like being failures. The last case appeared looking ill after 48 hours, but it passed off next day, & he has been well ever since. The psorosperms were given at all degrees of freshness & in large numbers; so that it certainly looks, as was to be suspected, that they are not the thing. But I will

watch & pray, & try a few more experiments; reverting meanwhile to the thread, I took over the Civil Hospital yesterday & immediately found a case of eye-forms & a summer-autumn - only a few crescents as yet. The eye-forms are certainly something funny. Though there is a true vacuole like an eye-form (which must not mislead) the real eye-form is something organic & living. I saw only two (in the same corpuscle) in the case (a baby from a malarious district with irregular fever). These had exactly the appearance noted before & were dancing about continually in the corpuscle with a brownian-like movement, but when they turned sideways the central dot always vanished. What can they be? - the youngest of spores perhaps; but then I could find no older forms; nothing else in fact. The summer-autumn is not yet fit for experiment. I am going to Ooty[1] for a weeks leave in three days & when I come back I expect to have numerous cases as the rains are in. Then I shall settle down to real work. Of course I have been dissecting mosquitoes a great deal & shall attack the pursuit of the flagellate spores with three times the confidence I had last year. I can extract a blood-filled stomach, *wash it* & examine. If the spores occupy the perivisceral cells, I shall find them, because they are sure to keep wriggling for a long time within the cell. But the belief is growing on me that the disease is communicated by the *bite* of the mosquito - what do you think? She always injects a small quantity of fluid with her bite, I believe - what if the parasites get into the system in this manner. I shall experiment in this direction & shall also dissect the head. Well, I ought to have about 2 hours a day to spare when I return; I have got my Health Department to work in well-oiled grooves. Between dissection & experiment I ought to get at something soon. I will also send you numerous specimens I hope; though I have my doubts about the sectioning, because I fear the flagella are too fine for the process. I have noted your advice about formaline, etc. Your method of making specimens with tissue paper is a first rate idea. I shall try it tomorrow I hope. The second method (that of making thick smears & washing out with acetic acid) I have tried already practically in the two specimens which I sent you and in which you said that you could find nothing. I shall try tomorrow an extension of it to liquid specimens for finding crescents. As I have now several very intelligent assistant surgeons, I shall train them in Laveranity & set them to work to assist me. We are proposing too, a regular fever-hunt & hope to get some statistics as to malarial & non-malarial fevers. Time, only, is wanting.

By the way, Dobson (Surgeon Colonel - he is very particular)[2] who has made all this fuss about sanitation here is on his way home & is going to see you. He will thunder on the subordination in which the profession is held in this country & the state to which sanitation has fallen: He is really a very strong man and I hope he will be listened to. As a matter of fact I know very well that the Govt. Resolution of which the British Medical wrote so much (Resolution of Oct. 26th 1895)[3]. will stand or fall by what he and I are doing here. It is a question whether sanitation will be executively in the hands of the medical, or civil & military services; & there will be a great fight, because executive sanitation in India means half the patronage & expenditure of municipalities. I have got it in my hands here - and this forms a precedent which, if it fails, will ruin the Resolution of Govt. I sincerely hope therefore that Mr Hart & the British Medical will take up Dobson and my report (which I sent them some mails ago without a covering letter). I told Dobson that I am sure you will help him.

28th. I must close abruptly - to continue in my next - by next mail. I have lots to say and to thank you for. With kind regards

Yours sincerely

R. Ross.

1 Ootacamund: One of the Indian Hill Stations. See Dane Kennedy, *The Magic Mountains. Hill Stations and the British Raj* (Los Angeles: University of California Press, 1996).

2 Surgeon Colonel A. F. Dobson, (1848-1921), Residency Surgeon (ie Medical Officer to the Resident, the civil staff and the Bowring Civil Hospital). Ross became officiating Residency Surgeon while Dobson returned to England on furlough.

3 'Resolution regarding the reorganisation of the Sanitary Department in India', *Indian Medical Gazette*, (Dec. 1895), 506-508.

Letter 44
02/017

21, Queen Anne Street,
Cavendish Square,
London. W.
May 20th., 1896.

My dear Ross,

I duly received your letter of the 29th of April. I gather from it that you are the victim of overwork, that you are suffering from the despondency of exhaustion; but take heart, the wheel will turn again and you will feel better by and by. You are quite right to take a holiday; it will give you time to think and time to forget. It seems to me a great misfortune that the best men in your service are the hardest worked; that is to say, that their energies and abilities are directed into such base utilitarian channels as practical sanitation of cities and the charge of big establishments requiring more administrative ability than brains. I suppose Government wants to get what it pays for and a little more. Your idea of training a young hospital assistant to work for you is a good one, and I think if you apply to the British Medical Association for help, you will certainly get it. The sum you mention is a very modest one and if it leads even to one step forward, it will be the best investment the association could make for the funds it has at its command for the forwarding of pathological research. Do not despair about your application to Cleghorn and Hankin. The application will keep you before the authorities and you may be pretty sure that when they want a man, they will pick you out; so I think; at least, I should. Very likely, the first man they get will prove a failure, and certain it is that much time will be wasted before he can thoroughly grasp the real situation of the investigation and acquire the knowledge and technical skill, which are necessary to carry the question to its next stage. I have read Lawrie's paper with astonishment.[1] The cheek of the man is something gigantic; fancy his assurance in placing himself alongside with Golgi[2] and with dozens of other men, highly skilled histologists and zoologists, whose boots he is not fit to black. I can imagine the good men of your service covering their faces with their hands for very shame. What is the man's idea? Is it to curry favour with the populace or is he mad? I have got another batch of mosquitos, but I can make nothing out of them as yet, perhaps, in a little while light may dawn on them too. I think glycerine and water two to one, is really the best preservative for the mosquito, at all events, I find that it has given better results than the osmic acid which is a dead failure, or the formaline. Should you chance to see Maitland,[3] tell him we had a case of varicose groin glands and lymphscrotum which was operated on at the urgent request of the unhappy sailor. The glands in one groin were completely removed and the greater part of the scrotum, the glands in the other groin, it was deemed prudent to leave alone for a while at least. The case has done well so far. No chyluria; filaria are abundant in his blood; the operation has made no difference in this respect. I shall watch the progress of events after the man gets up and is on full diet and working, with great interest. It is proposed in a short time to remove a considerable part of the scrotum that has been left and also the groin glands of the other side. I see Maitland has been showing filariated mosquitos; I wish he could spare a few for me.

Yours very sincerely
Patrick Manson

The B. M. J. wanted me to review Lawrie in detail. I declined to do so. He is too personal for my taste & moreover he does not begin to know his subject. I had to write them a short letter however.[4]

1 E. Lawrie, 'An address on the cause of malaria', *Lancet* (16 May 1896), 1334-1338. Lawrie's article, based on an address that he had delivered at the Grant Medical College, Bombay, castigated the stance that Hart and the BMJ had taken on the state of the IMS and of sanitation in India. He was critical of Manson ('that devoted worshipper of parasites and foreigners') and, on the basis of experiments with frogs and microscopical and clinical observations on fever patients, argued that Laveran's 'bodies' were actually diseased white blood corpuscles. Although Lawrie defended several IMS doctors, including Crombie, Cunningham and Bryden, he made no mention of Ross's work.

2 Camillo Golgi, (1844-1926), Professor of general pathology at Pavia University. See **Biographical Appendix**.

3 Maitland was especially interested in filaria, for example, J. Maitland, 'Removal of adult filariae in cases of lymphangitis', *BMJ* (2 Oct. 1897), 903.

4 Letter from Patrick Manson, *BMJ* (30 May 1896), 1355. 'I have not the slightest fear that the opinion of anyone who has really studied [the malaria parasite] will be changed by anything Dr. Lawrie has advanced.'

Letter 45
02/091

Bangalore
21 Sept. 1896

Dear Dr Manson,

I think it is now three months since I wrote to you on the subject - the reason being that I vowed to myself that I would not bore you any more with my letters until I had done some work worth writing about. Lest you should be disappointed I may tell you at once that I have been able to do nothing but six experiments to produce fever - all negative. When I last wrote I was going up to the hills, not feeling well, for ten days leave; but I had to return in five days in consequence of cholera breaking out in the station. Cholera lasted off & on until the end of last month & kept me, when taken together with sanitary & medical duties, on the rush all day. Nevertheless I have had time to examine most of my fever cases, but during the whole period have got only one case with a fair number of crescents. From this I obtained some mosquitoes which I am sending you (killed at about 1/2 an hour & put in strong formaline) - they ought to have been sent some time ago. I am also sending one or two attempts at specimens. Of these, I can make no good ones. Both in dried & in mounted specimens the spheres look more like spent pigment than anything else. I tried Farrant's solution,[1] but it makes the spheres shrivel up. Smearing mosquito blood seems to me to be hopeless - I believe it bursts the ripe spheres - but I will try again. Of course my work in this way was carried on during occasional half hours disturbed by other business.

Now for the experiments. Mr Appia[2] the assistant surgeon of my hospital volunteered to be bitten by mosquitoes which had been fed on the good case (one of triple infection with quartan, tertian & summer-autumn fever). I let loose on him 18 mosquitoes fed 3 days previously & six mosquitoes fed on the previous day. This was on the 13th August. Again on the 17th he was bitten by 15 of the mosquitoes which had already bitten him & remained alive & also 5 mosquitoes fed on the malaria case on the 15th. He said he was determined to get fever if he could, but he did not.

At the same time two other men were treated in a similar manner - Ramasami by 10 mosquitoes on one occasion, & Kristnasami by numerous mosquitoes, also on one occasion. Results negative.

These negative results appear to me to suggest that the bite of the mosquito is *not* the means of infection. In all three cases the number of malariated mosquitoes loosed on the subjects was much larger than is likely to be the case in the ordinary course of events, & yet the result was completely negative.

Three more persons drank the water in which all these insects had been kept - negative, though the doses were very large. I have now done 24 such experiments, with three or four successes or partial successes, and intend to send a brief account of them to our Branch. Unfortunately I have lost my record of Lutchman's temperatures of which I sent you a copy.[3] Do you think you could let me have it back? - it was my first case you may remember. Did I tell you that the five experiments done in May all failed?

22nd. Sept. Just found a good case of crescents this morning & am going to look at various species of mosquito at noon. The man's fever ceased a week ago, when I & a man who came down from the Central Provinces to study the parasite, found only two crescents in many specimens. Today 1 in about 3 fields - so must set to work. With kind regards.

Yours sincerely

R. Ross.

I have reasons for thinking that crescents don't proceed to flagellation in the speckled variety of mosquito - namely those I am sending you. Such points must be chased.

23rd. Hope I haven't missed mail. I must send specimens by next mail. New case very good.

1 Farrant's Solution, see Letter 22, note 3.

2 Mr K. N. Appia, Assistant Surgeon of the Bowring Civil Hospital at Bangalore.

3 Letter 8.

Letter 46
02/092

Bangalore
30 Sept. 1896

Dear Dr Manson,

I enclose registration receipt for a parcel of specimens which I despatch today. They consist of mosquitoes (crescents) at 1 hour - mosquitoes (spring tertian) at 1 hour - mosquitoes (crescents) at 1 day & 2 days, all for section - preserved in formaline. I also send some cover-glass specimens of mosquito blood done in various ways - (1) dried, (2) dried & treated with acetic acid (3) run into Farrant's Solution. In all the number of spheres appears to be nil or too small because these bodies appear generally to break up (except when just formed from the crescent) under the process of drying or in glycerine. Hence the parasites will all look like spent pigment, only that the spheres are represented by a circular cluster of pigment, while spent pigment is generally drawn out  & . Some of the specimens ought to show very numerous parasites in certain places, but the beautiful clear glass-ball-like appearance of the spheres in mosquito blood is entirely lost. They shrivel away in Farrant's Solution. Anyway I don't think you will find many crescents in the lot.

I have been doing 2 hours a day with the case & have improved my former method. Now I draw out the whole stomach & intestine etc (as you will see in one of the specimens I hope) and then examine with oil immersion. One can readily see spheres in the bulk of the blood in this manner. Thus I saw a small "manifestation" of flagellate bodies (7) in a part of the stomach *through the walls*. I have fixed on the process of exflagellation which must be worked out more carefully. It is a fixed & absolute rule that *all crescents shortly become spheres in the mosquitoes stomach*; but when, how, why the spheres become flagellate is now being tackled. I am on the search for some clue to this, as I think there is a law beyond what I have thought yet, namely that it depends only on the length of time the parasite has spent in the stomach. Yesterday I saw what I have not observed before 8 or 10 free flagella in proximate fields. I watched them for 3/4 hour during which they wriggled about like trypanosomes. Two appeared to attack some leucocyte debris. The motions seem to disappear gradually.

Must leave off as I want to get to work. With kind regards.

Yours sincerely

R. Ross.

Letter 47
02/093

Bangalore
14th Oct 1896

Dear Dr Manson,

Just a line to tell you that the case of crescents "dried up" two days after my last letter. The crescents disappeared very suddenly, & the disappearance was followed by a slight return of fever. I then expected a reappearance of crescents but this did not occur. The day before yesterday however the patient had a smart attack of *dysentery*. I examined the blood & mucous very carefully & could find neither amoeba coli nor any sign of pigment or crescents. I shall have another look tomorrow however, which is an office holiday. Not a single other case to hand.

You will be pleased to hear that there is every chance of my being put on special duty in a month or two to investigate the mosquito theory further. A Planters' Commission[1] has been sitting here & I got them to recommend to Government that a special investigation should be started. Govt. immediately asked me for information which I sent

& which would probably have been shelved but that Hon. Mr. Bliss[2] member of council has been here. I went to him & asked him to help. He promised to do so and as he rules the medical service & is a strong man & appears to have taken up the idea with some interest I think it will be carried through. I shall probably have to wait until I am relieved here, which may not be until January. What I propose is that I should be sent to the most malarious spot known & there study. I should like a place where there is only *one* source of water & where the malaria is very prevalent. There I would take stock of the species of mosquito abounding. This seems to me the unknown quantity which I must first obtain because it may well happen that the parasite does not develop in the ordinary species seen in most stations, so that all my experiments on the 2nd stage may have failed for this reason. By the way do you want back your Thayer & Hewetson[3] (which has been very useful to me)? Somebody stole my Mannaberg.[4] Do you think also that, unless I trouble you too much, you could ask the Scientific Grants Committee[5] to lend me a 20 or 25 inch apochromatic oil immersion with two suitable eye-pieces? I also write to the General Secretary by this mail but must have the lens as soon as possible if I am to use it when on special duty which may last only three months. I have referred him to you. The lens is wanted (or may be) for watching flagella. You cannot imagine how glad I will be to get back to real work after this endless organisation business. With kind regards

Believe me yours sincerely

R. Ross.

1 A meeting of the United Planters' Association in August 1896 resolved "that the secretary be instructed to move the Government of Madras to commence an enquiry into the development of the malarial parasite on somewhat similar lines to the investigation undertaken by Surgeon-Major Ross and others …", *Memoirs*, 201. See Letter 76, note 3.

2 The Hon. Mr H. W. Bliss, (1840-1919), member of the Madras Executive Council.

3 Thayer and Hewetson (1895).

4 Mannaberg (1894).

5 The Scientific Grants Committee of the BMA. Ross received a reply from the General Secretary, Frances Sowke, saying that the money for the year had been allocated and adding that the Association did not possess such a powerful microscope. **RA** 06/027 (Gibson, 1983).

Letter 48
02/018

21 Queen Anne Street,
Cavendish Sq.
12 October, 1896

My dear Ross,

I was very pleased to get your letter of 21st Sept two days ago and look forward to the consignment of mosquitoes in the course of another fortnight for I suppose they travel via Gib. I enclose Lutchman's temperatures as you request. I do not send the letter as there is no saying how soon I may have to refer to it now that attention is being directed in Italy and France to this matter of the mosquito in Malaria. Bignami has criticised our theory in Il Policlinico and has started a mosquito theory of his own.[1] I send you a translation of his article said translation having been prepared for the Lancet in which it is likely to appear soon.[2] I thought you would like to get early information of what is going on. Bignami is wrong in many things and blinks all my arguments nearly. I propose to answer him as soon as the paper appears.

Have you tried my paper dodge of spreading malarial blood? I have an improvement. Use clean uncrumpled gutta-percha[3] tissue instead of tissue paper. The results are better and more uniform. I get splendid films in this way and as many as I like in a few minutes.

I read your critique of Lawrie in the Madras Trans[4] and nearly split my sides laughing. You had the Hyderabad savant on toast properly. After this he should for ever hold his peace. I wish you had sent this paper or letter to the English medical papers. It would have clenched the matter with all objectors for ever and a day. I dont know if you meant it for satire but such it cannot fail to appear to Lawrie and I guess he will not love you for so thoroughly pricking his wind-bag. Let him pass.

Your experiments on mosquito biting are interesting although negative. It may be that the mosquito conveys the parasite in biting but I do not think so - at all events.I do not think that it does so directly; for the habit of the mosquito is to bite once only and the normal evolution of the parasite is sure to correspond and to run parallel with the normal habits of the insect. I think you are more likely - assuming that the parasite is conveyed by the bite of the mosquito - to find that it is conveyed by the offspring of the mosquito that has bitten the malariated individual - that it is conveyed by the children and not by the parent seeing that on the flagellum hypothesis it has to evolute in the insect that has bitten and swallowed. You might try feeding mosquitoes on a malariated man, keeping them, rearing their young and setting these to bite an infected subject. There is more natural logic in such an experiment. But I would reiterate the advice I always harp on - Follow the flagellum. Next case I get of crescents I mean to try to demonstrate nuclear elements in the flagellum. It is very difficult to get them so prepared as to be available for staining purposes. Were I in a hot place I would try to work this point out in birds rather than in man and I am not so sure that you might not be able to get along in this way yourself seeing that there would be no lack of material and opportunity and you could get native assistants to work for you. You could easily get some bird with flagellated forms in its blood, stick it in a cage and the cage in a mosquito house and set mosquitos to bite and have no worry about searching for crescents, squaring the man, accusations of homicide and so forth.

Do you find - as I gather from your letter you do - that mosquitos feed more than once. My experience was that if the mosquito gets one good undisturbed drink of blood she is satisfied and does not bite again but proceeds at once and invariably to develop her eggs. Is this not so?

By the way I think glycerine and water a better medium for keeping malaria charged mosquitos in than formaline. Some I had from Demerara in the latter were a failure.

Write me whenever you get a chance. I like your letters. No fear of boring me and dont mind asking me to do anything I can for you or anything to help forward the good work in England.

It is evident that the Italians are now on the scent. I do hope you will run into the quarry before them. Bignami is a clever little fellow and ambitious. Laveran is working up the Frenchmen. I do not hear that the Germans are moving but they will and so will the Russians. Cut in first.

Yours very sincerely
Patrick Manson

1 A. Bignami, *Il Policlinico* (15 July, 1896).

2 Amico Bignami, 'Hypothesis as to the life-history of the malarial parasite outside the human body. (Apropos of an article by Dr Patrick Manson)', *Lancet* (14 Nov. 1896), 1363-1367; (21 Nov, 1896), 1441-1444. Bignami's article, thought important enough to translate into English, reviewed the variety of theories regarding the

causation of malaria. Rejecting on both experimental and epidemiological grounds the view that malaria is transmitted by air or water, he implicated the mosquito, and, drawing on the work of Smith and Kilborne on the transmission of Texas Cattle Fever through the bite of the tick, concluded that it was likely that malaria is 'a disease of inoculation'. Manson's reasons for rejecting this view are mentioned later in this letter.

3 Chambers' Dictionary (1993 ed.): a highly resistive, waterproof substance, like rubber but harder and not extensible, obtained chiefly from the latex of the Malaysian trees of the Sapotaceae (*Palaquium*, *Payena* etc).

4 Untraced.

Letter 49
02/094

Bangalore
31st Oct. 1896

Dear Dr Manson,
I have sent in my official application to be put on special duty next February to work at the mosquito theory, and think that everything is in a very promising way to permission being granted. I hear from a friend in the Secretariat that Mr Bliss,[1] the member of council who presides over the medical department, is distinctly favourable to the investigation, so that, if I can only get Sibthorpe[2] to back me up, I think it is pretty sure to be carried. I have lately been thinking that the first thing necessary to further investigation is to be sent to a place where I can be pretty sure that the species of mosquito is a malaria-bearing species. I was much struck on reading again the Gulstonian lectures by the supposition that each species of parasite may require a different species of mosquito & it is indeed otherwise likely that only certain species can harbour the malaria. Here, for instance, though mosquitoes are plentiful, there is but little malaria. This may obviously be caused by the species of insect, the brown & the brindled, being not of the right kind; and if such be the case I cannot expect the flagellated spores to live in their tissues, so that I cannot hope to find malaria parasites in their tissues nor to produce malaria by means of them. You may remember too that I have seen no marked "manifestations" in the mosquitoes here, such as I saw in Secunderabad on several occasions. Indeed here, while all crescents become spheres, the second step, namely that of spheres becoming

flagellate seems to be much delayed, while spent pigment seems to be comparatively rarer.

What is to be done then? My peons don't seem to be able to get any but the brown or brindled mosquitoes, & as these, especially the latter, swarm in every house, while yet there is but little malarial fever, I don't suppose that they are a malaria-bearing species. The only thing to be done is to go to some very malarial locality, say a malarious village at the foot of hills, where there is only one source of water-supply, & there "follow the clue", especially taking note of the various species of mosquito. This accordingly, is what I have asked government to do with me. The place is to be selected after consultation with the Surgeon General. I have also asked for an assistant surgeon to help me. Mr Bliss said that I should have liberty to do as I like; & my programme will be

(a) To note the various species of parasite infecting patients in the locality.

(b) to note the various species of mosquito present.

(c) to compare the above with each other & with the neighbouring water sources.

(d) to try to find the malaria parasite in the mosquitoes, looking especially for the crescent form which will be most unlike the mosquito's natural cells.

(e) to "follow the clue".

I shall try to get a village or cluster of villages, at foot of hills, where the population is small. The end of February is the beginning of the fever season in such places here, the planters tell me. I shall probably take a party of five persons with me, & it will be a part of the investigation to see whether we can exclude malaria by boiling all drinking water & using mosquito nets. What do you think of the programme?

Now we must begin to get ready at once, because even if Government refuses to send me on this duty, I shall try to get three months' leave for the purpose. What I first want is your advice especially in regard to (d) above. I suppose I am most likely to find the parasite in the mosquito's perivisceral cells - but how am I to differentiate it from the numerous perivisceral cells which look just as if they have malaria parasites in them? Such cells are common enough. Do you think that any method of staining will do? - preferably wet staining? Would it be worth while trying coccidia stains? If so, what are they? Of course if I can hit on any body like crescents in the tissues of the mosquito the theory will be nearly proved. Secondly I want books - especially on the comparative anatomy, large & small, of insects; also on classification of mosquitoes. I see by Mr Thomas's book on Tank Angling in India,[3] which contains a chapter (not very useful) on the mosquito, that a Dr Christopher Johnston has written in a detailed manner on their anatomy in the Quarterly Journal of Microscopical Science[4] - a book which is out of my reach - Thomas does not give the date of the article.

If you could ask H. K. Lewis[5] to send me any books & Baker[6] to send any stains, etc, putting the cost to my account, I shall be extremely obliged. I have got Blanchard,[7] & Neumann,[8] & Leuckart[9] - none of them very useful in the matter. In my last I wrote about a strong oil immersion lens.

No cases since I wrote last, but one remittent fever just turning into crescents - I have had a good case swarming with eye-forms which worry me greatly. I believe they are some kind of parasite but cannot make sure - Fever very irregular; but no time to write about it now. With kind regards, yours truly

R. Ross.

2nd Nov. Just got your letter dated 12th & also translation of Bignami's article for which many thanks. I note contents of letter & will try second generation of mosquito (bites) with my crescent case which is just coming on. About birds, I forgot to tell you that I have tried several pigeons, doves & parroquets with negative results. This place is 2700 feet above sea level remember. However I will look again - I have not been working with animals. I am dying to get away to some regular hotbed of malaria & am now beginning to think of getting leave & going off somewhere, even for a week or two - I really think I shall but can't get away for about one month. However there is fever in Mysore during the cold weather. If my new crescent case gives only very small "manifestations" with the mosquitoes I shall be almost certain that the species here are not malaria-bearing, in which case I shall certainly be off on ten days leave to look round. I told you that an article on malaria-producing experiments has been sent by me to the S. I. B. of B. M. A.[10] This will contain the "bite" experiments on my assistant surgeon Mr Appia. These would go conclusively against Bignami if I could be sure that the mosquito used was malaria-bearing. *This* is the point, I really believe. But also give me suggestions as to how I am to distinguish parasite bearing cells in mosquito from ordinary cells - there will be no pigment remember.

R.R.

[Manson's writing]

Quart J. of Mic. Sc.

Christopher Johnston. Auditory apparatus of culex mosquito

iii o.s. 97-102 - pl i-v[11]

Archives de Zoologie experimentale et generale
3e serie Tome II
Parasites endoglobualires du sang du vertébrés[12]

1 Above, Letter 47, note 2.
2 Charles Sibthorpe, (1847-1906), Surgeon-General (civil) at Madras.
3 Henry Sullivan Thomas, *Tank Angling in India* (Madras: Higginbotham & Co, 1887).
4 Christopher Johnston, 'Auditory apparatus of the culex mosquito', *Quarterly Journal of Microscopical Science*, O.S. 3 (1855), 97-102.
5 The medical bookseller and publisher on Gower Street, London.
6 The manufacturer of Ross's microscope. See Letter 7, note 9.
7 Blanchard (1889-90).
8 L. G. Neumann, *A Treatise on the Parasites and Parasitic Diseases of the Domesticated Animals*, translated and edited by George Fleming (London: Ballière & Co., 1892).
9 Leuckart (1886).
10 R. Ross, 'Some experiments in the production of malarial fever by means of the mosquito', *Transactions of the South Indian Branch of the British Medical Association* (Dec. 1896), 93-106.
11 Note added by Manson - reference to note 4 above.
12 Note added by Manson - reference to Labbé (1894).

Letter 50
02/095

Bangalore
15th Nov. 1896

Dear Dr Manson,

I have been doing some interesting experiments with leeches yesterday & today. The case of crescents which I mentioned in my last ran away after the first mosquitoes were put on; but I found three others immediately afterwards. Mosquito experiments give same results - hardly any flagellate bodies found & spent pigment masses comparatively rare. I really believe that these brindled mosquitoes are of no use, and the brown ones here refuse to bite. Yesterday I put a leech on & took it off at half an hour, putting it into salt water. The vomited blood mixed with slime & salt solution was examined from 36 minutes after the leech had commenced to suck. In three specimens I found only four parasites - all *unchanged crescents.*

Today I put two leeches on, one on same patient & the other on another patient.

2nd leech had salt rubbed on its nose & vomited 55 minutes after beginning to suck - blood not much changed in 1st specimen, when I found by a rapid survey 12 parasites, 8 of which were crescents, 3 spheres & 1 oval. A second specimen made at same time as the first but examined 40 minutes later gave 1 crescent, 1 oval & all the rest spheres - blood much changed.

3rd leech. 1st specimen made 1hr & 20 minutes after leech was put on showed blood viscid - 1 crescent & all the rest spheres - a few spent pigment masses.

2nd specimen at 1 hr 45 minutes 1 oval, the rest spheres & a few pigment masses.

19th Nov. I have not been able to get leeches on again for one reason & another but will repeat experiments as soon as possible. From those given above it appears to me that the change does not go on nearly as briskly inside the leech. This will be a telling fact if substantiated by further experiments.

I have written a paper on Bignami's criticism but shall not send it for publication until I have worked out about the leech. The man's attempt is quite clear - he thinks that *he* is going to take credit for the theory - but you will see what I say. By the way could not you work the leech in London? Leech blood is very similar to mosquito blood but appears to me to become viscid much more slowly the reason being that the mosquito passes the water of the blood by her kidneys while she is still sucking. Hence I deduce that the evolution of the crescent is started not by chilling of the blood, but by change of specific gravity consequent on loss of water either by evaporation (ordinary specimen) or by osmosis (mosquitoes & leeches - the latter *sweat* while sucking).

I hear that the special malaria duty is *almost certain* to come off at end of February 1897.. Everything must be ready for it. But I hope to take a preliminary canter next month. With kind regards

Yours sincerely
R. Ross.

Letter 51
02/096

30th Nov. 1896
Bangalore

Dear Dr Manson,
If you have not published your reply to Bignami I will strongly suggest your holding it over till you get my paper on Observations on the Transformation of Crescents[1] which I am sending by *next* mail to the B. M. J. containing my views on Bignami's paper & also some new &, I think, important results which I have obtained during the last fortnight - results which appear to me to smash the degenerationists completely. I have discovered the *exact condition* which the crescents require to become spheres; it is *abstraction of water from blood.* I can check completely or produce their evolution at will. Hence of course it *must* be a vital process & not a degenerative one. In the last week I have had a case containing twice as many crescents as Abdul Khadir! [sic] & with it I have proved the point completely.

1st Crescents develop in leeches just as in mosquitoes only perhaps more slowly. Hence stomach of mosquito has nothing to do with it (don't be frightened).

2. Development of crescents does *not proceed at all* in blood drawn under vaseline & kept occluded from air for *any* length of time. They die in this position, but *none* of *them* become spheres. Hence degeneration theory is false.

3. In blood exposed to air for 1, 2, 3, 4, 5 minutes, more & more crescents become spheres & flagellates. In blood exposed for 5 minutes development is almost as complete as in mosquito & leech (though not quite so). I have seen beautiful manifestations of flagellates both in 5-minutes-exposed blood & in leeches.

What is the explanation of these phenomena? It cannot be exposure to air because this does not occur in mosquito & leech. It must be abstraction of water. Now this is the *only condition* which exists in mosquito blood & does not exist in ordinary blood, at least at first after the mosquito begins to suck. Hence (do you follow me) the transformation is a vital process & one intended for the stomach of suctorial animals where abstraction of water takes place directly the blood is ingested. Please try the experiments yourself as soon as you can. Do you follow their drift? The vaseline experiment is *immense.* How can they get over it! If you don't expose the blood to abstraction of water for an instant no crescents will change! This completes my mosquito work on the first step by showing exactly the *why* & *how*. Will write next mail with paper on Bignami. Am just off to Mysore for two days with the Resident (bad luck to it) but think that my splendid case will keep. I congratulate you on this additional strong support to your theory. With kindest regards, Yours sincerely

R. Ross.

1 Ronald Ross, 'Observations on a condition necessary to the transformation of the malaria crescent', *BMJ* (30 Jan. 1897), 251-255.

Letter 52
02/097

Bangalore
7th Dec. 1896

Dear Dr Manson,

I have finished my paper entitled "Observations on a condition necessary to the Transformation of Crescents" & shall dispatch it by this mail to the B. M. J. whose Editor will I hope send it to you for approval.[1] I have repeated the experiments over & over again since I last wrote & have experienced the same results; so that I can wish you a merry Xmas with a good conscience. You will gather from the paper the reason for this gross self-satisfaction - if you have not already gathered it from my last epistle, hurried as it was. Conceit is a vice of the discoverer of nature's little tricks. When I first saw nothing but spheres & flagellates in my fourth leech I was much alarmed I confess; but then the question came "why should they *not* transform in the leech as in the mosquito?" And then the question "Is there not some necessary condition?" Exposure to air was out of the question; next came abstraction of water from serum, and the vaseline experiment was tried. Complete success. Then the exposure experiments - also successful - what a muff I was not to think of them before. Evidently Sacheroff [sic][2] has worked it partially.

I think you will agree with me that the "necessary condition" knocks the involutionists into a cocked hat & also puts the theory one plane higher, because *that condition* is just the one which obtains in the mosquito - no other difference that I can see, at first at all events, between blood in vessels & in mosquito. Why then should the crescents select this very condition as the signal for change? Eureka!

Now I have taken the plunge into the investigation of the *conditions most propitious to exflagellation.* First condition - abstraction of water, of course. Second - I think exposure to air from 30 to 120 seconds, not more or less (in finger-blood specimens); that is an exact condition of density. In numerous 4 & 5 minutes-exposed specimens hardly any flagellates; in numerous 1 & 2 minutes-specimens, sometimes almost all spheres becoming flagellate between about 11 & 17 minutes. With my splendid new case the "manifestations" are splendid - maddening because I can't see all the flagellates at the same time. As soon as I have knocked a certain spark of induction out of the flint of barren facts, there will follow another paper on exflagellation. The thing comes on with an *aura.* Here we are - they are all going to become flagellate here in a minute or two - 9 minutes, 10 minutes, 11 minutes - now it comes - here's one, there's one, the specimen is alive! There follows the wild hunt after free spores. They are all lumped in the middle,  or ; but why do so few of them actually escape & if they escape, why do so few travel to any distance? - fibrin perhaps - I have seen them strangle themselves with fibrin. Is there so much fibrin in the mosquito? I am coming to that. Have *not yet put mosquitoes* to my splendid case - tomorrow I expect to do so - what shall I see?

Why have I been failing to get flagellates all these months? another law - because I have been working with *cinchonised patients.* Eureka again! My splendid case shall not come within a mile of a grain of quinine.

Bignami is a pure villain; he wants to secrete a mosquito theory of his own. He is wild with you. He wants to bite into the heart of your theory, suck its juices & then bloat & swell into a discoverer - or rather until he is thought to be one. You will see what I have said about it. He is welcome to his epidemiological inductions; they will only lead him face-to-wall against somebody else's. But he must be dealt with at once with clear distinctions because he is quite capable of spreading his six legs over your work & calling it all his own; next he will say that he knew about the flagellate spores all along, & so on. If you have not squelched him already you ought to do it.

Do you think it possible for the spores to get into phagocytes in the mosquito's stomach & live in there for a while? But I must cease now - dining out.

8th. These wretched brown mosquitoes refused to bite today but I have a brindled brood of stingers which will be ready by tomorrow. The best exposure to turn all spheres (or almost all) into flagellates is about $1^1/_2$ minutes (Temp. 68°F, air humid). I get numbers of flagellates now in every specimen with that exposure. Have been hunting flagella all day as long as eye-sight lasted, & am getting new views. Why don't the spores leave the sphere & dart away at once?

Because it is not their instinct to do so.

First, the sphere itself is easily capable of attaching itself to the cover-glass. Next the spores can do the same. I have seen them hold red corpuscles by the extremity of one flagellum. This many times; they can pull red corpuscles along. I have also seen a spore go to a distance & then *return* to the parent body where the other spores were still struggling. I have also seen spores when their movements have relaxed moving like *leeches*, crawling from point to point. Here it is then. The spores don't want to rush away at once; were they to do so they would probably be lost in the rapidly-becoming-viscid blood (German style!). They are not struggling to get free; they are *reaching out* in all directions while still holding on to the sphere. Why? They are waiting till the sphere is drifted by blood-currents in the mosquito's stomach within touching distance of the walls of the stomach. They catch, hold on, & presently all the spores do the same. Then they worm into the cells of the stomach. Thus every spore belonging to a flagellate body finds its location much better than if they had all gone wandering in all directions.

Now what is the meaning of the very long flagella sometimes seen.

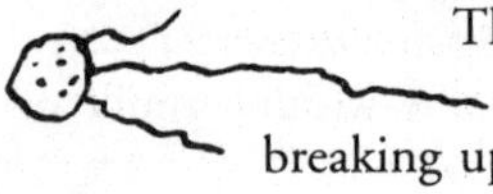

They are several spores holding hands in order to reach out. I have just seen one breaking up into three spores still

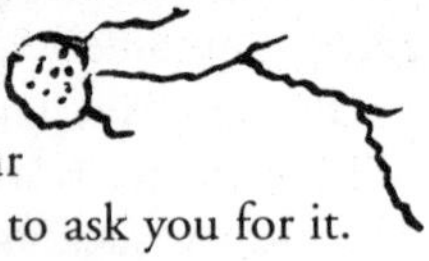

holding on.

Will you remember to send me your telegraphic address; I have long been intending to ask you for it.

9th. No time to work today. Have sent off my paper.

Kind regards & a merry Christmas.

Yours sincerely

R. Ross.

1 Letter 51, note 1.

2 N. Sakharoff had already found chromatin in the flagella, a point which Bignami (Letter 48, note 2) had noticed. *Memoirs*, 194, denied this.

Letter 53
02/019

21 Queen Anne Street,
Cavendish Square,
27th Nov. 1896

My dear Ross,

I ought to have written you some mails ago but have been so rushed with work of one kind and another that I sometimes dont get sleep enough and never any leisure when awake. As you know pay is often in inverse proportion to the amount of work done.

I am very pleased to hear you are likely to get away for a continuous spell of work on the mosquito and under government auspices. I have very little doubt you will learn a very great deal and I hope will run the flagellum to earth. I believe you will. But dont be cast down at difficulty and temporary failure. You wont fail if you stick to the flagellum. The more I see of this wonder and the more I think of it the more I am convinced of its importance and that it is the extracorporeal spore of the plasmodium. How these men can say it is anything else passes my understanding. It is simply damned nonsense to say it is degenerated protoplasm. The other evening I had some under observation for an hour or longer and when I lost sight of the thing it was as lively as ever. One I saw attacking a leucocyte just as you described.

Your scheme of work is a good one. I have a feeling that the ordinary mosquito is an efficient host but that the reason for the absence of malaria in certain mosquito haunted places does not lie in the inefficiency of the mosquito but in the presence of something inimical to the plasmodium in it. The plasmodium is only one of innumerable organisms fighting for life; sometimes and in someplaces it can get its head up; at other times and other places some other competing organism has the ascendancy. Otherwise it would over run the earth. I would make my experiments as laboratory-like as possible. I would grow my mosquitos in boiled water and in conditions as simple as possible with the idea of keeping out contending organisms. Just as with bacteria; those of decomposition can overpower many pathogenic bacteria when they get into a culture. So when the plasmodial spore falls on the belly of a mosquito it may get worried by a previous or more potent competing form. The belly of the mosquito or the pool in which it breeds is qua the plasmodium as a sort of garden in the wilderness in which many weeds may grow unless the gardener - yourself - takes care to clear it. You catch the idea. So keep your experimental conditions as simple as you can; clean mosquitos and clean water.

I would be inclined to still continue watching the flagellum in mosquito stomach; giving it the offer of different kinds of cells from the mosquito; trying to see if it attempts to enter some particular kind of cell. The epithelium of the stomach is the first cellular structure it brings up against. Try it. It looks juicy and comfortable in some of my sections. Then I should try the ova you will easily find them.

You saw Walker's paper in the Lancet[1] about the effect of a droplet of water in hurrying exflagellation. I believe he is right, for I have repeated his experiment lately in a somewhat different way and can now secure ex-flagellation very rapidly. I speak from the experience of one case only so that I may not be right to generalise from this. I find if I merely breathe on the slip and coverglass before applying the blood, flagella appear very quickly and the dilution of the blood favours observation very much enabling one to trace the flagella in the many clear spaces the mixture of water vapour and blood secures. Try this. I also find if I prepare a number of slides in this way, place them at once in a vapour of steam from a hot sponge under a bell-jar that I can remove the coverglass when flagellation (ascertained from a similar specimen kept near) has begun and secure good specimens for staining purposes. My case was not rich in crescents so that I could not get slides enough for a lengthened series of observations but I believe next time I get a good case of crescents I shall be able easily to stain flagella. The cover glass can be "kicked-off" with the point of a needle, dried, fixed, and stained. Try this and on such speicmens experiment with stains.

I think logwood[2] will be the best but methylene blue will also do or gentian violet. Doubtless you have got all these so I shall not send them out. When you have got a good method for flagellum staining then try sections of mosquito at intervals from the time of feeding. Best harden your mosquito either in glycerine or in formaline; then soak over night in acetic acid to dissolve out the haemoglobin; section; and then stain.

I would therefore recommend you to try two lines of experiment. First endeavouring to feed or rather provide a house for the living flagellum; second, having found this, to prepare slides of a permanent character showing the flagellum in his cell. Dont forget to search the ova of the mosquito.

I think that the addition of a little breath vapour to your mosquito blood slides will help you very much; try it.

I shall see Lewis this afternoon about the Quarterly Journal of Microscopical Science[3] and try to get the number with the article on mosquito anatomy for you. I have been at a good insect man but beyond the anatomy of the cockroach and the blow fly there is very little known about the microscopical structure of insects. These two insects have been fairly fully described but that is of very little use to you. I shall also get Lewis to send Labbé[4] to you. This you should have. Dont return Thayer and Hewetson:[5] I have another copy now. Very fine plates and bibliography. Is it not?

I hear there is to be a lot about malaria in the forthcoming scientific memoirs of the off. in India[6] and that you are contributing a paper. I shall see it but if there is anything in local journals worth reading I wish you would try to send it to me. I see the Indian Med. Gaz and most of the Indian medical journals but may miss some of them.

Take care of your health when you go to that village which I hope you will immortalise.

If you send me mosquitoes I shall get them sectioned and carefully examine them. The last batch turned out many of them very well and the slides you sent me with one exception showed well. But I cant get further than the sphere although I think in one I found flagella. I am going to have a long Sunday over them again and hope to find out something more from the sections which are already made and stained.

Be sure to post me of progress.

Yours very truly

Patrick Manson

What a rigmarole of rot from Hehir in today's Lancet.[7] Mad.

1 Not Walker but Marshall - see Letter 55, note 1.

2 Letter 34, note 3.

3 Letter 49, note 4.

4 Labbé (1894).

5 Letter 47, note 3.

6 J. Murray, 'Notes on the malarial parasite as observed in the blood during life, and in the tissues post-mortem, at Lahore, Punjab', *Scientific Memoirs by Medical Officers of the Army in India*, 10 (1897), 29-52; L. Rogers, 'On the influence of variations of the ground-water level on the prevalence of malarial fevers; , *Ibid.* 53-58.

7 Patrick Hehir, 'The haematozoon of malaria and its discovery in water and soil', *Lancet* (28 Nov. 1896), 1514-1518. This was continued in issue of 5 Dec. 1896, 1589-1595. Hehir's long-winded paper described his investigations (9 years and 7250 slide preparations) in detail, but offered no new insights into malaria.

Letter 54
02/098

Bangalore
15th. Dec. 1896

Dear Dr Manson,

I have just got your letter in which you mention that one Walker has published a paper in the Lancet to the effect that the *addition* of water to the blood hurries up ex-flagellation. No, I have not seen the paper as I don't take Lancet in, & what is worse can't find it though I have hunted through three months' borrowed Lancets. Must hunt again. As soon as I got your letter however I rushed off to hospital & tried the things. Of course water makes all crescents swell up just as it swells up corpuscles & leucocytes & *excess* of water *stops* exflagellation; but I now tried a trace of water; which I *have done* before. There were three of us at work & we made many specimens. Result for 1st day's work - trace of water converts nearly all crescents & allows many spheres to become flagellate but flagellation was *not* accelerated, nor were flagellates more numerous than in 3 minutes exposed blood. I added the water in two ways - by putting a drop on the finger & pricking through it (so as to avoid evaporation from the outset) & by mixing on the cover-glass - same results. It appears to be a sort of mechanical action of the water; but I must do it over & over again & must repeat my other experiments, often as I have done them.

In the meantime will you kindly *keep back my paper* to the B. M. J.[1] I wish I had heard of Walker's experiments before!

We have been working all the week at the exact steps taken in the ex-flagellation process. There are four stages in all.

1. The crescent becomes a sphere with a thick greenish outline. This may take from 2 to 10 minutes or so - generally 5 minutes.
2. The thick outline, due to the shell of the corpuscle, is *suddenly* discharged with a slight movement of the sphere or oval - generally done at about 8 minutes.
3. The pigment which was massed together now begins to be dispersed through out the cell which swells visibly - completed at 10 minutes at quickest.
4. The pigment begins to *move* not *oscillate*; this lasts for 1 minute. Then the flagella break out; not suddenly but like this: -
& so on.

Ex-flagellation begins *almost always* between 11 & 17 minutes; & those spheres which have not flagellated before 17 minutes rarely flagellate at all. Spheres in which the pigment remains massed never (that I have seen) become flagellate & when the pigment begins to oscillate quickly flagellation is generally checked.

These are new observations of mine & concurred in by the other men working with me.

Thus the process of ex-flagellation occurs between 11 & 17 minutes & is a simultaneous & very brief action of the parasites. In the water experiments the earliest exflagellations began at 13 minutes, the usual time. I am trying hard to find the subtle law which regulates exflagellation. In some specimens almost all the spheres become flagellate; in others hardly any. Exposure to air from $1^1/_2$ to 3 minutes turns nearly all crescents; but still further development may be checked. I think it is necessary to take a large drop of blood, so as to avoid pressure on the parasites, or at least sudden compression. Hundreds of specimens must be examined; but I swear to find it. In the meantime Walker's experiment seems to go just counter to mine; it is very odd indeed! How explain the vaseline experiment? I ought to have tried traces of water more frequently before. Tomorrow I shall try breathing on the glass & giving only 15 seconds exposure. Perhaps breathing acts merely by giving time to the blood to evaporate somewhat while you breathe on the glass. Again, for perfect exflagellation a certain degree of warmth may be necessary. I want to see if I cannot convert *all* spheres by some means. I am wild over it all.

16th. No, I have not been mistaken. We have made numerous experiments today. Here are some: -

1. An ordinary specimen made as quickly as possible so as to expose the blood to the air hardly at all. Actual exposure within 10 seconds.
   Examined after half an hour & 53 parasites counted. Of these 50 were crescents & only 3 were spheres (*all of which were near air-bubbles).*
2. Another similar specimen with less than 10 seconds exposure. Examined after 45 minutes.
   36 parasites found, of which 31 were crescents & only 5 spheres, all near air-bubbles.
3. A specimen made of a drop of blood which had been allowed to stand on the finger for 2 $^1/_4$ minutes.
   Examined at once & for one hour. *Not a single crescent remained unchanged* after the first 10 minutes or so.

We agreed that it is useless to go over such experiments again since they have already been done so often. Exposure to air (abstraction of water) is *necessary* to transformation. This is a law.

You will observe that the presence of numerous air-bubbles in a specimen always encourages transformation, & that crescents near them are oftenest transformed. You will also see that every second of exposure almost, increases the number of transformations.

Now for the addition of water. We *steamed* four slides & laid 30 seconds exposed blood on them. All gave the same results, namely about 30 or 40% crescents transformed, the rest remaining unchanged. In all flagellates were fairly numerous & in our parasite exflagellation occurred in 8 minutes (I have seen it occur in 7 in an ordinary specimen). The usual time was 13-17 minutes, the average in ordinary specimens. Here I suggest that your success with breathed-on glasses is due not to the breathing but to the *delay* in making the specimen caused while you breathe.

Now for the addition of a drop of water. If in excess it makes all crescents swell up & *die*. In many crescents the pigment is extruded in a mass.

If the water is in such small quantity that the shape of the leucocytes & corpuscles is not affected, the transformation is not affected either (?)

If so much is added that the leucocytes swell up & the haemoglobin is extravasated, all crescents too swell up, many die & a few become flagellate at the usual time (?)

We shall attack these latter experiments again tomorrow. But so far as I can see water has merely a mechanical effect. It swells the crescents at once & enables them to burst their sheaths; then a few proceed to exflagellation if there is not too much water. At the same time it shows I think that abstraction of water is required only for the first stage of transformation & that after this stage we may add water without stopping further development. Water too may encourage ex-flagellation by increasing the bulk of the blood & so preventing crushing. We are going to try crushing experiments presently. In fine, however I deprecate the addition of anything to blood; it alters the whole condition of it & is not a fair mode of estimating the natural facts of the transformation.

I have written to the Editor B. M. J.[2] & asked him to send you my paper & not to publish it. I propose to send you a note on the water experiments as soon as completed to add to the paper. Do you think it would be better to publish in the Lancet? It is most unfortunate, but I cannot find Walker's paper at all.

The fact that flagella come only from spheres with scattered pigment suggests that they are at first contained in an interior cell which swells up & pushes the pigment to the periphery - that is that they consist of nuclear substance.

Have noted all the remarks in your last. Will try staining presently - have already tried it. Will you repeat the experiments in my paper? King[3] has addressed Government about putting me on malaria duty & has found a suitable place. Hehir's paper[4] is worse that rot - charlatanism.

Yours sincerely
R. Ross.

1 Letter 51, note 1.
2 Ernest Hart was then badly ill and editing the *BMJ* from his home in Totteridge. He died on 7 January 1898. See P. W. Bartrip, *Mirror of Medicine: A History of the British Medical Journal* (Oxford: Clarendon Press, 1990), 91.
3 Surgeon-Colonel Walter Gawen King, (1851-1935), Sanitary Commissioner at Madras.
4 Hehir (1896).

Letter 55
02/099

Bangalore
23rd Dec. [1896]

Dear Dr Manson,
Just a line to tell you that I have at last found *Marshall's* paper in the Lancet Oct 24 & not Walker's.[1] We have been hunting everywhere for a year back among the original articles, etc & have now found the thing required, but too late for the mail. I will send you a on the subject to add to my paper next mail. The *abstraction* theory holds; so to some extent does the *addition* theory; the results are rather complex.

Experiment I. A drop of blood on the finger is exposed to warm *not* hot steam for one minute & these compared with one-minute-exposed blood - much fewer transformations & then nearly always in the presence of air-bubbles. The steam may even add water & not only prevent evaporation; but it checks transformation to some degree.

Experiment II. An excess of water is added. All crescents swell up but *die*.

Experiment III. A small quantity of water is added; numerous crescents swell up & a few proceed to exflagellation - not so many I think as in one-minute exposed blood, and these generally near air bubbles.

Now what are we to say? The water experiments have no real bearing on the mosquito theory because there is no water added in the mosquito's stomach - just the reverse. The abstraction theory is I think absolutely proved; but so apparently is the fact that addition of water swells up the crescents. I think it is really mostly a mechanical effect. But the following question remains: if a crescent is never exposed to increased density but is at once exposed to *decreased* density, will it transform? I don't know.

Unfortunately all my cases are drying up & are almost useless now. Many thanks for the Journal of Microscopical Science - I hope it did not bother you much to get. Must leave off to catch mail.

Yours sincerely
R. Ross.

1 Robert J. Marshall, 'The Malaria parasite', *Lancet* (24 Oct. 1896), 1187; above, Letter 53, note 1.

Letter 56
02/100

Bangalore
27th Dec. 1896

Dear Dr Manson,
I enclose a note to be appended to my paper on a Condition Necessary to Transformation of Crescents, which I asked the Editor of the B. M. J. to send to you.[1] I have had to dispatch it very hurriedly as must start for Madras this evening to get a Health Officer for this town. I leave the disposal of the paper to you - perhaps you may think it best to publish in Lancet instead of B. M. J. I think that the note puts the addition of water business in its true colours. We cannot call the effect of water exactly a mechanical effect. Change of density must have some influence on the corpuscles which is at once felt by the crescents. We have been carefully considering the various steps of the change; one of the most interesting facts is the rupture of the thick outline which occurs at about 5 minutes. Another is that the flagella are almost certainly contained *in the nucleus*, the scattering of pigment which occurs invariably before exflagellation being due to the swelling up of the inner sphere pushing the pigment to the periphery. All our cases have dried up &

it may be some weeks before I can set to work again. In the meantime it is of the *greatest importance* that Bignami & Marshall should be refuted *at once*, because the Govt of Madras have *approved* of the malaria investigation & have referred to Govt. of India, who, unless Bignami is put out of the way, may reject everything. I therefore strongly advise publication immediately of my paper &, what would be still better, an article from you.

I want to put in a "provisional specification", with you as witness, for a theory, namely that the eye-form-fever is a fever akin to *Texas Cattle-fever*.[2] The parasite, if it be one, is remarkably like the cattle-fever parasite. I had a splendid case of it some months ago. The eye-forms disappeared as the fever declined.

Must now leave off with numerous good wishes for next year which I hope will be "big with fate" for malaria. My kind regards to Mrs Manson & to your son.

Ever yours sincerely

R. Ross.

1 Letter 51, note 1. Ross's note was included in the published article.

2 Letter 48, note 2.

Letter 57
02/020

21 Queen Anne Street,
Cavendish Square,
25th December, 1896

My dear Ross

Your letter of 30th Nov. interested me very much more especially as I was working at the same subject as yourself namely exflagellation and the causes of it. But our conclusions - or rather results are diametrically opposite for I find that I get exflagellation by moistening my slides. The fact is that neither hydration nor dehydration of the blood has anything to do with it. Something else is at work, something that takes place no matter whether the blood is dense from evaporation or light from the addition of water. At the same time exflagellation does not take place if the blood is rapidly transferred to a perfectly clean and dry slide with a minimum of exposure to the air. Try this experiment. Breathe on a slide; prick the finger; take up blood on the breathed on slide; apply cover-glass; ring with vaseline. In a very few minutes you have exflagellation - at all events almost all crescents have become spheres. Therefore drying of the blood has nothing to do with exflagellation. I shall do your experiment next opportunity and doubtless will find exactly what you describe; therefore wateriness of the blood has nothing to do with exflagellation. I fancy some fibrinogen ferment which is liberated on the blood leaving the body and coming in contact with organic matter of some sort is the stimulant leading to exflagellation. When I got your letter I went to the Brit. Med. Jour. office and asked them to delay publication of your paper until they heard from you.[1] I took this liberty as I was sure you would be glad to have an opportunity to go over the ground again. I am sure you will pardon this liberty. They told me there was no chance of the paper appearing for a good many weeks to come so that there will be no damage done should you wish it to come out in its present shape.

I have succeeded in staining the flagellated body. Modus operandi. Breathe on slide; take up and spread out blood; invert over a blotting paper cell; wait for half an hour; remove dry and fix in alcohol. Remove haemoglobin with very weak acetic acid; stain with carbol fuchsin. I have not yet arrived at the best strength of the latter but I have got several wonderful slides with full strength. One body is simply perfect and shows about five flagella one of which is beautifully fine and carries a leaf shaped bulb at the free end. I shall have them photographed and send you a print. It is very fine indeed.[2]

I was working at staining the flagella so as to get a method for the mosquitoes when they come. But it is very difficult. This fuchsin after acetic acid is the best I have struck yet. Only I want more material and I dont often get crescent cases.

By the way my section cutter[3] says the best medium for preserving mosquitoes in is far and away pure glycerine. The formalin did not turn out well making the insect too hard and brittle under the knife. So when you send the mosquitoes send them in glycerine. ***Don't forget. Glycerine.***

This week I had a case of filariasis. I diagnosed the presence of the filaria in a small tumour on the arm. It was cut out and the filaria - female - was found in the tumour. It lived for 12 hours after removal swimming about in normal salt solution like an eel quite actively.

Be sure to go over the addition of watery vapour to blood before sanctioning publication of the paper you have sent home. I am certain you will modify your opinion about the cause of exflagellation when you do so. I shall try the leech next case. This is a very interesting point and we must try to clear it up for it, if found, will convey a useful hint I am sure.

Wishing you a happy Christmas I remain
Yours very sincerely
Patrick Manson

1 Published in January. Ross (1897a).
2 Manson published these experiments: 'A method of staining the malaria flagellated organism', *BMJ* (10 July 1897), 68-70.
3 Possibly Richard Muir, Pathology Department, Edinburgh University, whom Manson thanked for making the slides reproduced in the article, note 2.

Letter 58
02/101

Bangalore
11th Jan. 1897

Dear Dr Manson,
I have just got yours of Xmas day & see that when you wrote it you were in the same stage of perplexity as I was when you told me of Marshall's law. I hope by this time that you have been able to confirm *my* law. If not there are four of us here, Dr Srinivasa Rao B. Sc.,[1] Dr Chowksi,[2] Mr Appia & myself who will stand on our heads (!) with astonishment - or rather we will be astonished if you cannot confirm our facts, namely that transformation does not proceed in blood *drawn under* vaseline & proceeds more with increased exposure. The first point I should like you to note is that crescents lying near to air-bubbles, or in blood full of air-bubbles, generally become transformed. You will note this even in the breathing experiment. Hence ringing with vaseline after the specimen is made has no effect; hence also the very smallest exposure to air (or, as I think dehydration) is capable of starting transformation. Again pricking the finger under water has the same effect as dehydration. Again, exposure to air saturated with moisture seemed to me, working with numerous crescents, not to have the effect of exposure to dry air; though this experiment is difficult to do (a) because water is apt to be added by condensation of steam & (b) because there will be air-bubbles in the specimen. The breathing experiment causes transformation in two ways first by a few seconds' exposure & next by addition of water.

The facts being granted (after confirmation by you) what other conclusion are we to come to but that *change* of density is a condition necessary to transformation? Of dehydration & hydration, the first, I conjecture is the natural provocative & the latter acts accidentally in the same way by affecting similarly the shell of the corpuscle. This is hypothesis of course, but reasonable. For *all* bodies which we have *watched* become flagellate, the following stages have been passed through - crescent - thick-outline crescent - thick-outline sphere - sphere without outline - spreading of pigment caused (?) by swelling of the inner cell containing the flagella - a brief stirring of pigment - exflagellation. There is therefore always *excapsulisation* as you have said in spite of Labbé's statement (for whose book thousands of thanks).[3] Now I think that both hydration & dehydration act in the same way - by facilitating excapsulisation, the capsule being probably the shell of the corpuscle, in the same way as both facilitate extravasation of haemoglobin. You say that neither hydration nor dehydration have anything to do with it - "something else is at work, something that takes place whether the blood is dense ... or light..."[4] Precisely; is not that something a something which affects the shell of the corpuscle, & may not that something be *change* of density? I shall wait anxiously to hear what you will say after reading my paper, with the additional note which I sent in my last. I think that the cases of the crescent & filaria are exactly alike as to excapsulisation; in both extravasation of haemoglobin or commencing extravasation, is the change required to cause excapsulisation; and in both extravasation is *naturally* caused by condensation, though it may be produced artificially by hydration in the one case and cold in the other case. I shall also be anxious to hear what results you obtain from my experiments, especially the vaseline one which seems to me so conclusive against the degenerationists. I forgot to tell you that Srinivasa Rao says he found two flagellates in a vaseline experiment though all other parasites remained crescents. He may have included an air-bubble. Of all the experiments I am least certain of the steam one, which is hard to do. *Please keep back my paper as long as you like*, until you feel that the facts are sound. I have however already sent notes on the matter to the South Indian Branch where they were read on the 8th inst. so that there is no hurry.[5]

I gave over sanitary duties today to my new Health Officer & will now have time for work. Of course, not a case of crescents to be got!

I went down to Madras for a few days after Xmas & saw Maitland who says he had seen you;[6] also Sturmer[7] who is getting filariated mosquitoes for you which he proposes to take to you about April or May next. He gets a lot of filaria where he is, & I begged him to take you a number of mosquitoes.

12th. It is very important to trace exactly the steps of exflagellation. Compared with your description in the 1st Gulstonian Lecture we have noted the following differences

1. There is always (?) at first a thick outline which may be (?) *within* (?) the shell of the corpuscle. It is discharged suddenly at about 5 minutes. I think it is given in your drawings but the first crescent (B. M. J. page 644 fig 11-7)[8] should not have had a thick outline; this should have been shown as the *second step* (?). Also 10 may require some alterations (?). But what I think requires such special note is that exflagellation is always (?) preceded by slow spreading, *without boiling*, of pigment & a simultaneous expansion of the whole cell, as if an internal sphere were dilating & pushing the pigment, lying on its *external* surface, to the outer wall of the cell. Next exflagellation is preceded by a few seconds *slow stirring*, not boiling, of pigment & often indeed by a complete momentary pause of all pigmentary movement. True boiling is (?) a sign that exflagellation will *not* occur, & is generally only found when the time for exflagellation (11-17 mins) is past. If the flagella are contained in a cell within the pigment the bodies on p. 646 will need some other explanation(?). Exflagellation never occurs, that I have seen, unless the pigment has first spread; & careful focusing appears to me to show that spreading of pigment is not general but peripheral. But I shall work at these points and at your method of staining flagella with my next case. Sturmer spreads blood with tissue paper with great success.

Yours sincerely
R. Ross.

1 A Mysore bacteriologist who assisted Ross in his research.
2 Not identified further.
3 Labbé (1894).
4 Letter 57.
5 Subsequently published as 'Further observations on the transformation of crescents', *Transactions of the South India Branch of the B.M.A.*, 7 (1897), 118-123.
6 John Maitland, IMS Madras, (1852-1907). See **Biographical Appendix.**
7 See Letter 28, note 3.
8 Reference to an illustration in 1st Goulstonian Lecture.

Letter 59
02/021

21 Queen Anne Street,
Cavendish Square,
London. W.
Jan. 21st., 1897

My dear Ross,
Your first paper arrived two mails ago, the addendum last mail; both I have read with very great interest and have sent them to the British Medical Journal for publication.[1] I have told them to hurry with it. As soon as I know when they are to be published I shall probably, if they do not ask me to do so, suggest a leader on the subject.[2] In the following journal I may have a short paragraph describing my method of staining the flagella. I am not quite sure if I described it to you; you will find it an excellent plan and I am in great hopes it will be of use in helping us to demonstrate the flagellum in the mosquito. I proceed thus:- Breathe once - not more - on a slip. Take up on the slip the droplet of crescent-blood; spread out with a needle; invert it at once over a moist chamber made of blotting paper with a little square hole to take that part of the slip covered with the blood; see that the slip is well pressed down in the blotting paper and that the latter is not too wet. After from half an hour to three quarters or 1 hour remove the slide; allow it to dry; fix with alcohol; dissolve off the haemoglobin by half an hour of 20 per cent. acetic acid; wash thoroughly; dry again and stain with carbol fuchsine - 25 drops, & water - half a watch-glassful; leave the stain on for *six* hours; wash; dry and mount in zylol balsam. The flagella and flagellated bodies are clearly stained. I have got some very fine specimens showing the bulbous extremity in flagella. The bulb is much larger in some of them than one would suppose from examination of living flagella. I am glad to hear that the government has taken the malaria matter up. I have no doubt that you will solve the problem yet, but you must be prepared for no end of work and many disappointments. For example, yesterday afternoon I spent in the hospital trying to get some crescents to exflagellate and exposed the droplets à la Ross for 40 seconds and for one minute, and yet, although nearly all the crescents became spheres I did not get one flagellated body. In some of the spheres, I could see the flagella endeavouring to break through. Strange to say, the house physician whom I had instructed to experiment on your lines got them by the dozens the previous evening. The matter of the cause of exflagellum

is evidently exceedingly difficult and complicated; however your experiments prove that exposure somehow brings about favourable conditions. I am very anxious now that I know how to procure and stain flagellated bodies to procure the flagellates of tertian and quartan fever in the hope that I may find in the stained preparations some specific difference between them and the flagellates of the crescent forms. Go slowly about the eye parasite. Have you stained it? If not, wait, before publishing. To-day I saw a similar appearance in the blood in the case of septic infection from a rat bite. The bodies were very distinct although very minute, eye-shaped and with the central brownish dot. Dont forget to send me infected mosquitos preserved in ordinary glycerine. I find there is a lot of nonsense written about the malarial parasite; the writers as a rule, have no knowledge of the subject and do not know the parasite when they see it. Your vaseline experiment is an admirable one; if it is confirmed it proves that exposure is necessary somehow. Dont be seduced into going away to work at plague;[3] there are plenty of men there already. If I were Surgeon General Cleghorn, the first thing I would do would be to bring a Jehad against the rats and I would kill every rat in and about Bombay and all threatened towns. Plague has a feeble hold as an infective disease on a human community and if the chances for the bacillus were to be diminished by only one tributary agent, such as the rat, I believe the disease would quickly die out.[4] Have you seen Lingard's Surra papers?[5] They are interesting though abominably dull or rather abominably badly written. Just now there are some investigations going on in London on the similar disease in South Africa. I know both the men[6] who are working the subject and hear occasionally of their results. The trypanosoma, like the malaria parasite, passes through various phases in the blood and also in the serous cavities; it encysts itself and, I believe, divides into many minute spores. In one experiment they find that the blood of an infected animal, although the trypanosome may not be visible in the preparations, is infective; and, sometimes, that the blood containing trypanosomes in great numbers is not infective. The small spheres which they also find free in the blood are most likely the infective agents. I believe that the trypanosome, like malaria, has a life history outside the human body. Please let me hear of progress from time to time; you cannot write to me too often.

Yours very sincerely
Patrick Manson

Microphoto of stained flagellated body, à la Manson, enclosed. Original is of course much more distinct, being transparent reeling with malaria granules very distinct.

The larger kidney shaped lump at the side of the sphere is really the bulbous end of a flagellum. This is seen in the preparation.[7]

1 Ross (1897a).
2 [Patrick Manson], 'A neglected responsibility of empire', *BMJ* (30 Jan. 1897), 289.
3 For the Indian plague epidemic, see David Arnold, *Colonizing the Body: State Medicine and Epidemic Disease in Nineteenth-Century India* (Berkeley: University of California Press, 1993), and Mark Harrison, *Public Health in British India: Anglo-Indian Preventive Medicine, 1858-1914* (Cambridge: Cambridge University Press, 1994).
4 In the mid-1890s, several workers implicated the rat flea in the transmission of plague. These included Alexandre Yersin, Masanori Ogata and P. L. Simond. For a discussion, see Leonard Fabian Hirst, *Conquest of Plague* (Oxford: Clarendon Press, 1953).
5 Alfred Lingard, *Report on Horse Surra*, vol. 1 (Bombay: Government Central Press, 1893). Vol. 2 was published 1898-99.
6 Unidentified.
7 Probably from Manson. Letter 57, note 2.

Letter 60
02/102

Bangalore
8th Feb. 1897

Dear Dr Manson,
I have just received yours of Jan. 21st in which you say you will publish my paper; but please remember that, if you have any doubts as to the facts, it would be best not to publish until the question is settled. You say that you tried to get flagellate bodies by 40" & 60" exposure. That was not enough, especially in a cold damp climate. I should think the specific gravity must be increased or decreased to a certain point. Try two to three minutes exposure & use a fairly large drop of blood. I say in my paper that some other condition applies to exflagellation because we frequently observe out of two specimens made in the same way, flagellates in one only. This condition is I think *absence of any sudden crushing of the crescents*, but I am by no

means certain. I am wild with rage because I can't get another case anyhow. I have even written down to Mysore for malaria cases without result. Occasionally a case with one or two crescents or spring tertian parasites; but nothing fit to work with. I believe there are better opportunities in London. Your photo of a flagellate body is very fine & you may be sure I will try to stain in your way as soon as I can. I would have tried it before but was busy doing my own experiments. I do not think that the bulb is at the extremity of the flagellum but in the middle, because such appears to be the structure in all free flagella. In your photo, the other end of the flagellum was possibly twisted round the attached end, thus 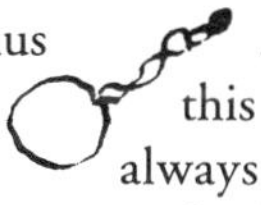 . It is only with free flagella that one can make out this fact (if it be one). In my experience flagellation almost always begins between 11 & 20 minutes after the blood is drawn. I wish I had seen Labbé, especially pages 175 et seq., before I wrote my article because I should like to have dealt with some of his statements, especially those on page 182.[1]

I hope that by the time this letter reaches you you will have tried the vaseline experiment. You can keep crescents unchanged for three or four hours & then produce flagellation by exposure to air; so that the experiment will be useful if you want to examine flagellates at leisure at home. I obtained swarms of flagellates after three hours the other day by this method, but I think the crescents begin to die after four hours, perhaps earlier in a cold climate.

Have you heard of the row that Hehir has got into in Secunderabad over a case of criminal abortion?[2] The magistrate commented very severely on his evidence & I expect he will get his *congé*. Some time ago I sent a letter to the Lancet on his Malaria work,[3] but I see that you have reviewed him in the B. M. J.[4] I really cannot believe that he continues to believe in his bloodplates & don't understand him at all.

You advise me to "go slowly" about the eye-forms. Precisely; I cannot understand them at all and have not succeeded in staining them yet. I had a very curious case in which I found eye-forms at first (a few) & then swarms of summer-autumn tertian - largish unpigmented amoeboid bodies - with tertian fever. Oddly enough not a single crescent was found afterwards though I gave only 10 grs of quinine in 2 doses & watched the man for a fortnight. Crescents ought to have been numerous.

My work here is finished & I shall probably leave my present acting appointment at the end of the month on Dobson's return from England. The work has given me great experience in sanitation & you will be pleased to hear that I have carried through all my sanitary measures after a year of fighting, abuse in the newspapers, anonymous letters, etc. It has been a regular campaign for me & I have defeated them in a score of pitched battles! I must send a full account to the British medical because these things don't happen every day.[5] The next thing is I hope, the malaria investigation, but I fear that Govt. will postpone it because of plague & famine. They always take such opportunities to oppose or postpone everything. If so I shall take leave (if I can get even that) & go off on my own account. When I am in the thick of it I shall get Mr Bliss the member of council who backs me up to worry Govt. to let me remain.[6] I am sending my wife & family to Ootacamund in anticipation. What must be done, & at once, is to see whether mosquitoes in malarious localities do not contain something like the parasite. If I don't do it some Italian will suddenly come across a crescent or a sporulating body in a mosquito & it will all be over. I have got my malarious localities (men - rather walking spleens than men) waiting for me. I hope to begin in about five or six weeks. Meantime we have heard nothing from Government. Your advice about not going to work at plague very reasonable. I may however take 10 days in the meantime to get & look at it. Our plague committee sits tomorrow & I advise powers to cause any house to be vacated at once. I shall read them your remarks about rats, which exactly accord with my advice formerly given. In fact we are killing rats by thousands here. Tomorrow I am going to hunt for surra parasites in the corpses. No I have not read Lingard's papers. Lancet, I suppose. Why don't they work on sewer rats in London? We have no plague here yet.

With kind regards
Yours sincerely
R. Ross.

1 Labbé (1894). Page 182 discusses the effects of oxygen, temperature and mechanical stimulation on flagellation.

2 Hehir was particularly interested in Indian medico-legal issues, but this case is not referred to in his *Outlines of Medical Jurisprudence.* P. Hehir and J. D. B. Gribble, *Outlines of Medical Jurisprudence for India*, 4th ed. (Madras: Higginbotham, 1898).

3 Subsequently published as an undated letter from Ronald Ross 'Surgeon-Captain Hehir and the parasite of malaria', *Lancet* (20 Feb. 1897), 551-552.

4 Presumably the anonymous review in the *BMJ* (9 Jan. 1897), 87, of Hehir's *Lancet* articles (Letter 53, note 6) published as a pamphlet *The Haematozoon of Malaria and its Discovery in Water and Soil.*

5 If he did, his communication appears not to have been published.

6 Letter 47, note 2.

Letter 61
02/022

21 Queen Anne Street,
Cavendish Square,
3rd February 1897.

My dear Ross,

Your paper appeared in last week's B. M. J.[1] After receiving your addendum I had no hesitation in urging them to publish. The paper is a splendid one and will give a fresh spurt to the study of the flagellate forms. I had hoped to have my microphotographs and drawings ready soon but I have such a lot of odds and ends work that my time is frittered away sometimes in a most depressing way. However I have all the preparations ready and most of the photos and the drawings are in hand. In many of the preparations I can see the flagella as you describe, ready-formed inside the limiting capsule of the sphere and I have more than once seen the flagella in active movement in the living sphere. You are right about their being derived from the central mass which grows visibly smaller as the flagella come off or out of it.

On Monday I repeated your vaseline experiment and found that your description is correct. There is no exflagellation so far as I saw until the bleb of blood is broken up and exposed. I kept a man with vaseline blebs on his fingers for an hour and then laid them on the slide. On first looking I saw one or two crescents; transformation was very rapid and in a very few minutes I had flagella in full swing. Tomorrow I mean to repeat the experiment and kill the crescents with heat as soon as the bleb is transferred to the slide.

I have now some specimens of stained blood with free flagella but I cannot make out any nucleus and believe that the chromatin is diffused through out the flagellum. Possibly now I know how to get free flagella in a condition suitable for staining I may be more successful with some other stain. I have set my man on the mosquitoes again sectioning as before but using the slow staining with dilute carbol fuchsin instead of haematoxylin. I hope for some result. I have promised him a fiver when he shows me a flagellum inside a gastric cell and I shall have much pleasure in paying him the money. I have not time enough to work at this myself being burdened with my book[2] and other men's books.

That picture of the circle of clear spherular-like bodies given in my lectures was drawn from nature. Can it be that these bodies are flagella which, after being liberated from the central mass, had failed to burst the outer capsule and had curled themselves up around the central sphere. It was a very striking object but I confess its explanation is difficult.

I look for an interesting letter from you soon. Thanks for putting your friend on getting filariated mosquitoes for me.[3]

Yours very sincerely
Patrick Manson

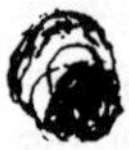
sketch of stained sphere before eruption of the flagella: flagella evident caught while wriggling about inside outer capsule.

1 Ross (1897a).
2 His *Tropical Diseases*, published the following year.
3 Dr Sturmer, see Letter 28, note 3.

Letter 62
02/103

Bangalore

7th March 1897

Dear Dr Manson,
I haven't had time to write and thank you for getting out my article in the B. M. J. & for giving the very appreciative little paragraph on the same.[1] It will probably clinch matters so far as the investigation goes, if the famine & plague do not prevent Govt. from indulging in such a modest *luxury*! Unfortunately another complication has arisen, namely that Dobson, who is the incumbent of the appt. now temporarily held by me has been transferred to Rajputana so that I must continue to act for him. There are two reasons why I should not give it up namely that the Resident in Mysore has specifically asked for me to be allowed to have the appointment because of

sanitary work, and secondly because this place suits my wife & children & the appointment is one of the best in the service. If I am now put on malaria work I may have to forfeit my chances here, because Dobson has been transferred only temporarily as yet. Red tape of course! but I hope that I shall be gazetted to act for Dobson in about a fortnight, when I think I can arrange about the malaria investigation without risking my anticipated appointment here. When fixed here permanently I shall be able to do really good work all round, so that I do not wish to throw away my chances.

Since last writing I have had no good cases except a few wretched tertians & quartans; but have now got a splendid remittent tertian, & another remittent just yielding crescents, & hope to be on again in a few days. But I have not been idle. I have taken to other parasites with startling success. A patient came in from Kolar Gold Fields, feeling ill & having enlarged lymphatics inside left arm. I guessed F. nocturna;[2] sure enough, there they were. But this patient had to go away immediately. Next, another case from the *same* gold mine with dysentery. I found the following pretty list of parasites in him. Amoeba Coli & ova of anchylostoma, trichocephalus, ascaris & oxyuris in motions. He had also tender glands in the neck. "My friend" I said "you have so many parasites that you may also have F. Nocturna, especially as you come from the same gold mine as my former case." Sure enough, filaria nocturna! Unfortunately, only one or two in a specimen - in the other case they were numerous.

I have also found amoeba coli in three other cases, two of dysentery & one of fatal diarrhoea without any lesions in the large intestine. Good for about a fortnight's work! Also three cases of *cercomonas*[3] of different species, & one more of anchylostoma! This isn't bad for a beginner. I fed a dog on amoeba coli (without croton oil) - no result. Give me time.

The amoebae were generally among red & white blood corpuscles, except in the case of fatal diarrhoea where they were in faecal matter. I saw also several cercomonas *worrying red corpuscles*. Am hot on the scent of these.

9th March. Two more cases of amoeba coli, in one of them cercomonas also. One a case of hepatic abscess with profuse diarrhoea (a native). Amoebae both in pus & in motions. Not in the laudable pus, but in sanguineous pus produced by probing the abscess & scraping its walls with the end of the probe - just as you said. The amoebae are numerous but very sluggish (Temperature 80°F). The other is a case of rather chronic diarrhoea in a child aged 4 years, one of a family of three all suffering from evident parasitism. (Coin me a word for the disease produced by numerous parasites - *parasitiasis.*) Amoebae very numerous but sluggish (motion passed three hours) - also cercomonas. I have written to Dr Cunningham[4] asking him to lend me a copy of his work on these animals. Crescents have not set in yet in my two malaria cases - hope they won't fail again. Will try the other two cases of "parasitiasis" tomorrow.

10th March. Have had little time for microscope work today but must leave off in order to catch the post. Again many thanks for the notice in the B. M. J. I am very proud that you should think my paper to be a good one. They worry me to death here about plague quarantine, new hospitals, sanitation, etc, to such an extent that I am obliged to refuse private practice & can't look at more than a dozen specimens daily.

With kindest regards
Yours sincerely
R. Ross.

1 [Manson] (1897a).
2 Filaria nocturna.
3 One of a group of parasitic flatworms.
4 David Douglas Cunningham, (1843-1914), FRS, Professor of Physiology in Calcutta where he had carried out medical investigations for the Indian Government for many years. See **Biographical Appendix**.

Letter 63
02/104

Bangalore
17th March / 97

Dear Dr Manson,
Just a line to tell you that all the arrangements detailed to you in my last have been upset by Dobson having determined, after going to Rajputana to return to this place, whereby I am thrown out of employ & have "no work to do". Govt. of India have wired down & asked what they can do for me. I replied "*Put me on malaria investigation.*" I also sent your article "a neglected responsibility of empire."[1] So there they have it plump, and if they refuse I shall be so

disgusted that I shall not care to serve much longer.

Of course the affair is unfortunate for me in one sense & especially so for my wife & children, because I lose a permanent independent appointment in the best Indian station. I also have to give up just at the moment of fruition the hard local labour of one & a half years. On the other hand *I am free for the germ.* No more patients, office work, etc - nothing but pure investigation. I must have a few weeks rest at Ooty[2] where I have taken a house & whither my wife has gone. This will enable me to make preparations - tents, servants, etc & then, sanction of Govt. or not, I am off to the nearest malaria breeding ground. If sanction does not arrive within two months I shall probably take general leave (on reduced pay) & continue the work on my own hook. It must be done; and I want to get as forward as possible before mosquitoes begin in Italy. I ought to get two months ahead of Europeans. Perhaps this is the most fortunate thing that could have occurred.

Yours very sincerely
R. Ross.

1 Letter 62, note 1.
2 Ootacamund. Kennedy (1996). Ross, *Memoirs*, 292, described Ootacamund as 'a bit of England placed on the rounded tops of the Nilghiri Hills, about 8,000 feet above sea-level.'

Letter 64
02/105

Blenheim[1]
Ootacamund
13th April / 97

Dear Dr Manson,
Here I am within a week, I hope, of going into the jungles after the malaria parasite. Dobson relieved me a fortnight ago at Bangalore & I intend now to devote my future to real work. The government investigation has not yet been sanctioned, but I believe it will be sanctioned. I enclose a little fillip I have given them in the Pioneer (9th April).[2] But I have no intention of waiting for them to make up their very sluggish minds, and have applied for two months' leave, so as to be able to start work at once. The Surgeon General tells me that

he will give the leave. My apparatus is ready packed for jungle work, & as soon as I get my leave definitely I shall commence work at the foot of these hills at a place where I hear fever is very bad. This place is at the bottom of the Sigur Ghat[3] (Cañon) the top of which is only half an hour's run from my house here (on a bicycle). I think however that I shall go & live at a dâk bungalow[4] lower down the ghat & just above the malaria. However I intend to make no definite plans until I have looked about a bit. Some weeks will be occupied, I expect, in such "looking about"; and I must probably buy tents & get right into the haunts of King Malaria. Tippoogadoo is the name of the place I have heard of. Will write more next mail, if things go well. Am dying to be off, but can't start till definite orders come. With kindest regards

Yours sincerely

R. Ross.

1 Blenheim was the name of the house Ross took for himself and his family.

2 In an anonymous article Ross wrote that it was high time that the mosquito-malaria theory was investigated in India and cited Manson's 'Neglected responsibility of empire' (see letter 59, note 2). He went on to mention that Bignami had studied the subject in Rome and despite opposing some of the observations and deductions of Manson and Ross, arrived at the same conclusion - that the mosquito is the carrying agent of malaria. **RA.** 02/106.

3 A ghat is a mountain pass.

4 A house for travellers.

Letter 65
02/107

Ootacamund

21st April 1897

Dear Dr Manson,

Just a line to catch the mail to tell you that the long-wished for investigation begins *tomorrow* the 22nd inst. when I am off to Kalhutti in the Sigur Ghat. It is not official at present but I have obtained (with some difficulty) two months leave to carry it on (at my own cost). The reply of the Govt. of India to the Govt. of Madras in respect to the official investigation is doubtful. The Gov. General recognises the importance of Dr Manson's theory & that Surg. Maj. Ross is the man to do it (doubtful) but says he is thinking about a Public Health Institute[1] for India (he will probably go on thinking for the next ten years) & so on. At the same time if the Govt. of Madras still wants to start the enquiry they can do so but must remember that there is a great paucity of officers owing to plague (they are as thick as blackberries here *on leave*). Everybody here is very keen & the planters will do everything to help me; but the big officials think that the best way to do the thing will be to start it on private leave & then if things look promising to apply again for the official enquiry. Hence I am off tomorrow. Kalhutti is just above a deadly place & out of fever range. I shall stop there & go down every day if possible. If not possible I shall descend to a house lent me by a planter Mr Richard Kindersley.[2] There are however numerous fever *holes* all over the place & if I find Kindersley's house not appropriate or too dangerous (it won't do for me to get fever) I shall try some of these. Generally planters' houses are situated just over fever range so that I can sleep in them & descend every morning for work. So here goes. Wish me good luck!

The first thing is to try to find our little friend in the mosquitoes' tissues. I think perhaps I shall now be able to spot any mosquito parasite like the malaria parasite. It is not unlikely that I may come across the analogue of the crescent in elderly mosquitoes - don't you think so.

With kindest regards
Yours sincerely
R. Ross.

I will write every mail but I wish you would give me a telegraphic address.

1 See Letter 80, note 1.

2 A coffee planter. See John Weatherstone, *The Pioneers 1825-1900: The Early British Tea and Coffee Planters and their Way of Life* (London: Quiller Press, 1986).

Letter 66
02/108

Ootacamund
28th. April 1897

Dear Dr Manson,

My reconnaissance has had rather an unexpected ending. I went to Kalhutti on Thursday the 22nd. On the 23rd I went down to the bottom of the ghat (4 miles) & then 4 miles across the spur of a mountain to another valley where there is Kindersley's coffee estate Westbury. We had had early tea at 7.30 a.m., started from Kalhutti at 8 a.m. & reached the coffee estate at 10.30 or 11.0 Then we had tea which I noticed was coolish, while the milk seemed watered (?). Then we examined a boy with fever (finding malignant tertian) & went to look at the source of drinking water, a puddle fed by a mountain stream or rather trickle. The puddle was full of frogs & water beetles, etc. Next we walked on the estate which was under irrigation, the ground & air teaming with life & seething with heat & moisture. We had breakfast at 1.30 (whisky & soda). More coolies examined afterwards; many with spleens; another with same parasite. Started back at 4.15 & above fever range at 6 p.m. On Saturday I examined specimens & on Sunday 25th did the same with several walks in the upper part of the ghat. At 10 p.m. I was seized with a severe go of fever & had to come back here yesterday.

The fever was bad at night beginning with a sudden pain in liver followed by 2 hours' rigor & then 2 hours fever with aching in bones & gradual defervescence. I slept from 4 to 6 a.m. on the 26th & woke feeling all right. I had taken 5 grs quinine on the 22nd, 23rd & 24th but 10 grs on Sunday the 25th. As soon as I knew what was wrong I took 20 grs more at once. Hence on Monday morning I found only one small amoeboid body (quite typical & moving) in two excellent specimens. I don't know the species. At 9 a.m. fever began to come on again without rigor & very slightly. I slept till 3 p.m. when I woke in much perspiration & have not had fever since. Liver still hurts on a deep breath but I gave the parasites such as warm reception with quinine that I don't think they liked it. I shall be off down to ghat again in a few days. Unfortunately had no thermometer with me at Kalhutti, but the fever must have run very high because I felt twitchings all over & was a trifle light headed I think for a little. Had no phenacetin,[1] etc.

Now I slept every night at Kalhutti inside a mosquito net & with closed windows & doors. At Kalhutti there is a planter, Nash, with a few coolies two of whom had been ill lately with fever. In the dâk bungalow where I was the native servant & his wife had both had fever lately. He had a large spleen but no parasites. In front of their hut was a puddle full of mosquito grubs which I am still examining. Neither of my two servants who also slept at Kalhutti have had fever yet. We all drank boiled water & milk religiously.

I must watch developments before judging where I got the fever but think I got it at Westbury, Kindersley's estate at the foot of the ghat on Friday the 23rd. This gives about 60 hours incubation period. Anyway the incubation must have been under 72 hours. Kalhutti is 5500 feet above the sea & Westbury about 3000 feet.

29th. I fear this letter has missed the mail. My case gives useful data to go upon. Assuming the incubation period to have been 48 hours, then with the most rapidly developing species of parasite, no more than two generations could have hatched in that time; in other words on average one parasite admitted on the 23rd could scarcely have become more than 100 parasites on the 25th. Again on the 25th I suppose that quite one in 10,000 of my corpuscles must have been infected, probably many more. Now I have about 25,000,000,000,000 corpuscles;[2] so that on the 25th I must have had about 2,500,000,000 parasites in my body. Dividing this by 100 we get the number of parasites which I must have taken on the 23rd namely about 25,000,000.

I think you will admit on consideration that this line of reasoning is really quite sound, fantastic as it may seem. We can roughly estimate the rate at which a quotidian parasite can breed from the number of spores it has & the period of the cycle. All this considered, I think that 25 million parasites or spores must have been the least number admitted on the 23rd.

Now on that day I spent nine hours in the malarious region & breathed about 30 inhalations a minute, each inhalation containing about 25 cubic inches of air (vide any physiology text-book).[3] Hence I breathed about 405,000 cubic inches of air during the nine hours. Suppose all the air to have been equally impregnated with malaria germs then the 405,000 cubic inches must have contained 25,000,000 germs; or 1 cub. inch must have contained no less than 62 malaria germs.

This is something unheard of, especially as I was in the malarious region only during the day. The largest number of bacteria found in air is I believe something like 1 bacterium in 10 cubic inches. Here we have 62 sporozoa in one inch! If however I contracted the infection while walking in the coffee plantation (one hour) the number of germs there must have been nine times as large namely about 558 a cubic inch!

On the other hand if I contracted the infection by drinking the tea, of which I consumed about $1^1/_2$ pints, we should still get a large number of germs per cubic centimetre of water but nothing unheard of. Anyway the air or water of the locality must contain large quantities of the material which causes malarial infection. I may add that my case of attack after 48 hours agrees perfectly with report & tradition which speak of numerous persons who have died straight off a day or two after having passed through the lower ghat.

All this appears to me to have a most important bearing on the great problem because it makes us expect to find large numbers of the free form of the germ, whatever it is, in the air & water, & ought to facilitate the search. I examined the Westbury water carefully. It did not contain a single mosquito grub not did I find a single psorosperm in the mud. Beside numbers of diatoms, infusoria etc, I found only one creature more closely allied to the sporozoa and that was a beast exactly of the size & shape of the mosquito gregarine but coloured *bright green* with a *scarlet* nucleolus & a long single anterior flagellum.

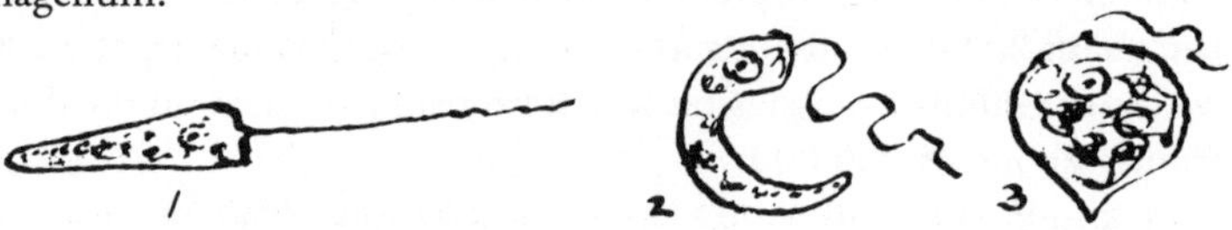

1 2 3

When slowly crawling about it licked things with the flagellum & had the shapes given above; then suddenly the flagellum would disappear & the creature would go skimming along with the shape of (1) without the flagellum & *exactly* with a motion size & shape (especially the square shoulders) of the mosquito gregarine. On drying movements became almost amoeboid & finally the shape was spherical. There were no cilia. The green colour I attribute to the animals' food. These creatures did not live so much in the mud as in the open water which seemed to be nearly a pure culture of them.

I have found nothing like the m. parasite in the mosquitoes at Kalhutti which moreover do not contain gregarines nor the rectal fungus which I think I mentioned to you.

I must also tell you that on Sunday morning (25th) I searched down the stream in the upper part of the ghat & up many of its tributary streamlets, & though I found many entirely stagnant pools, in *not one* of them did I find a single mosquito grub. On the 18th however some heavy rain had fallen which in all probability had scoured out all the ravines. On Monday the 26th I had proposed to examine similarly the lower part of the ghat, that is to hunt there for mosquito grubs. It is curious that though mosquitoes were found near dwellings at Kalhutti at the top of the ghat they were not found at all in the natural pools below that point, or at Westbury (I did not search round the servants' huts at Westbury).

Must leave off now
With Kind regards
Yours sincerely
R. Ross.

1 Phenacetin was still a relatively new drug, introduced in the 1880s.
2 In a footnote in *Memoirs*, 205, Ross amends this figure to 15,000,000,000,000 red corpuscles based on new data. He defends his reasoning, though the numbers have been described as 'untenable'. (Nye and Gibson, 1997, 66).
3 Augustus D. Waller, *An Introduction to Human Physiology*, 3rd ed (London: Longmans, Green, 1896), 122, says 30 cubic inches.

Letter 67
02/109

Blenheim Ootacamund
Monday 3rd May 1897

Dear Dr Manson,
I have had no more fever but found a typical C 8[1] in my blood on Thursday last. Am feeling quite well (20-30 grs quinine daily) & propose to start for the ghat again tomorrow or on Wednesday. I have been examining my specimens over & over again & have been sedulously reading Labbé & Ray Lankester's splendid article on protozoa in the Ency. Brittanica [sic].[2] This has given me a revelation simply. Why, the crescent question becomes quite clear & in accordance with some examples of protozoa. I propose in future to call the ordinary spores (and young m. parasites) "amoebulae", and flagellate spores "flagellulae" in accordance with Lankester's terminology. Taking, as Labbé says, the ordinary sporulating forms as a monosporocyst giving rise to amoebula, the crescent becomes a monosporocyst giving birth to flagellulae.

I have also been thinking hard at the whole question. You must confess that an incubation period of two or three days as often reported taken in conjunction with the fact that at the onset of fever a man's blood must contain on a reasonable count, some hundreds of thousands of millions of parasites, simply implies to mathematical demonstration an access or ingress of many millions of parasites at the moment of infection. Now whence does this invading host come? Are they at the moment of infection (a) multiplying free in nature or (b) parasitic in some other animal. Taking (b) first & assuming the m. germs to be parasitic, we must confess that either the hosts must be very numerous or must each contain enormous numbers of parasites. Since the parasites have a definite & not very small size, this means that the hosts must be small, very numerous & ubiquitous (each containing a few parasites) rather than few or large. Suppose for example that the mosquito grub is the host & that each grub contains 1,000,000 m. germs (too large a number surely), then I must have swallowed 25 mosquito grubs or the equivalent of mosquito debris. Now I did not find a single grub at Westbury; while supposing even that there had been millions of grubs there, the *forces of dilution* in the immense quantities of air & water on the estate make it *almost impossible* that I could by any accident have breathed or swallowed so concentrated a dose as the debris of 25 mosquitoes even if mosquitoes had been very plentiful there. On the contrary in the mud of the Westbury drinking water I have not found a single mosquito feather or other sign of mosquitoes. The same reasoning applies to other large & few hosts - these are so few & must contain comparatively so few parasites that considering the *forces of dilution* in nature it is extremely improbable that a man could ever acquire from them such an enormous dose as 25 million germs.

Hence it appears to me that we are driven to believe that the m. germ is at the moment of ingress either (a) parasitic in infusoria, or other very numerous protozoa, or (b) multiplying free in air or water as proteomyxa, mycetozoa or flagellata. Or, if we cannot necessarily arrive at (a) we may submit to the possibility of the m. germ being at the moment of infection in the state of spores lately derived from parasites of infusoria, etc.

To put it in another way, the number of animal parasites in small hosts does not by any means vary as the body-weight of the host. Thus a mosquito grub is 1000 times as long as a small flagellate organism & is therefore 1000^3 = a thousand million times as heavy; but it certainly is not calculated to have the same ratio of animal parasites. For example a grub contains only a few thousand psorosperms while a flagellate organism may contain several protozoal parasites. On the other hand the numbers of the smaller animals do vary roughly *inversely* as the body weight; thus for one mosquito grub in nature I suppose there are certainly 1,000,000,000 flagellatae of one species. Hence if the m. germs are *very* common in certain parts they are much more likely to exist either as free protozoa or as parasites of the small & very numerous protozoa than as parasites of the few and by-few-parasites-infected larger animals.

To put it in a third way, if in the small amount of air or water breathed & drunk by me while I was at Westbury I took in 25,000,000 germs, what must be the total number of germs in the air or water of the locality! And, since on the mosquito-parasite theory every few thousand of these germs would require a mosquito host, what must be the number of mosquitoes in the locality! — But I did not find a single one. Of course instead of living mosquitoes we may talk of the debris of dead mosquitoes; but this will not affect the calculations since I found no debris in several samples of water.

However I hope to go down again to Westbury & also to the pools at the bottom of the ghat & have a regular hunt for mosquitoes & mosquito-debris. If no adequate numbers can be found, the only conclusion which seems possible to me will be that *whether the malaria parasite is capable or not of being parasitic in the mosquito it is also capable of leading either a free life, or a parasitic life in some other animal found in large numbers in malarious localities.* Continuing to grant the cogency of the arguments which suggest a parasitic life for a time at all events in the mosquito as well as in man, the most plausible theory may possibly be that *the malaria parasite multiplies freely in nature but is capable of an optimal parasitism either in man or in the mosquito.*

After my next letter you will be able to consider the question on a firmer ground of facts & will, I hope, let me know what you think. The whole thing, considering the crescents on one side & the absence of mosquitoes in the Sigur Ghat on the other, is so perplexing that I don't know what to think. It will probably end in having to work out the subject in frogs, lizards & birds. I began yesterday on flies & frogs — in the former I found a worm; in the faeces of latter psorosperms, embryo worms & an infusorian, but no parasites in blood (brown frog). The chlorophyll-bearing flagellate found in large numbers of the Westbury water belongs to sub-class Lissoflagellata; order, Monadidea; family Rhizomastigma - Lankester. If you are passing Lewis in Gower street will you very kindly ask him to obtain some or all of the works on the accompanying list & put them to my account, addressing Blenheim Ootacamund.[3] I have had a fine case here of amoeba coli &

cercomonads-rectal dysentery & hepatic abscess.

Yours sincerely

R. Ross.

Lankester says spores of flagellates stand *boiling*, hence my tea at Westbury was not safe.

1 See Manson's Chart, Figure 3.

2 E. Ray Lankester, 'Protozoa', *Encyclopaedia Britannica*, 9th edition (Edinburgh: Adam & Charles Black, 1875-89), vol. xix, 830-866. For Edwin Ray Lankester, (1847-1929), see **Biographical Appendix**.

3 List is lost.

Letter 68
02/023

21 Queen Anne Street,
Cavendish Square,
20th April, 1897.

My dear Ross,

I am very glad to hear the plasmodium is to the fore again and that you will be on his tracks so soon. Stick to him. Sooner or later he will do much more for you than sanitation work at Bangalore, although I should have liked for your immediate comfort's sake that you had been confirmed in your appointment there. This is one of the ill winds that is going to blow good to you.

I have sent a short note to the B M J on staining the flagella.[1] I suppose it will appear soon or some day. I had a case of quartan at the hospital lately but the parasites were too few to do anything with. I am anxious to try to stain the flagellated phase of both the quartan and the benign tertian but material is so scanty here that I may have to wait a long time. I fancy that could we get them stained we might be able to make out some distinguishing differences and thereby supply an argument for or against difference of species. These bodies like the rosettes should be to the zoologist as the flower is to the botanist.

Lately I have found out where the filaria goes to in the day time. A filaria patient committed suicide with prussic acid at 8.30 a.m., that is just when the filariae have left the peripheral circulation. I found him post mortem in thousands in the lungs and arteries. Devil a one in liver or spleen or bone marrow and only a very few in the brain - just the opposite of what happens with the sporulating malaria parasite. Strange is it not. When I publish I shall send you reprint.[2] They want me to send it to the Royal Society. Nous verrons.

I have also found filaria perstans and filaria de marquaii[3] in blood of Indians from the back country of Demerara. Or similar filariae. Strange to say I heard of one case of a sleeping sickness, whether it was or was not the sleeping sickness I cannot say, among these Indians. If it was SS it is another argument for a pathological relationship of filaria perstans to that disease.

Be sure to write me of the progress of events. By the way by staining the plasmodial sphere in some cases I could see the flagella inside the capsule of the parasite as you describe and I have had it photographed and drawn.

I hear of no fresh malarial developments. Lawrie and Hehir are extinct but old Fayrer[4] is inclined to pooh pooh the parasite. He is a Thomas and wants to handle the thing before he can believe.

Yours sincerely

Patrick Manson

1 Manson (1897b).
2 Manson-Bahr and Alcock (1927), 48.
3 Manson (1898a), chapter 31, summarises contemporary knowledge of filaria infections.
4 (Sir) Joseph Fayrer, (1824-1907), see **Biographical Appendix**. Fayrer did not publish anything on malaria in obvious journals in the 1890s, but Manson would have seen him regularly at medical meetings.

Letter 69
02/110

Ootacamund
12th May 1897

Dear Dr Manson,

Another five days in the jungle have reversed the position of affairs in favour of the mosquito theory but only just as I was beginning to give it up. I started to Kalhutti again on the 5th. On the 9th I went to Sigur, the bottom of the ghat, & spent the whole day there hunting for mosquito pools & examining dew puddles, etc. Not a mosquito grub to be found. There is a rest-house there & in it I found a native with fever. He said he had arrived on the 27th April

& had been attacked with fever 4 days afterwards (he may have contracted it on the way). On my intimating that I wanted to examine his blood after breakfast he disappeared. I found however a family of 9 Kusbahs living all their lives at Sigur in a spot supposed to be absolutely deadly; not one of them had ever had fever, they said, & certainly none of the 7 men & children had spleen. They drank river water. I encamped at this spot during the day on the 6th & 7th inst. returning 4 miles up the ghat to Kalhutti in the evening. I found not a single mosquito grub anywhere but caught a mosquito full of blood in the rest-house. The mosquito was small with wings striped *brown* & white.[1] The Kusbahs (aborigines) informed me that sometimes mosquitoes are so numerous at night that fires are required to keep them off.

On the 8th I descended again & went to Nash's estate two miles out in the plain beyond Sigur. Here 13 out of sixteen people had large spleens or fever. They drank out of irrigation streams & lived in the midst of jungle. Even here I could not find a single mosquito pool. The same evening I went on to Westbury, 3 miles from Nash's plain estate, with intent to live there for a few days (this is where I expect I got my fever at first).

On Sunday 9th. I examined water of puddles, mud, everything - not a sign of a mosquito. There was not a mosquito in the bungalow either. I then offered a reward for every mosquito alive or dead, brought to me & went to bed feeling that mosquitos could play no essential part in the propagation of malaria.

On the 10th. (Monday) I returned to Nash's estate & examined bloods - one case of malignant tertian; looked about a little more & went back to Westbury. Here about 80% of the people have spleen. Out of 19 Kusbahs I found about half with spleens or fever (women would not be examined). Hence the Kusbahs are by no means immune, though they are partially so compared with other natives on the estates who had come from distant parts. Hence again the fact that the nine Kusbahs at Sigur are free from fever appears to show that that part is free from fever though Nash's estate & Westbury close by, are so bad. The river at Sigur, from which the 9 Kusbahs drink, is however a mountain stream running over stones & sand; the streams at Nash's & at Westbury run through rotting vegetation.

After breakfast on the 10th an intelligent native brought me 5 very small mosquitoes. I jumped with astonishment at sight of them & told him to take me where he had found them. Instead of taking me to the servants' huts he led me into the neighbouring jungle. It was then midday. He sat down; in one minute four or five mosquitoes had fastened on his black legs & arms, one was on my hand & several were prospecting my trousers. I let the one on my hand bite me, which it did in a few seconds, giving a sharp pain like a bee sting. One on the native's legs filled itself in about a minute. These insects abounded in the darkest parts of the jungle, which however was not large jungle but rather thin scrub & thorn. I searched everywhere for the grubs but could not find a pool of water anywhere, though it had been raining over night. Anyway the adult insects swarmed everywhere in the wood. In the evening we looked again for grubs, & at last discovered some in a small pool in a rocky ravine almost entirely sheltered from the sun by thick overhead vegetation & fully half a mile from where we had first found the mosquitoes.

Hence enter Culex Silvestris or Nemoris![2] - which I ought to have thought of before. Oddly enough there were none under the tree at Sigur where I encamped. The fact is they do not frequent single trees, but shady glades. They appear to fix on one with voracity morning, noon, evening, or night. They do not enter houses - at least well-made ones - though the natives say they come into their huts at night. They breed apparently only in the darkest & most secluded woodland pools in dried up water courses & are quite different from the ordinary house-mosquito.

The adults are very small with brindled bellies & very formidable suctorial apparatus. The grubs are also small, brindled & with very long air-tubes. The adults contain swarms of psorosperms, but in the few which I have yet examined I have not found anything very unusual. I am arranging to be supplied with relays of grubs & will examine more thoroughly & let you know result.

On the 11th I had to return here.

Now about my own case of fever. On the 10th. I found an old well close to Kindersley's cook house; the water was solid with mosquito grubs of the house variety & it is more than possible that our tea (which was called for hurriedly) was made out of this water slightly warmed up. More about this hereafter.

Well then, the Culex Sylvestris has entirely altered the state of affairs. When I was just about to give up on the theory owing to the absence of mosquitoes I find that mosquitoes are swarming. *If then malaria occupies the mosquito at all it occupies the Culex Silvestris*,[3] and I must find it there by hook or by crook. Besides this you will perceive that the habits of the Silvestris are such as exactly to suit the facts we know about malaria. The example the women at Westbury & Nash's generally deny having fever, the men & children almost all

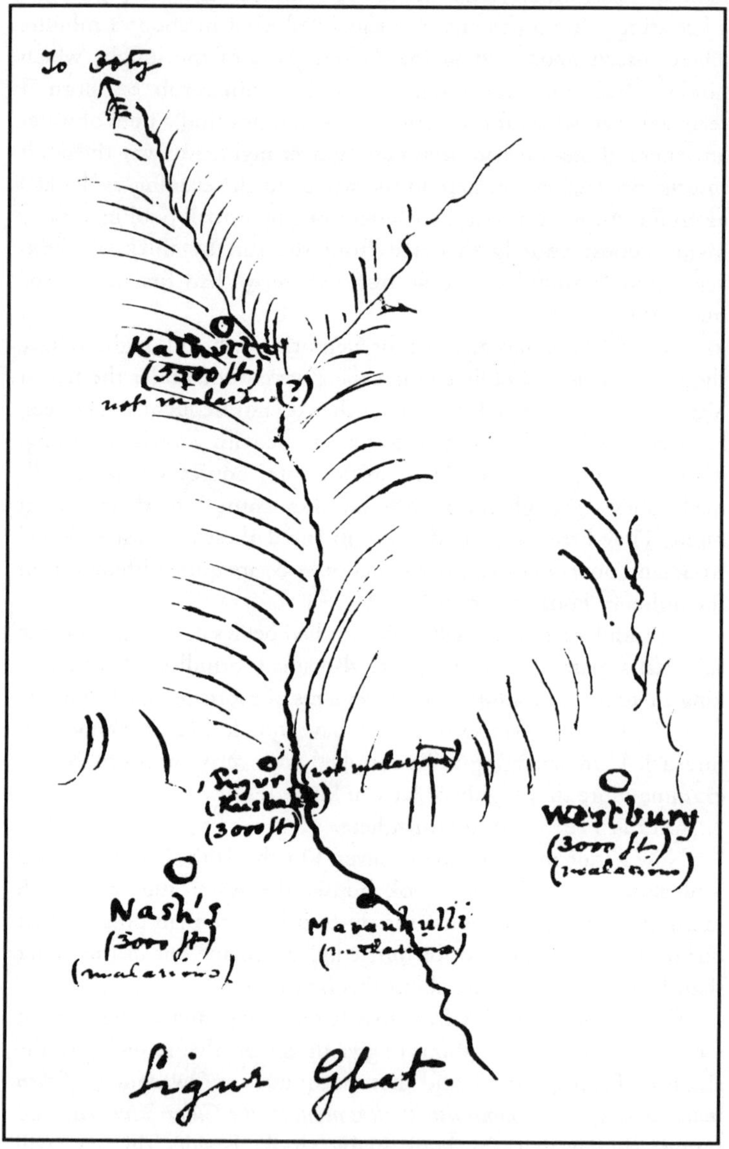

Figure 7
Ross's map of the Sigur Ghat.

get it, probably because they are continually in the jungle looking after cows or working, while the women mostly cook at home or work only in the gardens where the silvestris does not live. It looks also as if the bite does it in some way,[4] it appearing to me very questionable whether the forces of dilution in air or water would not reduce the chance of infection almost to an impossibility even granting that the woods are full of the Silvestris. It appears much more likely that infection is brought straight to men (as a rule) by the insect itself.

I shall see Kindersley today or tomorrow & will make complete arrangements with him to be supplied with numerous grubs of the Silvestris. He is keen on the subject. I shall also experiment with Silvestris water.

My best congratulations on your most remarkable find respecting the filaria embryos. It is indeed interesting, & by what a fortunate stroke (in a way)[5] were you enabled to ascertain the point! But how do the embryos, which cannot swim, manage to hold on in the arteries?

Many thanks for yours of 20th April. Someone who calls himself "sceptic" has been denying the parasite again in the Pioneer.[6] I have gone for him.[7] If he pokes up his head again I shall give him something. It is rather fun.

My next excursion will be in the direction of the Bhawani Valley where I want to combine science with fishing. I must track the habits of Silvestris a little more.

With kind regards
Yours truly
R. Ross.

1 *Memoirs*, 208, notes that this mosquito actually had spotted, not striped wings, and that it was Ross's first *Anopheles*.

2 *Memoirs*, 209, comments that these were probably a small variety of *Stegomyia scutellaris*.

3 *Memoirs*, 210, remarks on the irony that the 'single spy' *Anopheles* was actually the culprit, rather than the 'battalions' of *Culex*. cf. *Hamlet*, Act IV, Sc. 5.

4 Letter 48, note 2, for Bignami's suggestion that malaria is a 'disease of inoculation'.

5 i.e. by the patient's suicide. Letter 68.

6 A letter to the editor by a Sceptic, 'The cause of malaria' *Pioneer* (25 Apr. 1897), 7. **RA** 05/006. The author states that not only does he

not support Manson's theory that mosquitoes convey malaria, but he also doubts the existence of the parasite. He stresses the influence of environment and climate on the presence of ague.

7 R. Ross, 'The cause of malaria' *Pioneer*, (6 May 1897), 6. **RA** 05/007. Ross countered the writer's argument saying that despite the writer's claim to having read all the relevant literature, he showed an 'immature knowledge' of the subject.

Letter 70
02/111

Ootacamund
16th May 1897

Dear Dr Manson,

A week of intensely exciting work over my samples from Westbury. I have not succeeded in finding any parasite exactly like the malaria parasite, certainly no crescents; but I have discovered two or three new protozoal parasites any of which may be the alternative form required. Of course in one week and with my limited material I have by no means arrived at definite conclusions, so that please note that the following sketch will probably need revision after further study & certainly requires much amplification.

I brought home two samples:-

A. Grubs, mud & water from the jungle puddle containing culex silvestris. Only 7 grubs remained alive after the journey & none of these have [sic] hatched out. I have dissected four of them.

B. Grubs, mud & water from the old well from which perhaps the tea was made which may have given me fever. Grubs numerous, & all hatched out & have been dissected.

The parasites found were

1. Spherical cells about the size of a grown tertian containing central masses of brown substance & numerous swarming & sometimes circulating granules. I doubt whether these cells are intracellular. They occur in large numbers in some tissues near the tail & have a greenish colour *en masse*. I have studied them but little & am not quite sure that they are parasitic, but they are roughly not unlike the m. parasite. 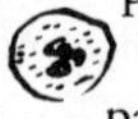

2. An intra- or intercellular parasite living in or amongst the visceral cells (or elsewhere?) found equally in the larva & imago, & forming sporocysts, also in both these stages, containing a few small chlamydo[1] spores. The bulk of these parasites equals a sphere

of about 40μ in diameter. Their shape is irregular. I have not observed amoeboid movement. They have the colour & granular structure of gregarines but appear to have no free & motile stage like the gregarine & produce spores which are quite different. The spores are oval, bright & hard (?), about 4μ in length and 2μ in breadth, & contain a clearer round spot at one end 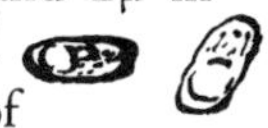. They are all pretty uniform in size & occur in clusters of eight or there abouts. There is no sign in them of Schneider's residue[2] nor of crescents, & they are not like gregarine psorosperms. The parasite does not seem to go to the malpighian tubes to breed, the sporocysts being found round the stomach, and, as I have said, all stages of the parasite occur during all stages of the host. As I have seen no free gregarine forms as yet I believe that the parasite is an entirely intracellular sporozoön allied neither to the coccidia nor to the gregarines. The following are rough sketches:-

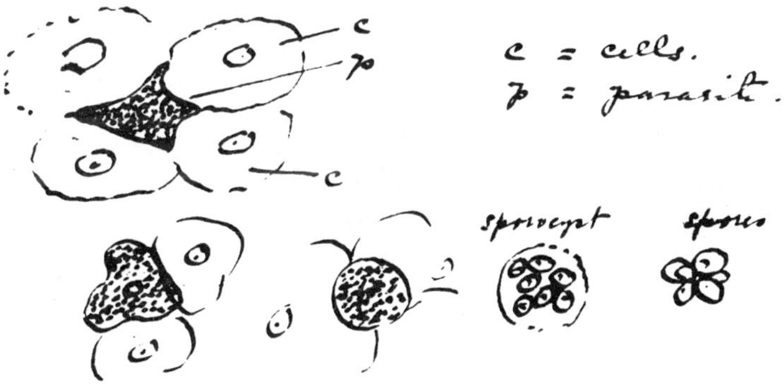

One insect does not contain more than say 500 spores. Much more work is however required on this animal.

3. My third discovery is something quite astonishing if my present views hold good on further observation - anyway it is interesting.

You remember the green flagellates with orange-red nucleus which I found in such large numbers in all the Sigur waters. I think there are several species of these, of which I will send you drawings & specimens if necessary. They form jar-shaped sporocysts in which the green chlorophyll becomes first a ball & then gives place to a number of oblong, bright, different-sized spores.

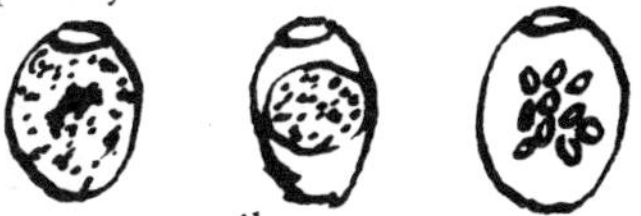

These sporocysts can easily be traced to the flagellates & often contain the remnants of the red nucleus. Well, when I commenced examining my grubs I found that their crops were stuffed with these flagellates & their sporocysts which abound in the water of my samples. Looking further I found that many of the sporocysts were burst in the grubs' stomachs & the spores scattered there and in the intestine. Then I found a grub the intestine of which appeared to be lined with these spores *or others just like them* (these spores are quite different from those of parasite 2 above). Then I took up an imago & found its intestine also lined with spores; & as I looked at the rectum I was astonished to see some of the spores moving. Taking another imago I found the stomach *literally crammed* with myriads of these spores which as I looked became active flagellulae just like the parents only that they did not contain chlorophyll. Imago after imago gave the same result, and I have spent most of my time watching this phenomenon. The spores appear at first as hard little bright bodies, then seem to become larger & to contain granules & at last on the addition of water get a single anterior flagellum.

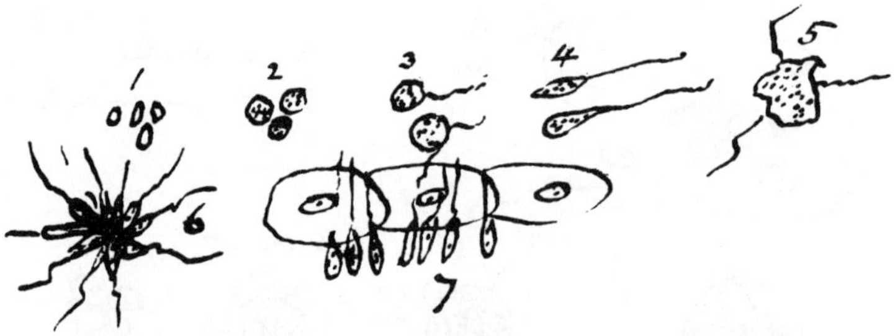

The spectacle is wonderful. The development from 1 to 2 appears to go on inside the mosquito; from 2 to 3 & 4 on the addition of water. Clusters of flagellulae like 6 are very numerous, and occasional large forms which appear to have many flagella (5) are common consisting perhaps of several flagellulae stuck together. The flagellulae grow under the sight until they reach about 10μ with flagella of 30μ or more, & they immediately begin to attack the tissues of the host, plunging their long flagella into the cells & *fighting for places* (7). I have kept them alive for 6 hours.

There is one point where this history is uncertain that is I am not quite sure that the spores of the green flagellates are the same as the spores from which the flagellulae arise, but I think so. The fact that the flagellulae have just the same shape as the green flagellates is another, but not conclusive, argument in favour of the view that the flagellulae are the children of the flagellates hatched out in the alimentary canal of the mosquito, &, I think, developed to some extent at the expense of the mosquito's cells. If I ultimately find such to be the case we shall be in possession of the extraordinary fact that a flagellate organism abounding in malarial water is capable of becoming for a time parasitic in the mosquito! I must also call attention to the possibility that these flagellulae are deposited on the human skin during haustilation[3] since they are found in the stomach of the young adult mosquito. Owing to their active progression they could easily find their way into the human blood either through the puncture made by the mosquito or through abrasions of the skin caused by scratching!

On the 14th inst. I gave the flagellulae of two mosquitoes in water to one of my native servants by the mouth, just as a chance experiment.

I have now exhausted my samples & am expecting another lot tomorrow. I propose to work out the life history of the new parasite & then to attempt to produce fever by means of them. As however none of my silvestris grubs are hatching out I must I think go to Sigur again after the adult insect. The adults of sample B were like the mosquito found by me in the rest-house at Sigur.[4]

If ultimately I cannot find a parasite just like the m. parasite in the cells of the silvestris I think we must be driven to the conclusion that the alternative form differs morphologically from the human form & that the changes between the hosts are of a complex nature - don't you think so? The sporozoa may undergo very marked transformations from one host to another or to external nature. The life-history of parasite 3, if given correctly above, may yield remarkable suggestions. If the flagellulae are not the children of the green flagellates they must proceed from some parasite of the grub. Possibly they may be connected with parasite 2, but I scarcely think so. I must track the matter out.

It seems to me that, whatever the alternative form of the m. parasite may be, we have cogent epidemiological reasons for supposing that it will be very numerous either in the mosquito or in external nature or in both. Hence I am paying especial attention to parasite 3 in spite of difficulties in the way of conceiving *it* to be the alternative form. In short, I think, complexity of transformation must be allowed to tell less against a theory than the existence of large numbers of the animal in nature or the mosquito must tell in favour of it. However we shall see.

I fear that the official investigation is not possible on account of the plague. I have only one more month's leave. No more fever but am feeling very cheap & the excitement of work is followed by much reaction. Going to take a holiday today.

With kindest regards

Yours sincerely

R. Ross.

What a splendid case was that last one of filariasis!!!

1 A unicellular, flagellate, green alga.
2 The significance of Schneider's residue is not clear.
3 The action of sucking.
4 Letter 69, note 1.

Letter 71
02/112

Ooty,
24th May 1897

Dear Dr Manson,

My scheme of getting up samples from Sigur and working here has failed; the men I sent down brought me up tadpoles instead of grubs though I told them exactly what to get. I have not returned there yet because my cook has rheumatism & because I found parasites I & II[1] in some mosquitoes up here & have thought it best to work at them before going back to the jungles. Consequently I have done a hard week's work at No II without however reaching conclusive results.

The first thing was to find the exact habitat of the clusters of spores. They lie, not in the digestive system, but in a vessel which extends from the head to the tail along the back & just under the scales. This vessel is, I think, the lymph vessel & has sinuses at every joint where it gives off branches, but it is very difficult to make out clearly. It has no very active circulating fluid but contains perfectly clear, non-nucleated cells with a very delicate outline. Similar cells are packed into all the interstitial spaces of the grub. They vary much in size & look like mere globules of some fluid. The spores of Parasite II are found in the sinuses of this lymph vessel in about 1 in 2 grubs & 1 in 7 adults. They occur in clusters consisting *invariably* of eight spores each; & fifty or a hundred such clusters are collected together in a group. There are three or four of such groups in one grub & these groups can easily be seen & studied roughly with the oil immersion in a *living* grub. They are found in grubs of less than 1/4 in. in length but not in smaller ones. I have not found them in pupae as yet.

On opening an insect & pressing upon the cover glass the clusters of spores travel along channels between the muscles & escape into the open after which the spores tend to break apart. I examine them as they squeeze through the channels and afterwards when they lie in the open, but have not succeeded in working backward with certainty to the parent sporozoon, though I have tracked them backwards some steps. I *think* now that these spores have nothing to do with the masses of gregarine-like substance described as their parents in my last letter, but believe (pending further research) that they are the spores of a cytozoon occupying the lymph cells of the mosquito. Here are the stages worked backward as far as I have seen hitherto.

1 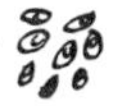 Scattered spores, each with a vacuole at one end.

2.  A cluster of eight spores.

3 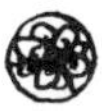 A cluster of eight spores enclosed in a lymph cell.

4. 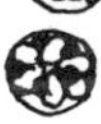 The same as 3, but the spores only outlines & with bright granules between, which stain brightly (chromatin?).

5 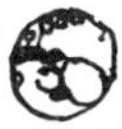 Indications of spore formation together with granules which stain well.

6 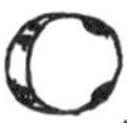 A circle with marginal masses of chromatin(?), and an inner circle of clear fluid.

Forms 5 & 6 are always found among the forms 1, 2, 3 & 4, but I have failed in tracing further back than this with certainty owing to the extreme delicacy of the lymph cells & also to the swarms of cells & nuclei of cells which are to be found in the mosquito & many of which simulate closely cytozoa. This morning however I found an adult mosquito containing large numbers of cells amazingly suggestive of cytozoa.

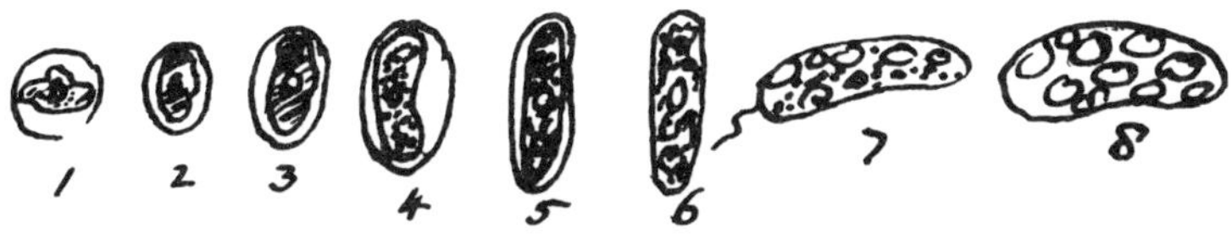

Of these forms 4, 5, & 6 are however just like cells or nuclei which I think are normal. So are 7 & 8; but on one occasion, I should tell you, I saw No 7 *moving* with a shivering movement of one end & also a slight movement of progression. It seemed to have a flagellum at one end; but I have not seen this again, nor any movement of any kind in these bodies except on this one occasion. The above forms are like either crescents or like Labbé's Danilewskya.[2] I expected to find young & mature cytozoa amongst the clusters of spores, but have not succeeded in doing so. The inference is that all the cytozoa mature at the same time like the malaria parasite. Then I examined minute grubs for the parent cytozoa but could not find them (as yet).

Parasite (?) I is very common. The cells contain greenish granules which swarm violently on the addition of water, the swarming often ceasing suddenly - just like the swarming of pigment in the malaria flagellulae-cysts. These cells are often contained also in the lymph cells of the mosquito & may have a connection with parasite No 2, but are present in every adult while the clusters-of-eight occur only in a small proportion of adults.

Now I must cease for this mail. The case to whom I gave parasite 3 on the 14th had an attack of fever on the 19th & another next day & then became spontaneously well. I could not find a single parasite in him & cannot understand these frequent partial reactions at all. The malaria investigation has been temporarily postponed - I may probably write you at length on the subject soon. The mosquitoes found here are of the same species as those in the rest house at Sigur & in the well at Westbury - we can call it C. putealis Siguri (!). The clusters-of-eight are of the size of a tertian flagellula-cyst; the intracellular crescent-like bodies reach a length of say 30μ. Parasite 2 may be the spores of Parasite I & these intracellular crescents may be the crescent form of the parasite, all occupying lymph cells - but this is a conjecture. I think however that we have certainly one or more cytozoa to deal with - that is, entirely intracellular protozoa. I find the spores in large numbers at the bottom of the mosquito bottle; so they must escape somehow, though I can't conceive how unless at the change of skin.

Yours very sincerely
R. Ross.

1 Letter 70.

2 Labbé (1894), 124-8.

Letter 72
02/113

Ooty,
31st May 1897

Dear Dr Manson,
Another week's work on parasites I & II has not led me much further. This is chiefly owing to the fact that these parasites, like gregarines, seem to disappear from grubs kept in bottles so that I have to spend half the day in hunting for infected insects. Meantime the puddle from which I got the grubs has dried up. I found another lot of mosquitoes of the same species as these containing I & II, which however did not contain I, so that I conclude that this *is* a parasite; but I have got no further. With respect to No II I can only confirm the first series of drawings in my last letter & have not again seen the crescent-like bodies. But I have made a curious discovery respecting the spores. I told you that these are found at the bottom of the bottle. On looking at the sediment after the lapse of a fortnight I found that the spores had grown to double the length (eight times the size) while retaining the same characteristics. At first I thought I had found an allied but different species; but on observing all intermediate sizes & on not finding the large spores in any insects I conclude that the spores have the power of growing in water. This is unusual or unknown I believe, but I state only what I see.

I have also found alterations of the spores & empty shells; here is the series

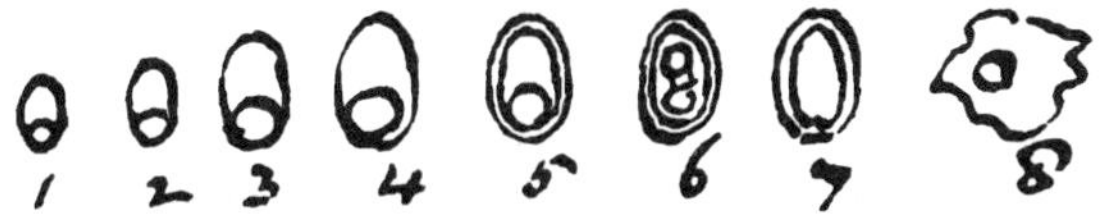

1-4 are spores increasing in size; 5 is the same as 4, only with a double outline; in 6 the vacuole gives place to an irregular marking of the yolk; 7 is an empty shell rather flattened at the ends; 8 is an amoeboid body with a contractile vesicle which *may be* an amoebula escaped from 7. From 1 to 7 is pretty certain, but I am not sure that 8 belongs to the series though it looks like it. The length of 4 is about 8 or 10µ, that is, not so much smaller than a cluster-of-eight. Hence I can't make head or tail of the life-history. At times I fancy I am dealing with a sarcosporidium like Miescher's Tubes;[1] but one of my specimens, which I have mounted shows the whole lymphatic duct, almost, crowded with clusters-of-eight not looking as if they belonged to separate sarcosporidia. I don't know what to think, and must investigate further. Unfortunately my leave ceases on the 15th June.

In spite of the very flattering orders passed by the Resident of Mysore on my work in Bangalore my prospects in the service are owing to the disgraceful rules of the service, so bad that I fear I shall be forced to apply for my pension at the end of the year unless I can get a good billet in the diplomatic medical service. Of this & matters respecting the malaria investigation I shall write at length shortly. I am disgusted at this service & don't think I can remain in it. Tomorrow I am off again to Westbury to look after the silvestris & will at all events do my best for the Great Problem. With kind regards

Yours sincerely

R. Ross.

1 Parasitic sporozoa reproduce through binary fission, forming cysts (Miescher's tubules) in muscle tissue, named after the Swiss pathologist, Johann F. Miescher.

Letter 73
02/114

Ootacamund

7th June 1897

Dear Dr Manson,

I spent three more days down at Westbury. Owing to the heavy rain which has fallen lately there (though the monsoon has not yet set in) the aspect of the country has changed. Everything is green & there is much more water both in streams & by way of puddles. In the latter however the green flagellates have almost vanished. The silvestris is much more scarce & I entirely failed in finding parasites 2 & 3 this time in Westbury. This is disappointing, especially with regard to No 3. I found No I however in a black jungle mosquito larger than the silvestris while it now appears to be absent from the mosquitoes of the Westbury well.

In one single adult out of the well (putealis) I found yesterday another new parasite & today have found the same in a second adult from the same source. Only one chrysalis remains to hatch out & perhaps I will find the new animals in it also.* It appears to me to be a coccidium occupying the cells of the stomach & is just a little bigger than the spore of the gregarine culicis. It is intracellular, lies close to the nucleus, is egg shaped, about 9μ in length, but does not contain psorosperms.

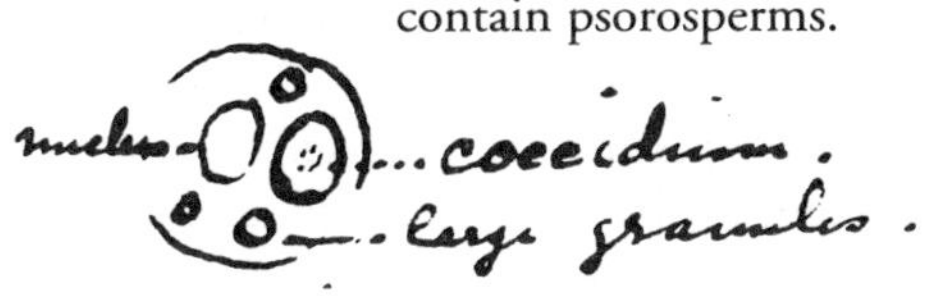

The cell containing a coccidium also contains several bright granules. The coccidium has a thick border & very refractive contents which are uniform with the exception of showing a very faint vacuole surrounded by indistinct granules. 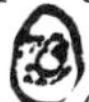. Of course this animal is quite different from the spores-of -eight (Parasite 2) which we may call octospores. On the addition of formaline these coccidia take a double outline, the vacuole vanishes, the contents tend to divide into two masses 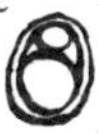. I fancy they are coccidia before the stage of segmentation into psorosperms. I noticed a cup shaped depression in the small end of one of them 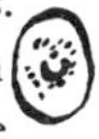.

I think I forget to tell you that some weeks ago I found three immature nematode worms in a large grub from the Westbury well. They were in its stomach wriggling about actively. I will send you the specimen. But I have never found the same before or since. Hence we have the following list of parasites in the mosquito.

I. The filaria sanguinis hominis.

II. A nematode worm.

III. Gregarine Culicis (several species).

IV. Coccidium (?) Culicis.

V. Octosporidium Culicis (Parasite II or spores-of-eight).

VI. Flagellulae of the stomach (Parasite No 3).

VII(?). Chlorosoma Culicis (Parasite I - the greenish cells described before).

VIII(?). Gregarine-like masses of which the spore formation has not been observed - described formerly in connection with the octospores.

IX(?). The intracellular crescent-like bodies described before in connection with the octospores.[1]

The first six of these are certainly parasitic; 7 & 8 pretty certainly so; & 9 doubtful.

I think I told you that I tried to infest mosquito grubs with guinea-worm embryos in Bangalore, but failed.[2]

I have only a very few specimens to send you. I will send one of the nematode, three of the octospores, & one or two of the coccidium, all mounted in formalin. In this medium the octospores become rather indistinct & show a dark spot in the centre of the vacuole (as I called it), which is therefore probably a nucleus. The green cells (chlorosoma) seem to shrivel up & disappear in formalin; & in my only preserved specimen of the flagellulae, these parasites have become indistinguishable. For the octospores, look between the air-tubes along the back. I have drawn out the alimentary canal (where they are not found) in order to give a clearer view. The coccidia & worms will be found in the stomach, also drawn out. The octospores can easily be distinguished from oil-globules by their containing the vacuole (nucleus).

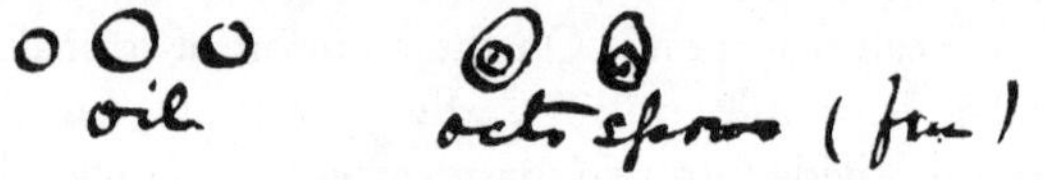

I think you will easily make these out though they are not nearly so distinct as in fresh specimens. I now think that what I described as the lymph duct is the spinal cord. I have been able to dissect it out sometimes.

Here then my work must end for the present as I have only a week's more leave & must get some walking & cycling for my health. I fear however that you will be much disappointed to hear that the present is likely to finish my microscope work for ever & a day, though I sincerely hope it will not be so. You said in your last that this work will be likely to do more for me than sanitary work in Bangalore. I think neither will do anything at all for me, rather the reverse if anything. The fact is that in spite of all my work & frequent official commendation, I now hold what may be described as the worst appointment in the service, namely medical charge of a native regiment; & so far as I see I should continue to hold it & not get anything better were I to do as much & as good scientific work as yourself, Laveran, Carter, Lewis, etc, etc, all put together. It is of course out of the question my continuing in such an appointment. It will never pay me at all to do so. On the other hand a novel I wrote some time ago[3] has succeeded quite enough to make it clear to me that I shall do better by taking my pension next year & attacking literature. In short unless I get a very good appt. of some sort in the next few months I must send in my papers. Some influential friends are however taking up my case, so that I still have some hopes. On receipt of certain letters which I expect daily, I shall send you a full account of affairs, including the malarial investigation fiasco, which will enable you, if you like, to take some action. Failing all this I must prepare to go; & literature must take the place of the microscope in my future life. Never imagine however that I do not abandon the *great theory* with much pain.

Yours sincerely

R. Ross.

* I *have* found them in it - 8th June.

1 In *Memoirs*, 211, Ross claimed that he had discovered five new kinds of parasite, in addition to the *Filaria bancrofti* ('sanguinis hominis') in his letter. These were his nos. II-VI. See, also, his retrospective article, 'Parasites of mosquitoes found in India between 1895 and 1899', *Journal of Hygiene*, April 1906, 101-108, in which he reviewed these findings in the light of continuing work on the parasites of mosquitoes.

2 Ross had made no mention of this in his earlier correspondence with Manson, but see Letter 62.

3 Probably *The Spirit of Storm. A Romance* (London: Methuen & Co., 1896). It was the only one of Ross's novels to make a profit (he eventually received £17.7*s* 11*d* in royalties). He had earlier published another novel, *The Child of Ocean* (London: Remington, 1889), but this one actually involved him in protracted disputes with the publisher and certainly never made him anything. Nye and Gibson (1997), 195ff.

Letter 74
01/099

Ootacamund
11th June 1897

Dear Dr Manson,

As certain letters which I referred to in my last as being expected by me have not yet arrived, I cannot send you the correspondence about the malaria investigation by this mail. When the matter is ripe, however, I shall send you the correspondence in the belief that you can act upon it with great effect. In the meantime I think I should let you know by this mail exactly how I stand in the service, in the hope that you may possibly be able to do something to help me in my present circumstances which otherwise may compel me to retire (as I told you before).

My position is this. After leaving Bangalore I was offered two appointments, one in Rajputana and the other in Berar, and was obliged to refuse both because I had every expectation of the malaria investigation being sanctioned. Shortly after refusing them I heard that the investigation was indefinitely postponed. At the same time I discovered that my prospects in the service are practically nil. The reason for this is that as I have never served in the Madras Civil Service[1] I cannot now enter it without beginning at the bottom of the list. (I shall send you the official order to that effect together with the investigation correspondence). Now this order excludes me from all the best appointments in the Madras service & prevents my ever becoming the head of the department in the Presidency. At the same time it can, mark you, be waived in my favour if Surgeon General Sibthorpe[2] here were to think fit to try to do so. This he is evidently not willing to do; for, though he is here, he has never spoken a word to me on the subject, nor even on malaria work; nor though I applied two years ago for an appointment in the Madras Civil Branch has he attempted to offer me anything. The truth is I understand - much to my surprise, for I believe I have offended nobody anywhere & have lately done some good work - that I am not wanted in the Madras Civil Medical Department at all. Hence, in the ordinary course of events, I must remain in the military branch of the Madras medical service. This means regimental employment for many years with a net salary of about R700 a month, foreign service in Burma next year with separation for years from my family, & with a final prospect of becoming principal medical officer of some Madras or Burma district or perhaps, if I am very lucky, of the Presidency Command.

You may say here that the malaria investigation is only postponed and that I may look forward to it. But you must understand that the investigation is not likely to last for more than six months or so, after which I shall find myself in just the same, or a worse, predicament than I am in now. As I mentioned to you in my last, I have an opening now in literature if I seize the opportunity at once or in a few months; I can take to it, and retire next year. But if I postpone this for the sake of malaria investigation my opportunity will be lost, perhaps for good. Hence I cannot afford to wait for the investigation, & I *cannot take it up at all* unless I am assured that I shall get something good afterwards.

The truth is that the circumstances described above strike me hard in two ways; first they compel me to remain in regimental employment; & secondly they suggest very strongly that no amount of work is likely to bring advancement in the service. Now regimental employment is for pecuniary reasons alone *out of the question* for me when I have a pension and an opening in literature as an alternative;

while for obvious reasons I can never be willing to remain in a service and give it the best work of the best part of my life, where I know that such work will meet with no advancement. I fear I cannot accept the prospect; and I don't think that you would do so in my place.

I don't mean to claim having done anything particularly wonderful! But I have a knowledge of the protozoal parasites perhaps greater than possessed by most men in the services - a knowledge acquired with some pains & likely to be of considerable use in the theory & practice of the three most important tropical diseases, malaria, dysentery and diarrhoea. I am a Parkes memorial medalist, have invented a microscope lately purchased by government for use in India, &, lastly, owing to my recent rather exceptional experiences in Bangalore, have a pretty thorough practical knowledge of Indian sanitation & municipal business. Not excessive as are these claims to consideration, they may still excuse me for asking for such a prospect in the service as will enable me to remain in it and do useful work in the future. My present appointment, namely medical charge of the 19th Regiment of Madras Infantry, may justly be regarded as the poorest kind of appointment in the Indian Medical Service.

The Madras Civil Medical Service being debarred to me, my only hope is to find a good prospect in the Indian Foreign (Diplomatic) Service. Colonel Robertson, Resident in Mysore, is very kindly interesting himself on my behalf in this direction.[3] An appointment in this service will place me directly under the Govt. of India instead of the Madras Govt. & will, I hope, enable me to do good work. Perhaps, if you see your way to doing so, you may be able to assist me with your influence at home. I may add that I naturally feel my present circumstance to be rather trying, as, failing the one chance open to me, I see before me only the prospect of beginning life again at the age of forty and of giving up the fruits of all my past work. With kind regards

Believe me

Yours sincerely

Ronald[4] Ross.

1 It was usual for Indian Medical Service officers to apply for the Civil Service after two years' duty. Although civil officers could still be called to active service during times of crisis, the life in the civil service tended to be more pleasant and lucrative than that of the

military. For a discussion, see (Sir) Leonard Rogers, *Happy Toil. Fifty-five Years of Tropical Medicine* (London: Frederick Muller, 1950), chapter 2. It is not entirely clear why Ross neglected to follow this usual path.

2 Charles Sibthorpe, (1847-1906), Surgeon-General (civil) at Madras. See **Biographical Appendix**.

3 **RA** 01/100 (attached to letter **RA** 01/099). Letter dated 2 May 1897 from Robertson to Ross saying he had sent on his letter to the Foreign Secretary mentioning that if the Foreign Department had any difficult work to be done they may safely entrust it to Ross adding that he had tact and discretion and was an enthusiast in his profession. Robertson hoped the recommendation might be productive of some good to Ross.

4 Except for Letter 2, this is the first letter in which Ross signed his full Christian name. He did so in moments of excitement or emotion.

Letter 75
02/115

Ooty,
12th June 1897

Private

Dear Dr Manson,

By this mail I fear I must inflict you with the business letter promised by last mail. You will find it enclosed. It is written in an official vein & may safely be shown to anybody you please. If you can see your way to giving me a helping hand in the matter I shall be extremely grateful to you as it makes me quite sick to think of throwing up all my work at this point. This however I literally *must* do unless I can be assured of good prospects in the service. A native regiment in some hot hole of a station with poor pay and a certainty of going to Burma is not possible to a man, especially a man with a family, who has any capacity of work in him; nor indeed is some second-rate civil appointment. Both my wife & myself are agreed upon this point - it is out of the question. £300 a year at home with a fixed home and complete leisure are worth much more than R700 a month in a hot & perhaps unhealthy station where it will be impossible to keep my children, necessitating the upkeep of two houses, one in India & the other in England. You will also be able to perceive, on reading between the lines of my letter, that a merely provincial career leading to no influence & to no professional opportunities is little to my taste

- in fact I won't have it. I want to be able to do good work, to push on sanitary & research matters, & not to lead a futile kind of life in looking after half a dozen patients in a military hospital. If I get what I want I know I shall be able to do a great deal; if not I should only get ill & do nothing, besides leading a miserably disagreeable existence. In addition I feel not a little aggrieved, & justly so. I have never received the good things of the service though I have worked harder &, really I think, done more lately than most men in it, & I don't see why I should have the very worst appointment in India as a reward. Besides this I now see clearly that, unless I make a stand of some sort at the present opportunity, I shall, while getting thanks for my work, never get anything else. I have been made to feel this very distinctly in the last two months. The appointments offered to me in Berar & Rajputana were only very poor ones & only officiating, & I was obliged to refuse them because the Surgeon General knew nothing of the malaria investigation (the correspondence regarding which was all the while lying in the Madras Govt. Office!). Nothing else has been offered to me & neither the civil surgeon general (Sibthorpe) nor the military (McVittie)[1] have deigned to utter a word to me either on my prospects or even about malaria work. A modest request to be moved from my regiment in Secunderabad to another in a better station (Bangalore) has even been refused while I cannot even get leave for continuing the malaria work, though a man in charge of the regiment next to mine in Secunderabad has been on leave for the last six months for racing purposes! Not a soul here, except some planters, has taken the slightest interest or even enquired about the malaria work. The fact is I have the extreme honour of belonging to a service which does not care a button about the most important scientific matters, and in which advancement goes simply by seniority, while the majority of its members actually I believe *resent* good work. I make this statement coolly & am not at all in a *hepatic* condition. So marked has been this attitude in the medical men here that I have thought at times I have done something to offend them; but I am sure I have not & have been most careful of my words & acts. As an example, a patient with severe diarrhoea & dysentery asked for me in consultation. I found swarms of amoeba & cercomonads & advised the other men to base their treatment on that fact. I got the cold shoulder all round for my pains, though I was most humble in my statements. Of course you understand that it would be quite impossible to represent these matters officially - I should only be snubbed & dispatched to Quilon[2] or some such place as a *reward.*

I think you will agree with me that under these circumstances it is high time to make a stand. It is a mistake, for the sake of general principles alone, to work on in the service without exacting recognition, as Vandyke Carter[3] did. They *thank* you, call you a fool behind your back for you pains, and when you are old & worn out make you Honorary Physician to the Queen. For the sake of our great medical science alone it is a mistake to submit to this kind of thing.[4] If I do good scientific & sanitary work I must insist on being rewarded step by step just as I should be rewarded were I to go on a military picnic up the Nile or to Chitral. If not I will be as good as my word & leave the service at all costs. That will not hurt *them* to be sure, but it will save my self respect. I do not care to go through life with a grievance; nor, for the sake of my family, am I willing to lose all my prospects in the service of a government that will show no gratitude for work done, or of a department that takes no interest in it.

Of one thing I am sure - that you will sympathise & agree with me in all this; and I may still be able to work at the great theory even after retirement & in conjunction with literature; but I don't know whether you can see your way to giving me any assistance. Yet I think perhaps that you can. You are well known to the Govt. of India at all events & a word from you, or leaders of the profession at home, goes a longer way with them, I believe, than many words from the leaders of the profession out here, whom, somehow, they do not appear to pay much attention to. If then you can give me a hand the way would be to tackle someone at the India Office, if possible not a medical man. If you don't know anybody there, it would be quite correct to send my letter and enclosures, backed by a letter from you to the Secretary of State for India.[5] But perhaps you may not care to do this; or it may be better to do it in connection with the question of the malaria investigation which I will send in a mail or two. A private correspondence with a man of influence at the India Office (not a doctor) will I think be sure to put me straight, especially as Colonel Robertson[6] & I hope Mr Mackworth Young,[7] Lt.-Governor of the Punjab, are interesting themselves about me. But if you find any difficulty in doing this don't trouble - I must depend on Col. Robertson.

Well, this is a very egoistical letter; but I shall not inflict you with any more of the same nature.[8]

Please remember that the opposition of the Madras Stars is certainly not owing to a single breath against my character, etc. Stupidity on their part, I think.

I return to Secunderabad on the 16th. Please address there. It is raining heavily here. No more malaria work possible.

Yours sincerely
R. Ross.

Specimens will be sent by this mail.

P.S. (13th June)
On second thoughts I think it best to send you the malaria business by this mail, and enclose it accordingly with some official remarks of my own & accompanied by some other documents. It is however no use to attempt to press on the investigation just yet, for two reasons: first the Govt. of India is not likely to do anything until the coming monsoon is so well established that the famine is sure to cease; and secondly, for reasons already given, I must first be assured that government is going to do something for me before I care to plunge into the investigation & risk my health & prospects in it. As soon as I see that I am all right in the Foreign Department then it will be time to force on the investigation I think. Besides as soon as I get an appointment, I shall set to work again on the flagellulae & try again to track them. I shall also keep a man to get me mosquitoes from malarious places & so on, so that no time will really be lost. If you can *first* help me to get the appt. in the foreign department & then some months hence press on the investigation it would be best. The letters attached to this are for the former purpose only, the malaria business is fastened together separately. When the time comes to act on it, it would be best for you and if possible several leading men in London to send it with your remarks to the Secretary of State for India. You will get it done at once.
R. Ross.

Please *return* enclosures when done with.

1 Charles Edwin McVittie, (1842-1916), Surgeon-General (military), Madras.
2 A small coastal town in south India.
3 See **Biographical Appendix**.
4 This is a theme which became an obsession in Ross's later life. See Eli Chernin, 'Sir Ronald Ross, malaria, and the rewards of research', *Medical History*, 32 (1988), 119-141.
5 Lord George Francis Hamilton, (1845-1927), Secretary of State for India, 1895-1903.
6 Donald Robertson, (1847-1930), Resident at Bangalore.
7 William Mackworth Young, (1840-1924), Resident at Bangalore before Robertson, appointed Lieutenant-Governor of the Punjab in March 1897.

8 Ross did, however, e.g. Letters 78 and 84.

Letter 76
01/126

[In margin Ross has written - Sent to Manson under my letter to him of the 12th June 1897.

R. Ross.]

Correspondence in respect to an Investigation into the mode of infection of Malaria

Ootacamund

13th June 1897

My dear Dr Manson,

Please read the following enclosures:-

1. Letter from the Prime Minister of the Patiala State referring to a malaria-investigation proposed by the Maharajah's Government, with a note adding that it was not sanctioned by the Punjab Government.[1]
2. Letter from the Surgeon General with the Govt. of Madras supporting an application made by me to be allowed to carry on a special investigation on malaria.[2]
3. An extract from the Madras Mail dated 19th August 1896 reporting a Resolution of the United Planters' Association of Southern India asking the Govt. of Madras to institute an enquiry into malaria.[3]
4. Extract from the Inspection Notes of the Sanitary Commission, Madras, recommending an enquiry & suggesting an appropriate place for it.[4]
5. Orders of the Govt. of Madras on 2 & 3 above, addressing the Govt. of India on the subject.[5]
6. Reply of the Govt. of India to the above, intimating that the Government of India is projecting a Public Health Institute &, for this reason and because of the scarcity of officers due to plague and famine, recommending postponement of the enquiry proposed by the Madras Government.[6]
7. Letter from the Madras Govt to the United Planters'

Association intimating that the investigation has been postponed but will not be lost sight of.[7]

8. My application dated 12th July 1895 to be admitted into the Madras Civil Medical Branch.[8]

9. A letter from me to the Surgeon General, Govt. of Madras asking whether if I enter the Civil Branch I must do so at the bottom of the list (under date 18th March 1897).[9]

10. The reply of the Surgeon General to the above, sending Standing Order No 60 of the Civil Medical Department, & also Standing Order No 149, showing that promotion in the Department must depend chiefly upon seniority in it.[10]

11. Orders of the Resident in Mysore on my services in Bangalore (under date 7th April 1897).[11]

2. From this correspondence you will perceive that a malaria-investigation has been proposed or recommended from time to time in India by the Patiala Government; the United Planters' Association; myself; the Surgeon General, Madras Govt.; the Sanitary Commissioner, Madras Govt.; & lastly by the Madras Govt. itself. You are also aware that the investigation has been repeatedly asked for at home.

3. Enclosure No 6 shows that the Govt. of India, while seeing the necessity for the investigation and recognising that it should be entrusted to me, recommends the postponement of the matter for the present.

4. This being so, I send you the whole correspondence (since in fact you have been really the originator of the proposal) in case you may like to take any further action in the matter. At the same time I should like to add some remarks which should be considered in case you decide upon doing so.

5. On the postponement of the official investigation I obtained two months' leave to do some preliminary research on my own account. The result of this preliminary enquiry, extending from the 19th April to the 19th June, has already been reported to you. It has been decidedly encouraging since it has shown that in the exceedingly malarious locality of the Sigúr Ghat near Ootacamund mosquitoes are sufficiently numerous to account for malarial infection by their means, while they contain protozoal parasites, one of which may be the alternative form of the parasite of malaria. These facts combined with your original inductions, based on scientific reasons, that the mosquito is the alternative host of the parasite, & with some later observations of mine, are so encouraging that they

appear to call for a full study of the subject in the interest not only of Indian Planters but of the Army in India and indeed of the Indian people generally. How pressing and important the matter is may easily be estimated from a study of the Annual Reports of the Sanitary Commissions with the Government of India, from which it will be seen that malaria is by far the most important of Indian diseases &, though not so fatal in individual cases as cholera or enteric fever, yet in the aggregate causes a larger mortality and an immeasurably larger amount of sickness. Thus amongst the general population of India in 1894 there were no less than 5,000,000 deaths returned as being due to fever against about 500,000 due to cholera; or ten times the number. In the European Army in India, numbering 71,031 men in 1895, there were 24,798 admissions for malaria and 259 deaths & men invalided for that cause against 1870 admissions & 500 deaths and invalidings for enteric fever and 44 cases and 32 deaths from cholera. This amount of sickness due to malaria very nearly rivals that due to venereal disease in the European Army, namely 32,489 cases and 363 deaths and invalidings, in 1895. Amongst native troops & prisoners, who are not much subject to enteric fever & venereal disease, malaria causes one-third of the total sickness. Though it is difficult to estimate exactly the mortality due exclusively to the parasite of malaria, I think on the whole that out of the Indian population of 400,000,000, it must cause, either directly or by implication, something like 10,000 deaths a day.[12] But, apart from this vast amount of sickness, malaria is of all diseases the most important in political, agricultural & military affairs, since it renders large tracts of fertile country more or less uninhabitable, impedes cultivation, planting & public works, & is often the most serious enemy which armies in the field have to contend against. On the whole then I think we are justified in claiming that the malaria-question is quite as important a matter as famine and plague.

6. The discovery of the form of the parasite of malaria outside the human body, which is the knowledge now wanting in our scientific comprehension of the subject, is required to enable us to devise adequate measures of prevention. It is the object of the proposed investigation to make this discovery; and in my opinion the solution of the question, involving as it will an exact knowledge of the means of infection, is not unlikely to cause an immense saving of life, sickness and expense both to the public at large and to the Government of India - a possibility which must justify almost any expenditure for the object of attaining the information required.

7. As a result of my preliminary investigation however, I must

now suggest that if the research be undertaken by government at all it be undertaken on more extended lines than proposed in Enclosure 2. At first I suggested only an enquiry into the theory of infection by the mosquito; but I am now of opinion that the whole question at issue should be thoroughly dealt with. In this, I venture to think, Government will concur. I may suggest then the following changes in the original programme as laid down in Enclosure 2:-

(a). The investigation should be under the Govt. of India instead of the Govt. of Madras, to allow of more various regions & climates being examined, and to permit the research to be under the direct orders of the Director General, Indian Medical Service.

(b). The investigation should be arranged for one year at least.

(c). The head-quarters of the investigation should be fixed at some town where there are an adequate library and laboratory, such as Calcutta or Agra.

(d). If my services are to be employed I should be assisted by a junior commissioned medical officer, if one can be spared, instead of by an assistant surgeon.

(e). The officers employed for the investigation should, while on that duty, be placed on somewhat the same footing as officers on active service. The object of this would be to enable them or their families to receive adequate pensions in case of the invaliding or death of the officers caused by malaria contracted while on the special malaria-duty. For example I contracted malaria before I had been three days in the Sigúr Ghat; and it may well happen that officers working for long in exceedingly malarious places may become permanently ruined in health or may even lose their lives in consequence; so that the contingency should be guarded against.

8. With regard to difficulties in the way of the proposed investigation, & first as to that given by the Govt. of India in Enclosure 6, that the Governor General deprecates isolated research and is considering the establishment of a Public Health Institute, I may perhaps be allowed to remark, owing to my experience in this particular subject, that the most obvious way to start such an Institute is to commence by isolated research along particular branches of enquiry. Owing to the highly specialised character of most Public Health research it will be impossible that one man will be able to undertake or even to supervise the whole. For example the study of the bacterial diseases is broadly different, both in methods & the knowledge required, from the study of animal parasites. Though to the public mind a Bacteriological and a Public Health Institute are synonymous, it may be remarked (a) that a bacteriologist

is not necessarily well acquainted with the animal parasites; & (b) that the tropical diseases due to animal parasites (malaria, dysentery, hepatic abscess, worm-diseases, forms of diarrhoea, etc) are just as important, if not more important, than those due to bacteria (cholera, typhoid, leprosy, etc). Hence Public Health Research work *must* split into various branches, each requiring different investigators. At least, I think I am justified in saying that few bacteriologists at present in India have paid any special attention to the malaria question.

Secondly, with regard to cost, it is evident that the expense of the enquiry as projected above will be exceedingly trifling and, since the medical officers required can easily be removed from other work without increasing the total establishment of the service, will amount to nothing more than their special & travelling allowances.

9. Lastly I should like to ask for one stipulation on my own behalf, if it be still proposed to employ me on the investigation; that is, I should like to be assured that my prospects in the service shall not suffer by my being placed on the special duty. This may appear a strange stipulation to make; but I am driven to asking for it by the fact that hitherto my studies appear only to have acted to my detriment in the service, inasmuch as, in spite of scientific & sanitary work on my part, I find myself after sixteen years' service to possess the poorest kind of appointment in the service, namely regimental employment. This is due to the regulations of the Madras Civil Medical Department (see Enclosure 10) by which advancement in it goes mainly by seniority in the Department - a regulation which, as I have never served in the Department, practically excludes me altogether from it. On two occasions (or more) I have given up opportunities of entering the Branch for the sake of scientific work, & the result has been, as already mentioned, much to my detriment. Hence I feel fully justified in asking that if I am to be placed on special malaria duty, my prospects shall not again suffer in consequence of it; and that I shall receive assurance to the effect that after the special duty is over, my position in the service will be such as to compensate for my labours in it and to allow me a prospect, equal to that possessed by others, of rising to the head of it. Otherwise, as I have prospects altogether apart from the service and cannot afford to remain in or return to regimental employment, I must, if I undertake the malaria investigation, do so at a considerable loss to myself which it is scarcely fair to expect me to undergo.

10. I may add, in conclusion, as my qualifications for the investigation, that I am a Parke's Memorial Gold Medalist for an

essay on malaria; that I have invented a form of microscope which has been purchased by the Government of India for the use of medical officers; and that I have made a special study of the malarial & other protozoal parasites. I also attach (Enclosure 11) some orders by the Resident in Mysore on certain sanitary work lately performed by me while on special deputation in Bangalore.

Believe me

Yours sincerely
Ronald Ross.
Surgeon Major
Indian Medical Service.
In Medical Charge 19th Rgt. Madras Infantry.

1 The following summarise the attachments to Ross's letter:
RA 01/127, 15 May 1895: Copy of a letter from Sirdar Gurdit Singh Gl. Prime Minister Patiala State to Surgeon Major Owen, Medical Advisor to HH the Maharaja of Patiala. forwarded to R. Ross.
Informs Owen that proposal regarding obtaining services of Ross for investigation of malaria was sanctioned by the Council on 11 May and the correspondence had been sent to the foreign minister to take early steps in getting loan of services of Ross. Asks Owen to mention this to Ross and expenditure of R1200 per month, stating that his services would be asked for by the State through direct channel through Govt of India.
Note on back by Ross saying that sanction refused by Punjab govt on ground that gov of the Maharajah of Patiala was not in a financial position to carry it on (13 June 1897).

2 **RA** 01/128: Copy of a letter from Surg General of the Govt of Madras to Honourable Chief Secretary to Government Public Department (30 Oct. 1896).
Supports Ross's application to be placed on special duty saying he is competent to carry out such an investigation and it is in the interest of science and invaluable to Government in dealing with the large question of the prevention of malarial diseases. Also says that on his relief from special duty he will revert to his permanent military appointment. He should draw the same pay with travelling and halting allowances and suggests that he might be granted an honorarium at the end in proportion to the value of the work he does. Also mentions an assistant surgeon or hospital assistant trained in microscopic work.

3 **RA** 01/129: "Madras mail" 19th Aug. 1896. Meeting of the United Planters' Association of Southern India held on 14th August 1896 at Bangalore. Speech by Mr J. G. Hamilton suggests that the "harmless, necessary mosquito may not be as harmless as he looks in fact he is distinctly charged with disseminating malaria. But a serious charge like this should not be made without carefully investigating, and it is suggested that we, as interested parties, should invite enquiry." Passed a resolution "That the Secretary be instructed to move the Government of Madras to commence an enquiry into the question of the development of the malarial parasite on somewhat similar lines to the investigation undertaken by Surgeon-Major R. Ross and others, and the Association trusts that the theory as further developed by Surgeon-Major Ross and explained in his pamphlet on the subject will be thoroughly investigated on the same lines as the investigation of cholera by Drs. Haffkine and Hankin."

4 **RA** 01/130: Extract from the Inspection notes of Sanitary Commissioner on the rural valleys in the South Arcot District - Pudupett, a hamlet of Vriddhachalam [W. G. King - sent to RR 13/12 96]. Discusses the location of malarious regions and the work of Manson and Ross and states "I would therefore advise that Surgeon Major Ross, who thus far has ably contributed to this enquiry and has made the subject a speciality, should be deputed to pursue the mosquito theory at Pudupett" which he considered the most favourable location in the Presidency.

5 **RA** 01/132: Copy of Proceedings from the Madras Govt. Public Department, 14 Dec. 1896, concerning the letters from the United Planters' Association and the Surgeon General (notes 2 and 3 above). Order: The Govt of India will be addressed.

6 **RA** 01/133: From J. P Hewett Sec to Govt of India, to Chief - Secretary to the Govt of Madras, 19 March 1897.
Reply to proposal about Ross and special duty. States that Madras Govt in event of Govt of India being unable to give effect to this recommendation, they would endeavour to find necessary funds. Govt of India in complete accord with Govt of Madras as to the advantages derived from such an enquiry, but Governor General in Council has a scheme of a Central Institute of Public Health and therefore averse to entrusting an independent authority with the duty of making it. Therefore not putting Ross on special duty. If Govt of Madras consider inquiry should still go ahead with Ross under the orders of the Governor in Council, they would raise no objection but present financial position and urgent calls on medical dept for other duties make present time inopportune for this inquiry.

7 **RA** 01/134: Copy of proceeding from the Madras Government Public Department
"Secretary of United Planters Association, Southern India will be informed ... that in view of the present financial position and urgent calls on the Med. Dept. for other duties, it has been decided to postpone for the present the proposed enquiry into the development of the malarial parasite, but that the matter will not be lost sight of."

8 **RA** 01/135: Letter from Surgeon Major Ross to the Principal Medical Officer, Her Majesty's Forces, Secunderabad & Belgaum districts.
Request to forward for registration his application to be admitted into the Madras Civil Medical Department. Claims for the favourable recommendation of his application:
Diploma of Public Health 1888.
Course of bacteriology under Dr Klein in 1889.
Three years service in Bangalore as staff surgeon where he was practically also civil surgeon of the station.
1894 special study under Patrick Manson.
Parkes memorial prize, 1895.
Mentions he is especially qualified in parasitology of malaria and dysentery and should like to lay his services at the disposal of the Surgeon General for any investigation or special work.

9 **RA** 01/136: Letter from Ross, 18 March 1897, to Secretary of the Surgeon General with Govt of Madras asking if elected to serve in civil branch would he have to enter at bottom of list. Needs information as there is a possibility of his gaining admission to the medical service of the Indian Foreign Department.

10 **RA** 01/137: Reply from D. Simpson to above letter enclosing copies of Standing Orders No 60 *Seniority of Medical Officers Serving in Civil employ* in which it states "the seniority of a medical officer officiating in civil employ shall be determined by the date on which he assumes charge of his first appointment" and No 149 *Positions of Medical Officers in Civil Employ Transferred from one Province to another.*

11 **RA** 01/140: Proceedings of the Resident in Mysore, No 1538, dated Bangalore, the 7th April 1897.
K D Erskine (First Assistant to the Resident). Records Resident's appreciation of Ross's services:
1) Special duty Sept 1895 - Jan 1896 in connection with cholera outbreak - examined sanitary condition of station and the constitution of the sanitary dept of the municipality and submitted proposals on how these might be improved.
2) Special duty Jan 1896 - May 1896 in order that he might initiate

reforms proposed by him in health report.
3) Officiating Residency Surgeon Bangalore.

Of Report on cholera and sanitation, late resident Mackworth Young requested that his best thanks be conveyed. Work led to a large measure of success, with zeal, thoroughness and tact. Resident confident that no more capable officer could have been selected.

12 Most estimates in the early twentieth century put the malarial mortality of India at about 1,000,000 per annum, or about 20-25% of the reported 'fever' mortality. Ross's figure is much higher, at about 3,650,000 malaria deaths per year.

Letter 77
02/024

21 Queen Anne Street,
Cavendish Square
24th May, 1897.

My dear Ross,
I intended writing to you last mail but I have been so busy I have had very little time for anything except the necessities of life. I have had my telegraphic address registered; it is *FINICALLY, LONDON. Finically, London*. And I hope the first message coming under that address will be from you to the effect that you have run the plasmodium to earth and that it is a parasite of the mosquito. Be very sure of your facts before making the announcement; but if you are quite sure of your facts dont hesitate to make the announcement. You must be ahead of Italians and Americans. They are working, or preparing to work, in both America and Italy.

I have treated myself to a new objective[1] and yesterday, being Sunday, I went over again some of the sections of the mosquitoes which you sent me. With my old lens I found plenty of spheres in the sections but only one body which I could swear to being a flagellated body; but with the new lens I found two more about the nature of which I had very little doubt. So there should be no difficulty in making permanent preparations to illustrate any discovery you may light on. The best preparations - in fact the only ones which can be worked up properly, are the glycerine preserved mosquitos. Bottle plenty of them therefore for future working up. The formaline mosquitos were too hard and too much shrivelled up for sectioning.

I have also treated myself to a new diagnostic microscope. The first pattern[2] had no coarse adjustment; consequently there was often trouble in focusing. Baker's have now put on a coarse adjustment and it is a great improvement although it adds a little to the cost. I advocate the "Diagnostic"[3] whenever I can and I believe a good many of them are now in use. It is a real boon to the man with a short purse and a light kit. I always carry it in my bag now and find it of very great service.

I had three malaria cases in hospital last week but they were all benign tertians and not suitable for flagella work. I hope soon to get another crescent case when I will again repeat your experiments. I sent a short note to the B M J lately describing my method of staining flagella & confirming your statements on exflagellation but they have not seen fit to publish it yet.[4] I have an idea that they have mislaid my illustrations. Be sure to try the plan I described to you lately. You will get a lot of useful information from it.

Wishing you good luck and personal freedom from the plasmodium I remain

Yours very sincerely
Patrick Manson

1 For his microscope.
2 i.e. model.
3 i.e. Ross's. See Letter 7, note 9.
4 Eventually published in the 10 July 1897 issue. Letter 57, note 2.

Letter 78
02/117

Secunderabad

20th June 1897.

Dear Dr Manson,
Here I am at Secunderabad & have just got your letter of the 24th May & note your telegraphic address. I am still awaiting letters about my prospects and have a great deal of writing to do on sanitation and malaria; after which I may be able to tackle the plasmodium again for a little. I shall hark back to the mosquito fed on crescent-bearing blood & examine after three days to see if I can find the developed flagellulae in the tissues, & shall also send you mosquitoes in

glycerine. There is plenty of fever in the regiment here but, as leave is now open, I may be sent off northwards any day. I am glad you like the diagnostic microscope with the course adjustment. Did I tell you that Govt. has bought a number, but instead of supplying them to the hospitals has given one to each command so that they may be called for when wanted - they never *are* wanted apparently. I said I would not bore you again with the question of my prospects in the service, but I think now that I should do so to the extent of one more letter in order to explain two points more fully so that you may not think I am hypochondriacal in respect to my present position.

First, as to the service not being worth stopping in unless I can get a first rate opening *now* - here is my record up to date.

I was appointed in April 1881. When I had been seven years in the service (three years of which were spent on unemployed pay) I applied for furlough due after five years. It was repeatedly refused. At last I threatened to resign; the furlough was granted. I went home, took the D. P. H., married & came out. I was immediately ordered off to Burma on 24 hours' notice (to punish me for threatening to resign). I was now at Govt.'s mercy & had a prospect of spending several years in the Burmese jungles & having to send my wife home again. Luckily, a friend, Surgeon Colonel Roe,[1] came to our rescue & I got the staff surgeoncy at Bangalore instead, being my first permanent appt. after 9 years' service. I had however to vacate it on becoming surgeon major on 12 years' service (according to the rule). On doing so, in 1893, I might have gone into civil employment but preferred to take a regiment at Secunderabad to study malaria with Hehir[2] - only an acting appointment. In three months a permanent employment fell vacant here, to which I was entitled by every rule. Instead of getting it however, I was packed off to Berhampur on the east coast. In these moves I was cheated out of part or all of my travelling allowances. In March 1894 I got furlough once more, came home, studied with you, "invented" the diagnostic, took the Parkes medal & arrived out again in April 1895 to Secunderabad whither my regiment had moved in my absence from Berhampur. On arrival I applied for the Madras civil. My application was filed & I think forgotten. In September I was sent on special duty to Bangalore, which I left in March 1897 after having done work which has made me pretty well known in the country. After this I might have expected Sibthorpe to have offered me at least something; but he has never said a word on the subject & has given me to understand that he will do nothing for me. In that matter the Madras Civil Service is scarcely worth entering, but Sibthorpe may as well have recognised my work in some way.

(The new laboratory which is going to be opened in Madras will be given to *Grant*).[3] Hence in the natural course of events I must remain in medical charge of the 19th Rgt Madras Infantry for many years. My pay after deducting subscriptions, etc, amounts to about R700 net a month. I can't keep my family here; the climate is not good enough, & the houses are tumble-down barns more fit for footpads than for a gentleman to live in; while the position and work are such that only half-castes & native doctors remain in such employment now-a-days. A modest request to be transferred to a better regiment in Bangalore has been refused on inadequate grounds. Hence I must remain here (and go to Burma next year) and must send my family home for an unlimited term of years. On the other hand at the end of this year I can apply for my first pension of R 292[4] a year, which will at least give us a house to live in, & work at literature & research (a combination which I like) at home. It may be remarked that R700 a month with two houses to keep up will leave me just as poor as with £292 with one house in ~~London~~ England - also that private practice is not possible to a man in regimental employment, who is looked upon by the public, & generally very rightly, as a fool. I cannot expect to become P. M. O. under ten years, & three years more service will give me only £70 a year more pension. Hence, as I think you will agree with me, my only possible choice under these circumstances is to apply for my pension. It would be sheer folly on my part to undergo all the disagreeabilities of life in India & to live apart from my family for years when I don't even get pecuniary remuneration for doing so. Further than this, it would be sheer folly to live in India at all, since I can get pension & literary employment in England, unless I can get work of such nature & with such a salary as will repay me for the disadvantages of doing so. I may add to all this, that I do not like the service, I do not approve of the manner in which it is being conducted, I find the greatest difficulty in getting anything done, and I believe (I think with some cause) that the Madras men want to "keep me down", and, lastly, that I have at least as much claim to get up higher as have men who notoriously & confessedly never open a book of medicine. The simple fact which I see quite clearly is that the present is a crisis in my life when I must decide either to start a new life in England or to take a position in India to which I am entitled. I feel I have every right to try & assert myself. If I do so with success I shall do good work in India, if not, I must retire.

Secondly, you may ask why on earth I don't represent all this officially. I shall do so, if necessary, just before my pension is due. If I do so now the official answer will be either a snub or an appointment to the worst civil surgeoncy in the Madras Government, which will certainly compel me to retire. It is in order to avoid this that I am writing to you & trying to work the matter unofficially.

Well, I won't trouble you again about it, but will of course let you know the course of events. I have never yet worried & teazed authorities for appointments because I have thought that it is their duty to see that their officers are properly treated. I was mistaken.

With kind regards - yours truly

R. Ross.

1 *Memoirs,* 86 says Surg-Gen W. C. Roe, presumably William Alexander Crawford Roe, (1847-1915), IMS.

2 Ross (1893b); *idem.*, 'Nodulated and vacuolated corpuscles, and the solution of corpuscles mistaken for parasites', *Indian Medical Record* 4 (1893), 213-214; see also Letter 1, note 1.

3 A . E. Grant, (1862-1903), Professor of Hygiene at Madras Medical College. See **Biographical Appendix**.

4 A slip for £292 a year.

Letter 79
02/118

Secunderabad

28th June 1897

Dear Dr Manson,

Just a line to tell you that I am sorry now that I have bothered you so much about "my prospects". I have just received a telegram from Surgeon General Cleghorn's Secretary saying that I am to be appointed under the foreign office *soon*, but he does not know when. So that puts the matter all right & removes my *grievances*. I fear my letters may have given you some trouble; but I felt that if I could get nothing at this juncture it would really be useless my staying any longer in the service.

I have been doing a little work here (can't resist it). There are no good cases in hospital, so I have been looking for my new parasites in the local mosquitoes. Can't find them as yet - only gregarines.

But I have taken another step as regards investigation. As I am not to get into the foreign department just yet, I have written to

Leslie, Cleghorns secretary, asking to be sent at once to *Assam* for a few weeks. I see that Rogers finds the malaria parasite in Kala-azar & thinks that disease is simply a virulent form of malaria.[1] I have my doubts as to whether it is not malaria & anchylostomiasis combined; but if it is malaria it seems to be an epidemic or communicable form of the disease, & hence the affair is of the utmost importance in respect to the malaria question, and I want to go there at once and look at the mosquitoes in the infected houses. I hope Cleghorn will send me, as I can't get any more leave. I shall also be able to confirm Rogers' work.

I have just been reading Cunningham on his protomyxomyces[2] & wish I had done so before sending a hasty paper lately to the In. Med. Gazette on the subject.[3] All the same I think that the amoeba, & perhaps the flagellulae too, are pathogenic & I don't see how his life history fits in with the presence of amoebae in hepatic abscess. How I long to be settled & do some steady work.

We were all nearly killed here by toxin poisoning the other day - five officers & three servants. I had cramps & was coming near collapse - am weak still, three days afterwards. Filthy brutes these native cooks are.[4]

Why does not your article on staining flagellulae appear in the B. M. J.?

Lawrie has challenged me to a tournament of the microscope.[5] I have made excuses (diplomatically) at present. He seems to me to be a man incapable of *thinking straight*, so what is the use of my endeavouring to convert him. But I suppose I must do as he wants. Believe me

Yours very sincerely

R. Ross.

Please *hold off* about the malaria-investigation for a little.

1 A Leader 'Kala-azar', *BMJ* (5 June 1897), 1434-1435, describes his work, subsequently published L. Rogers, *Report of an Investigation of the Epidemic of Malarial Fever in Assam, or Kala-azar* (Shillong: Assam Secretariat Printing Office, 1897).

2 Reference not traced, although one of his obituaries refers to his publications on parasitic *Algae* and *Fungi*: ('D. D. Cunningham', *Proc. Roy. Soc. London*, Series B, 89 (1917), xv-xx.)

3 R. Ross, 'Notes on some cases of malaria, amoeba coli and cercomonas', *Indian Medical Gazette* (May 1897), 172-175.

4 *Memoirs*, 214, allowed himself a black joke in mentioning that the

three servants who also suffered from eating the offending ice-cream pudding should not have done so for caste reasons.

5 *Memoirs*, 215, described the 'duel' with the microscope. Ross chose a patient with the early stages of *Plasmodium falciparum*. Unfortunately, by the time of the demonstration before the faculty and students of the Nizam Medical School, the man's blood was free of parasites. 'I was absolutely routed and did not even dare to describe my defeat to Manson.' Of Lawrie, Ross remarked that he was 'one of the many good surgeons and passable doctors who have no clear conception of what science means.' (*Ibid.*).

Letter 80
02/119

Secunderabad

13th July 1897

Dear Dr Manson,

I think I forgot to ask you to suggest provisional names for the new parasites of the mosquito; that is if you can make them out well enough from the few specimens I sent you. I should like to dedicate them both to you in the *specific* name, but perhaps we shall not be in a position to give *generic* names as yet. Coccidium (?) Mansonii, etc, may do provisionally! Nothing but tertian cases here & very poor ones. I can't find the new parasites in these mosquitoes at all as yet. A remittent case is coming on & I hope to get some crescents soon.

As soon as I know your opinion about the new parasites, I will, if you think it wise to do so, write a short article in the B. M. J. on my Sigúr experiences. I have reported officially to Cleghorn on the subject. My letter to his secretary, Leslie, asking to be sent to Assam to have a look at Kala-azar has received no reply as yet, nor have I heard anything further about my appointment in the Foreign Department.

The monsoon has failed almost entirely up to date, and unless it rains heavily soon the country will be in a frightful state, while Govt. will be so hard up that there will be no investigation work. At present however there are undoubted signs of a Public Health Institute being started. Govt. have written round to local governments asking them to mention men who have been doing research work, & certain Rajahs have come forward offering money for the institute.[1] I dont know however whether they will ever employ me; though I should of course like it immensely if I am given to understand that I shall not be relegated to this miserable regimental work afterwards. I fancy that secretaries and men like Grant,[2] that is lecturers on physiology & pathology, etc, will get everything, and I should not wonder if they make a muddle of the whole business.

I don't think the time has yet come for you to push on the investigation business, because Govt. seem already to be stirring themselves, and I should like to see what they will do after receiving my report on the Sigúr enquiry. But perhaps a letter from you to Cleghorn may be very useful at this juncture, that is if you feel at all that it would be appropriate. I am simply wasting my time here, as I feel so unsettled that I cannot do good work. Besides I hear that promises as to appointments are not quite equivalent to performances & am continually harassed with the fear that I shall soon have to send in my papers. This regimental employ is indeed out of the question!

My children, who are still in the hills, all have had whooping cough. Lawrie has made me go & discuss the parasite with him. He has certainly seen a good deal, but has not, I think, studied anything closely, while he is stuffed full of the most ridiculous theories. Red corpuscles arise from the nuclei of leucocytes - he has *seen* it![3] He is just leaving for England & will go and see you. I think he has sense enough to come right in the end in your hands; at all events he understands Hehir's work at its value.

With kind regards yours sincerely

R. Ross.

1 A number of research institutes and laboratories were established in late nineteenth- and early twentieth-century India; the Indian Medical Congress of 1894 had submitted a resolution calling for this. From a subsequent comment in Letter 106, it is likely that Ross was referring to the Laboratories established for W. M. W. Haffkine in both Calcutta and Bombay, the latter subsequently being named after him. The first Indian Pasteur Institute was established in 1900. For background details, see C. G. Pandit and K. Someswara Rao, *Indian Research Fund Association and Indian Council of Medical Research, 1911-1961* (New Delhi: Indian Council of Medical Research, 1961); Deepak Kumar, *Science and the Raj, 1857-1905* (Delhi: Oxford University Press, 1995); and Harrison (1994).

2 Letter 78, note 3.

3 Letter 79, note 5.

Letter 81
02/120

Sec'bad

18th July 1897

Dear Dr Manson,

I have been going on in the same way & have now examined very carefully a number of brindled mosquitoes, large, small, black & dark brown. I have found nothing at all, either in them or in their evacuations. I am now beginning on a large, voracious, light brown species with brindled legs and proboscis & three black bars on the wings - like one of the Sigur species - a kind which I have obtained here with some difficulty.[1]

If the parasite is cultivable in the brindled fellows it must become something very obscure & like ordinary cells. Of course so far as the phenomena of exflagellation warrant us in going, we have no very clear right to assume that the flagellulae must develop in the tissues of the mosquito - they may, for example, lose their flagella shortly after escape from the present sporocyst & remain in the mosquito's stomach-contents as motionless spores which will be capable of development only on falling with the insect's evacuations on a suitable basis. In this case such spores would probably be like fat-cells & debris in the evacuations & I may very probably have missed them. Such spores may grow into mycetozoa on damp ground. This theory will have to be worked out if I fail in finding parasites in malariated mosquitoes. We may call it the mosquito-*convection* theory as against the mosquito-*parasitic* theory, the flagellulae being supposed not to undergo any development, except the loss of their flagella, in the insect. The flagella would be given them at first in order to enable them to avoid leucocytes (?). I want to know what you think of the possibilities in this direction.

Have been examining a flea from a rat with trypanosomes & will work more with such as an instructive parallel study. Fleas have much the same anatomy as mosquitoes. I am collecting a number of malariated mosquitoes in glycerine for you. Have had no answer from Leslie to my letter of 3 weeks ago (!) Nothing likely to be done yet owing to this frontier war.[2] They are probably going for the Amir.

With kind regards

Yours sincerely

R. Ross.

1 *Memoirs*, 219, describes the various kinds of mosquitoes Ross was using.
2 At this stage the campaign was to suppress the uprising of the Mohmand tribe in the North-West Frontier Province. The Tirah campaign against the Afridi tribe, who had captured all the British posts in the Khyber Pass, needed more preparation and took place between October 1897 and April 1898.

Letter 82
02/025

21 Queen Anne Street,
Cavendish Sq
4th July, 1897.

My dear Ross,
I have been very much interested in your last three or four letters[1] and hoping that each one would add some clue to the problem you are trying to solve. This much they show that the problem is much more complicated than at first sight one would think. And this they also have made me feel that you wont get forrader[2] unless you hang on to the flagellum. Stick to it and try by all sorts of microscopical device to hang on to its tail and get, so to speak, dragged with it to its destiny. Working with these other forms is more or less blind groping; sticking to the flagellum is following the leader. I wait for another letter to hear if you have got any further before drawing conclusions from your present line of observation; but the feeling with me just now is such as I express.

Surely some temporary disappointment has sent the evil thought to chuck the service and profession for novel writing. Surely your better angel has crushed this thought ere this. Speaking as an outsider, as regards the Indian Medical service I would say that your success therein is already assured and that you are bound to step ahead soon. You must be wrong in saying that there is no reward for such work as yours. Administrators and surgeons are thick as peas anywhere, but a man like yourself, who is capable of original work, of discovery, is not to be picked up every day and no government in its senses would ignore persistently your existence or fail sooner or later to reward good work done. Have you enemies at head quarters? If you are able to give me any information about the outs and ins of official intrigue I might make it unpleasant for conspirators and better for you and workers like you. Persevere. You are bound to come up. Those papers of yours in the Indian Medical Gazette are excellent and are bound to tell. For very obstinacy and determination not to be beat I would stick to my last were I in your place.

Novel writing is no good. Unless a man is to the manner born[3] he can't go on drawing on his imagination year in and year out, and writing, as I have found, is a terrible weariness to the flesh. To write a book or two of that sort every now and again by way of pastime is one thing, but to make it the business of your life and the source of your income is quite another affair and is sure to end in worry and disgust.

I hope to hear from you next mail that you have changed your mind about this and are once more on the track.

Yours very sincerely
Patrick Manson

1 Letters 72-74.
2 Forwarder (slang).
3 *Hamlet*, Act I, Sc. iv.

Letter 83
02/026

21 Queen Anne Street,
Cavendish Sq.
7th July, 1897

My dear Ross,

Since my letter of the 4th I have received yours of 12th June. I immediately wrote to Sir Charles Crosthwaite as per enclosed copy[1] and await his answer. I do not know if he is in town. If he is not there may be some delay but so soon as it comes I shall forward a copy of his answer. I think he will help you if he can. He is a man of great influence at the India Office and if he cares to leg you up he probably can do so. At all events he will be able to put me on the track of stirring up a little dust if necessary. Nous verrons. However he answers dont do anything in a hurry. It is so easy to break a sheet of glass; so impossible to§ mend it. I dont believe that any government can ignore your work. I think it would be well to send to the Indian Medical Gazette some sort of memo of the work you have been doing lately. Keep yourself before the public.

Some details about those mosquito protozoa would not only be of interest in itself but would show that you are really in earnest and have been up and doing. Moreover it would show the people who have the selecting of a man for malaria work that they have in you the article ready made and that it would be almost hopeless to get another man in India who without a long preliminary training could possibly undertake it.

I shall keep this open till mail day in the hope of being able to give you some news from Crosthwaite.

8th July, 1897.

I have just received a letter from Sir Charles Crosthwaite in which the following occurs. "I saw Hooper yesterday about Ross. He recommends Ross to apply direct and in person if possible to the Home Secretary, J. P. Hewett,[2] at Simla and to ask for a civil appointment under the Govt of India in the Central Provinces Jabalpore for preference. I enclose a letter of introduction to Hewett for Ross. It is very hard if he cannot get this much done for him. I will also speak to Lord George Hamilton[3] but there is very little chance of his moving because all these appointments are left to the India authorities."

I also saw Hooper[4] yesterday and he advised in the same sense as above. He said if he wrote to Cleghorn it would damage your chances as he and Cleghorn are not of the same kidney exactly. I know Cleghorn very well but Hooper tells me he resents anything like a lead and rather advised me not to. I also know Leslie his secretary. Do you think it would do any good to write to him. Let me know at once and I will do either or both.

Wishing you good luck which I fancy is not far off if you act on Crosthwaites suggestion.

I remain Yours very sincerely

Patrick Manson

I will write if I hear from Crosthwaite again: he has not returned your papers - I suppose he is keeping them for Lord G Hamilton.

1 **RA** 02/027. Manson wrote to Crosthwaite of Ross's researches, his conviction in the theory and his wish to continue this work. He enclosed correspondence pointing out what Ross wanted and recommended him as the best man in India to carry on a malaria investigation. He asked Crosthwaite for help or advice on influencing the Indian Government to supply Ross's demands and added that he wanted England to get the glory of teaching the world how to deal with malaria. See *Memoirs*, 216-217.

2 John Prescott Hewett, (1854-1941), Home Secretary between 1895 and 1902, with an interval as member of the plague commission in 1898-99.

3 Lord George Francis Hamilton, (1845-1927), Secretary of State for India, 1895-1903

4 Surgeon-General Sir William Hooper, (1837-1921), President of the Medical Board of the India Office, 1895-1903.

Letter 84
02/121

Secunderabad

27th July 1897

Dear Dr Manson,

Having at last found some fair cases of crescents, I am in full tide of work again and am endeavouring to attack the last stage of the problem. The experience gained in the Sigur Ghat as to the new parasites has given me confidence & knowledge, as to parasites of the mosquito & as to their anatomy, which I did not feel or possess before; so that I now have hopes of working out the subject. I am of course sticking to the flagellulae again, but on a slightly modified principle. Owing to their extreme delicacy I doubt whether they can be directly followed into the insects' tissues; but this difficulty can be avoided in a simple manner. The question I have set myself to answer, & which I now feel myself able to tackle, is "Do healthy mosquitoes fed on malarial blood contain any parasite which similar mosquitoes fed on normal blood do not contain?" In other words can we cultivate flagellulae in the mosquito? To obtain a reply, I keep mosquitoes, after feeding on crescents, for one, two, three ... days & then examine, so as to allow the flagellulae time, by supposition, to mature into full-grown mosquito-parasites. After some days they should form spores, say like octospores, which should easily be found. Suspicious bodies being noted, I have only to compare with control insects fed on healthy blood in order to decide whether they have anything to do with the malaria parasite. Another question however must be held in mind - "Do mosquitoes fed on malarial blood *evacuate* any protozoa not evacuated under similar circumstances by mosquitoes fed on healthy blood?"

It may take weeks or years to obtain answers to these questions; but I am now working forward steadily. I dissect each malariated mosquito with the utmost care and then search every *micron* of it with an oil-immersion. Each mosquito takes about two hour's work. I have examined only a few insects as yet, so that it is not time to talk of results.

Yesterday I examined the evacuations of two freshly malariated mosquitoes, passed during two hours after feeding. It appeared possible that the flagellulae might escape directly in this manner; but I could not find them.

Thinking over the whole subject, I cannot conceive any other explanation of the exflagellation process except that it is meant for the mosquito. Hence the flagellulae *must* either develop in the mosquito or be evacuated by it at a certain stage of growth; the things are there & *must* be found! It is simply a matter of hard work. There is one great difficulty however which largely complicates the question - the flagellulae may be capable of development only in a particular species of insect.

28th July. Last night I received yours of the 4th & 7th with enclosures & don't know how to thank you for your great kindness & interest on my behalf. The only thing I fear about is that I must have put you to great trouble; and also - that I shall need all my energy to live up to the letter about me which you sent to Sir C. Crosthwaite! I felt indeed, when I found myself in the fix of six weeks ago, that you would do all you could for me. Well, I must now try & come up to your expectations. The only adequate thanks I can give you is to solve the problem!

I knew you would be surprised at my dreaming of abandoning the service & taking up literature; but you must remember, first that literature has been my Eldorado all my life, & secondly that both my wife & myself are quite determined that a home in England with poverty is better than life in a poor medical appt. in India, which would mean poverty in India without a home. Remember, during the last 16 years I have never been more than 3 years in one place. For the last 4 years we have had no home at all barring 6 months in a house with hired furniture & the expectation that we would be moved in a month or two. During the last 7 years I have spent two hundred pounds over my income though we have lived very simply & have not even kept horses. A poor appointment, or one in a hot disagreeable station, simply means a continuance of this kind of thing *ad infinitum* together with separation from wife & family. The thing is out of the question. I should simply be a fool were I to stay under these conditions. Of course some men do so. They are mostly bachelors, half-castes, men with huge families & lazy men. Dymott,[1] one of our smartest men, has just left on his first pension, & other men are doing so. I *know* that I could make double as much by literature as I shall ever make in India & I should also have a home & my family with me, and the English or Swiss climate.

With a leading appointment, a good Indian climate, or, say, work on the Health Institute, work in which I could take interest, the case is of course quite different. Even with this however, to tell you the truth, I really doubt, after carefully thinking the matter out, whether the advantage will lie so strongly with the good appt. in India as some may think.

Again, you must not think that I was hypochondriacal in my fears about not getting a good appt. I was indeed offered three appointments, but I have since discovered that they were all inferior ones. The truth is all the good appts. have been bespoken long ago & the service is so tied up with red tape that it is extremely difficult for a man to push himself in it unless he begins to do so when he enters it. In fact my present predicament is a great deal my own fault; but that does not make it any better. Hence I saw clearly at last that I must push for myself; it is no use leaving things to the justice or mercy of Surgeons General; they have their own favourites.

No; I don't think I have a single enemy in the country. Sibthorpe doesn't love me quite I believe - or else his manner is a very bad one - and Dobson[2] who travelled lately with Leslie tells me that the latter did not think much of my work, malarial or sanitary. But he is not of much consequence perhaps. A Madras man said to me "We I. M. S. men are not meant for research & so on - we are simply doctors." There is a certain feeling against not only research, but men whose names are seen in print - verb. sap.[3] I think that this & my own carelessness are chiefly the cause. Finally I really doubt whether good work in the service ever gets much reward. I could name a dozen men.

But enough. Things looks better. I have been promised my Residency Surgeoncy owing to Col. Robertson.[4] Moreover on reporting my Sigur work to Cleghorn (as I did the other day) Leslie wrote back for him to say that *as soon as the state of the service admits*,[5] Cleghorn will endeavour to give me special opportunities for my malaria work. Lastly I have written in officially urging my claims and demi-officially to Leslie hinting that I must go if I don't get something. With your efforts on my behalf to fall back on in case of need I ought therefore to do well now. Hence I don't think that any further efforts need be made at present - many thanks again for yours. I shall use Sir C. Crosthwaite's letter to Mr Hewett[6] if necessary if the "state of the service" (the old shiboleth) keeps me waiting too long. Meantime I have my work cut out for me.

Here's another long & tedious letter for you; but perhaps my next will be more interesting. I am putting up numerous malariated mosquitoes to send to you.

With very many thanks, believe me
Yours sincerely
R. Ross.

I enclose my letter to the Un.-Planters' association.[7]

1 Donald Frederick Dymott, (b.1856), IMS Madras, retired 11 May 1897.
2 Surgeon Colonel A. F. Dobson, (1848-1921), Residency Surgeon (ie Medical Officer to the Resident, the civil staff and the Bowring Civil Hospital).
3 *Verbum sapienti sat est*: a word is sufficient to the wise.
4 Donald Robertson, (1847-1930), Resident at Bangalore, 1896-1903.
5 *Memoirs*, 216, quoted Leslie as saying that Cleghorn 'considers the [Sigur Ghat] paper original and highly interesting, and that, when the state of the service permits, he will endeavour to provide you [Ross] with more favourable opportunities for carrying on your researches than are at present possessed by you.' **RA** 03/064 (20 July 1897).
6 See Letter 83.
7 **RA** 05/119. The letter was printed and circulated, *Letter to the Secretary of the United Planters' Association of Southern India* (Madras: Addison & Co, 1897).

Letter 85
02/122

Sec'bad

4th August 1897

Dear Dr Manson,

I have done ten days' good steady work over the malariated mosquitoes (barring one day when I was ill). The work has been very deliberate & thorough as you may judge from the fact that I have examined only 20 malariated & 4 non-malariated insects in that time, though I have worked 4 or 5 hours a day. I have also much improved my dissections in small ways (e.g. brushing off the feathers before dissecting) & in fact search all the tissues exhaustively. No parasite has been found. At one time I suspected some nucleus-like bodies & some amoeba-like bodies found under the skin in the same position as the greenish cells which I found in Sigur - but on comparison of mosquitoes fed on healthy blood these cells seem to be quite normal. Malariated mosquitoes dead at 5 days contain no distinct hard spores like pseudonavicellae or octospores.

Well, I must double or treble this work before making definite statements; but by my present methods I go over every micron with my oil-immersion & have seen nothing suspicious as yet. But again I have examined only three species of mosquito, the large black brindled; small black brindled; and large brown brindled. I have with regard only to brindled mosquitoes also examined continuously the evacuations of three malariated mosquitoes kept in inverted bottles in a moist chamber. No flagellulae or amoebulae - only bacteria. Lastly I have inspected three grubs just hatched out of the eggs of a malariated mosquito - nothing.

I see my course clearly now - it is to make an exhaustive search on these lines. I shall not miss a cytozoon, a spore, an amoeba, or a flagellum, believe me. When the brindled mosquitoes are done with I will try another species. The animal will be found if it is there, which it must be.

I saw a unique sight while looking at some developing crescents. One became flagellate in 6 minutes from pricking the finger; the flagellulae escaped entirely in one minute. Returning to the field a few minutes later I found *three or four free flagellulae attacking one small leucocyte* (lymphocyte)!

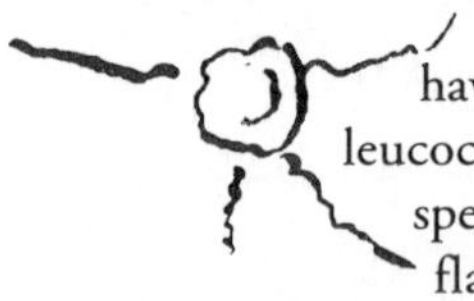

Since the "adventures of a flagellum"[1] I have not infrequently seen flagellulae going for leucocytes, but never anything like this. The spectacle suggests hypotheses. I wonder if the flagellulae pass through the mosquito's stomach & intestines inside the human leucocytes. The evacuations must be more carefully searched.

Your excellent paper in the B. M. J. of July 10th.[2] The photos are wonderful. If you get a chance you might look for flagellulae inside leucocytes by this means; and I will use the method later for some schemes I have in view. I may suggest two petty improvements - (1) expose the blood for 3 minutes before mounting on a breathed-upon slide (to make unstained specimens) & (2) mount between 20 & 30 minutes instead of between 30 & 45 - at least to get flagellate bodies & not free flagellulae. From a large number of observations I conclude that exflagellation generally occurs between 10 & 15 minutes & nearly always between 6 & 30 minutes. The flagella may escape entirely in one minute. Free flagellulae are commonest between 25 & 30 minutes, after which many appear to die. With care we could get stained free flagellulae by your method, which would be very instructive as regards their real form which is always 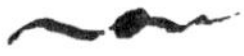 or  with a thickening in the middle.

The times are most unpromising for a malaria investigation. The monsoon will probably fail again in great part & we now have another Malakand war.[3] Govt. seize upon any & every excuse for stopping projects for investigations, etc. I showed a knowing man my communications anent[4] the Residency Surgeoncy & the investigation. He said they are not worth much because the "state of the service"[5] means any time up to two years. I have therefore written again to Leslie asking him to endeavour to give me a fixed time. If these "intrigues" fail I shall use Sir C. Crosthwaite's letter. Am feeling extremely discontented & anxious, the infinite dawdling about everything driving one nearly wild, while this regimental employ is unendurable. A lady asked me yesterday whether I had got into trouble after my Bangalore work that I should be sent back to a regiment! Nice, is it not?

My children at Ooty are better.[6] Suppose I shall see them again some months' hence. With kind regards, yours sincerely

R. Ross.

1 See Letter 15.
2 Manson (1897b).
3 The young Winston Churchill got himself attached as the *Daily Telegraph's* correspondent during the campaign, producing a volume on it in 1898. For details, see Lawrence James, *Raj: The Making and Unmaking of British India* (London: Little, Brown and Co., 1997), 402ff.
4 i.e. concerning. 'Anent' is one of the few Scotticisms in the correspondence.
5 Letter 84, note 5.
6 Letter 80.

Letter 86
02/028

21 Queen Anne Street,
Cavendish Square,
22nd July, 1897.

My dear Ross,

I was very glad to gather from your last that your chance of getting your heart's desire is now so good. I did not think that, unless the authorities were mad, they could long overlook your claims or, rather, their own interests. Sir C. Crosthwaite has interested himself a good deal about you and I fancy has stirred up Lord George Hamilton in the matter though of course, for obvious reasons, this must not appear. I return the papers herewith as there seems now no longer any good purpose to serve in keeping them. The B. M. J. had a paragraph about you in their last issue which may be of some use.[1] In the same number you will see the announcement of my appointment to the colonial office.[2] This should be an encouragement to you to work on, believing that in time your reward will come. I had no influence whatever with the authorities and made none. Hearing the post was vacant I sent in half a dozen testimonials and the thing was done. So that you see the casting of bread on the waters bears fruit though it may be after many days. This appointment means a lot of work I fancy; but it is congenial work and it is not without its pecuniary rewards. It will bring with it many opportunities and if I can see my way I shall do my best to give a leg up to the teaching and study of tropical medicine. As things are, in this important section of medicine, they are simply shameful.[3] If I can get my way no man shall be able to get a license to practise tropical medicine, at all events as a public servant, who cant demonstrate the malaria parasite and one or two others.

I am working just now at my book when I get leisure and am not dead beat; also at the new West Indian filariae.[4] They are cunning little devils - one of them very handsome. The B. M. J. had mislaid my illustrations of the flagellated bodies; they appear to have found them at last, and two numbers ago the note was published.[5] I enclose a reprint in case you have not seen the article. They made a mess of some of the photos.

The kala-azar business is a good idea. I dont much believe in the competence of Nicholl[6] - is it - to work up the malarial side of the question. Be very careful about arriving at a conclusion, in the matter of germ. A directly infective malaria germ is not likely and I would have a lot of proof before coming to such a conclusion. Be sure to keep me posted on progress.

Yours very sincerely
Patrick Manson

1 'The risks of the study of malaria', *BMJ* (17 July 1897), 163, reported on Ross's dose of malaria at Sigur Ghat, commenting that, despite his illness 'he has made some important and hopeful

observations in connection with the theory for which he has done so much.'

2 *BMJ* (17 July 1897), 163. See Eli Chernin, 'Sir Patrick Manson: physician to the Colonial Office, 1897-1912', *Medical History*, 36 (1992), 320-331.

3 For evidence of Manson's efforts in the field, see Patrick Manson, 'The necessity for special education in tropical medicine', *BMJ* (9 Oct. 1897), 985-989.

4 Manson (1898a) and his paper for the Sixty-fifth Annual Meeting of the British Medical Association held in Montreal, 31 Aug. - 3 Sept. 1897 'On certain new species of Nematode Haematozoa occurring in America', *BMJ* (25 Dec. 1897), 1837-1838.

5 See Letter 85, note 2.

6 Unidentified. Manson may have meant Rogers or Giles.

Letter 87
02/030

21 Queen Anne Street,
Cavendish Square. W.

Telegraphic Address
"Finically, London"[1]

23rd July, 1897.

My dear Ross,
I have just got a letter from Sir C. Crosthwaite. He writes "I have got the Secretary of State to send on your letter to me about Ross to Lord Elgin - & I hope it will bear fruit." I have no doubt it will. I pitched it in very strong about neglect of opportunities, of efficient & willing men, about the importance of the subject & the backward position of England in this matter, etc, etc.

Yours
P. M.

1 The first time Manson used new stationery with his telegraphic address.

Letter 88
02/123

Sec'bad

11th August / 97

Dear Dr Manson,

If I could believe it possible to live up to all the flattering things you have said about me lately I might have some hopes of thanking you in deeds for your kindness! No other kind of thanks appear to me likely to be adequate; but I must see what I can do in the other way. If you get an opportunity, will you kindly thank Sir C. Crosthwaite for me. As you say, the Secretary of State's action is sure to put the matter to rest, and has relieved me of considerable anxiety which anyone who knows India could not help feeling in my circumstances. But I must hurry, as I have numerous fever cases to examine today, & will write more about the malaria investigation by next mail. Owing to my case of crescents drying up & to extra duties I have examined only 12 more mosquitoes, 4 of them fed on a mild tertian after the attack; but these have been searched with, if possible, still greater care than the former ones. No definite results; and I expect that I must soon state: -

(a) that the brindled species I have been examining are not the hosts of the flagellulae of crescents or spr. tertian, or (b) the flagellulae develop in them into something very delicate, or very small, or very rare, or almost indistinguishable from normal cells or nuclei.

Dead & decomposed mosquitoes of the fourth day certainly do not seem to contain hard, bright spores such as pseudonavicellae or octospores. Yet if the haemamoeba escapes into external nature from the mosquito it should escape as spores in all probability. I have also examined fruitlessly the evacuations of two more mosquitoes & several grubs bred from the eggs of mosquitoes malariated on the 26th July. However this is evidently the line of research which must be successful in the end - I must discover America if I continue to sail along this parallel westward far enough.[1] But I intend to go all over the "first step" again when my next crescent case is ready.

The news of your appt. to the Colonial Office is great.[2] I only wish you were our Director General. Yes, I think we want a revolution in our methods in tropical medicine. I am teaching a couple of men here the m. parasite, but the rest don't care a button about it. I think that now with your assistance in regard to the Secretary of State, etc, I shall be able to help considerably in this matter. I shall of course now drop my second string, the Residency Surgeoncy, and do my best to be put on malaria research work. Kala-azar is promising. I *don't* think it is conveyed by infection, but through the mosquito. Well, I must be off to work, which is the best way to thank you for your prompt action. With kind regards

Believe me, yours truly
Ronald Ross.

1 In later years, Ross liked to compare himself to Columbus, having also given to mankind 'the godlike gift of half a world.' R. Ross, *Studies on Malaria* (London: John Murray, 1928), 58.

2 See Letter 86, note 2.

Letter 89
02/124

Secunderabad

22nd August / 97

Dear Dr Manson,
In my last I told you that I was going to abandon the brindled mosquitoes for a while & attack some brown ones. Now prick up your ears because the hunt is up again. It may be a false scent, but it smells promising.

Unfortunately it turned out that my mosquitoes (brown) were very few in number, but they bit well & kept well. I dissected the first ones without any result, but some were bad dissections, broken eggs, etc. On Friday 20th I had only two left.[1] One of [these] was very carefully dissected (4th day after being fed on crescents). I noticed at once some cells in the stomach rather more distinct than the usual very delicate stomach cells. Altogether there were a dozen of these lying mainly towards the upper end of the organ. They varied from 12μ to 16μ in diameter & were full of stationary vacuoles. The outline was sharp but fine & not at all amoeboid, the shape spherical or ovoid, the substance rather more solid than that of the neighbouring cells. There was no contractile vesicle; but one or two of the cells seemed to be contained in some of the large gastric cells. Now I am so familiar with the mosquito's stomach that these bodies struck me at once; & you may imagine how much more struck I was when, on focusing carefully I found that they contained *pigment indistinguishable in colour, shape etc from that of the haemamoeba*! It was black or dark brown (not blue, or yellow or greenish like the cell granules, debris etc), not refractive on up-focusing, consisting of little balls or rods, & sometimes oscillating rapidly with a small range in parts of the cells. This pigment was not however copious at all & the granules did not shift their place in the cell appreciably; though I find on comparing drawings that they alter their position after 24 hours. In some cells there were pretty large clumps of pigment; in fact the latter was *exactly* & *in every detail* like the pigment of the haemamoeba.

Now what do you think of this? Well, I irrigated with formaline, sealed with glue & labelled for you. Examining next day, the cells, as I expected they would under formaline, showed up more clearly & could now be made out easily with a 1/6th inch. The pigment had clustered more into clumps. In fact apart from the pigment, the bodies looked parasitic, though they were not nearly so bright as the coccidia I sent you from Sigur.

On the 21st I killed my last brown mosquito (5th day after being malariated) & rushed at the stomach. The very same bodies (!) only larger, more distinct & with a thicker, perhaps double, outline (sometimes). There were 21 of them, again in the oesophageal half of the stomach. The largest ones were 20μ, but some were only 12-14μ. Pigment & vacuoles as before. Formaline, etc again. I will send you the specimens when I can get some more (I want them now for comparison).

No more brown mosquitoes!

In their absence, I have taken a number of brindled malariated mosquitoes which I had ready & have examined them again to make sure that I had not previously overlooked the pigmented bodies. Not one in eight of them.

Hence we have (provisionally)

1. The pigmented cells appear to exist in malariated brown mosquitoes but not in brindled ones.
2. They are larger on the fifth than on the fourth day.
3. They occupy only one part of the stomach.
4. They become more distinct under formaline.
5. They are sometimes intracellular (?)
6. They have pigment exactly like that of the malaria parasite.

The remarkable thing about them is undoubtedly the pigment. I have never seen this before in any mosquito (I have now examined hundreds - or a thousand). It always lies in the cells & is not scattered outside them or in any other cells. In short it is as distinctive a feature of them as it is of the haemamoeba. *No other bodies but these two that I have ever seen contain such pigment; and it is the same exactly in both*. In some cells it even lies in a ring at the centre 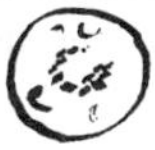 In others marginally 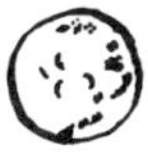. In others, again quite irregularly. In some cells after formaline I think I can see a central nucleus with the pigment round it 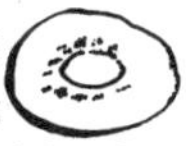. Wait now. You will say at once (as I used to think) that the parasite in the mosquito cannot have pigment, because this is known to be derived from haemoglobin, and the mosquito has no haemoglobin. Has it not though? Why its stomach is full of it, and these cells which lie in the wall of the stomach, perhaps almost touching its contents, could easily absorb unlimited haemoglobin. Anyway there's the pigment, just like what we see in our old friend.

Only one difficulty remains - to get more brown mosquitoes. I may add that it is a filaria bearing species. One of my patients has very rare filariae & I found one kicking in the *tissues* of a 24-hour mosquito.

I must first keep my mosquitoes alive for more than 5 days, by giving them a second feed, in order to see whether the pigmented cells develop spores. By their appearance on the 5th day, I imagine sporulation will begin at about the 7th day. If spores form, the parasitic nature of the cells is established &, taken together with the pigment, leads to an obvious inference.

Next I have to see whether unfed brown mosquitoes or the same fed on healthy blood do or do not possess these cells, and whether malariated ones always possess them.

All this is only a matter of a little work. Unfortunately I can't get any more of those brown devils.

Meantime the find of pigment is as encouraging as it is unexpected. It is of course quite unlikely that these cells are mere ordinary cells which have absorbed pigment granules from the stomach-contents by amoeboid action. The cells are too few & their pigment too scattered & scarce - not like that of a pigmented spleen-cell for instance. Besides, why should they not exist in the brindled insects?

23rd Aug. No brown mosquitoes yet. Am doing nothing else but look at my pigmented cells. They keep beautifully in formaline. The pigment, though much more scanty in comparison to the size of the cell, is absolutely identical in characters with that of the haemamoeba. I have never seen anything like it before except in the haemamoeba. Wonder if I am really on it at last! If not, what can these cells be? Something very unusual.

5p.m. Two brown mosquitoes caught in hospital ward, a male & female, the latter containing one day's blood. No pigmented cells. These then appear to be not a normal feature even in brown mosquitoes.

Two points must be proved; (a) that the cells are parasites; (b) that they are malaria parasites. Please note however that owing to the presence of pigment, (a) will really almost involve (b). Hence, if I can find that the cells *sporulate*, the thing is *morally* certain, though formal proof of (b) will be required.

24th Augst. No more brown mosquitoes bred from grubs; but I have caught 10, 1 male, 7 unfed females, & 2 females whose stomachs & ova show that they were fed 2 & 3 days ago. In none of these have I found pigmented cells, though all were examined most carefully. It appears then that these cells are peculiar to malariated brown mosquitoes.

With kind regards
Believe me
Yours sincerely
R. Ross.

1 Ross always celebrated August 20th as 'Mosquito Day'. See **Introduction**.

Letter 90
02/031

21 Queen Anne Street,
Cavendish Sq.
11th August, 1897.

My dear Ross,

I had no time to write you by last mail but got my wife to copy out two important papers which have recently appeared in France and which go a long way to support our view about the life history of the malaria parasite.[1] The writers dont seem to know about our particular views but that makes no difference to the views or to the value of their support. I fancy the Italians will shut down now on their degeneration hypothesis. The close correspondence with the spore phase and with the rosette phase of the coccidia is very remarkable. I am more convinced than ever that the mosquito is the alternative host and I hope you will soon be able to prove it.

Some time ago I had a crescent case from Delagoa Bay[2] in hospital and again repeated your experiment with the vaseline with complete success. At the same time I made a number of stained preparations of the flagellated body with excellent results. I have now many good stained specimens and among them not a few free flagella both near and at a distance from the parental sphere. But I cannot make out a nucleolus. The free flagellum seems sharper at one end than at the other. I hope to be able to send you a micro-photograph some day soon. Would it not be possible to watch the flagella in a crushed mosquito's stomach and follow it up to its destiny in some stomach or other cell. I still think you have got to hang on to the tail of the flagellum to be put on the right track. Once find out the cell and you are all right to trace it to its final stages.

I have been over your preparations, but, alas, with the exception of the filariae and the long gregarine 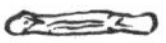 I can make nothing out of them. They have evidently perished for I see crowds of bacteria in them or debris like bacteria. It is a pity.

I think you should name the various organisms for your own use but not as yet for publication as it is just possible they may have been named already and I would advise you to see some European authority before committing yourself in this matter. Make good drawings in case the preparations perish - photos if it can be managed.

I am anxious to hear how the Government is going to fix you. I have no doubt it will be all right and if you could settle the Kala-azar question it would give you irresistible claims. I hear Lawrie is home en route for the Montreal meeting of the B. M. A.. I suppose to ventilate his chloroform fad.[3] I hear he is going to call on me. I hope he will. Apart from his untenable malaria views he is an interesting personality apparently.

I have a paper at the Montreal meeting. They dunned me into writing one and so I gave them a screed on the new American filariae thinking it would be interesting to Uncle Sam to know that he had a worm all to himself. I have also sent some specimens of malaria flagella.[4]

Thank God my book is out of hand. The manuscript went in on Monday. I already find I have a lot to add and must try to get in these new French discoveries.[5] I suppose it will have to go as a foot note or appendix. I have still a long article to do for Gibson's Practice of Medicine[6] and an introductory lecture to write; after which please the pipers I may have a little leisure to think. I have had a very hard summer and this appointment to the Colonial Office coming on top of the other activities has left me no time for the work my heart is in. It has even deprived me of my annual grouse-shooting holiday and now I have a dose of the gout to make me cheerful and pleased with the order of nature. However I try to think I shall get a fortnight in October.

I had a good case of liver abscess in a doctor today - a man from the Niger. It is the first case I have met with from abroad in which there was no history of dysentery. In the pus at the operation there were no amoebae but I may find them later on in the discharge from the drainage tube as I have frequently done in other cases.

If you have a lot of benign tertians try to stain the flagellated body in one of them on my plan. I am interested to know what they would look like.

Good luck to you. Have *nil desperandum*[7] for your motto and work on feeling sure of your reward.

Yours very sincerely
Patrick Manson

1 **RA** 02/032 and **RA** 02/033. 'Le cycle évolutif des coccidies chez les arthropodes' Note de M. Louis Léger, presentée par M. A. Giard; *Compt. Rend. Acad. de Sc., Paris* 124 (1897), 966-969. 'Recherches sur les formes de reproduction asporulée dans le genre coccidium' Note de M. le Dr. P.-L. Simond, presentée par M. Metchnikoff; *Compt. Rend. Soc. Biologie* (1 Mai 1897), 425-428.

2 Now Bay de Lourenço Marques, Mozambique.

3 The Sixty-fifth Annual Meeting of the British Medical Association was held in Montreal, 31st Aug. - 3 Sept. 1897. The rising number of deaths from chloroform anaesthesia had become a subject of much concern in the 1890s. Among several commissions and experimental groups examining the physiology of chloroform was a commission in Hyderabad, of which Lawrie was president. The Hyderabad group concluded (erroneously) that chloroform has no direct action on the heart, death coming from respiratory depression. See Edward Lawrie, 'Chloroform and the heart', *BMJ* (17 July 1897), 131-132; 'Partial anaesthesia with chloroform', *idem* (31 July 1897), 271-272. For a general discussion with references to further secondary literature, see Christopher Lawrence, 'Experiment and experience in anaesthesia: Alfred Goodman Levy and chloroform death, 1910-1960', in Christopher Lawrence, (ed.), *Medical Theory, Surgical Practice* (London: Routledge, 1992), 263-294.

4 Manson (1897d).

5 Note 1 above. He did not discuss them in the first edition of his book.

6 G. A. Gibson (ed.), *Textbook of Medicine* 2 vols (Edinburgh &

London: Young J. Pentland, 1901). Manson wrote several entries for this publication including 'Malaria and malarial disease', vol. i, pp 290-316.

7 Horace, *Odes* I, vii. 27.

Letter 91
02/125

Secunderabad

31st August [1897]

Dear Dr Manson,

Very many thanks for yours of the 11th. Will you kindly ask your publishers to send me a copy of your book with note of price.[1] I will return cheque. Am glad you have got it off & am anxious to read it. Please give Mrs. Manson my thanks & compliments for the copies of the very interesting articles.[2] They must have cost her a great deal of trouble to copy, especially the accents. I must get a typewriter (for my wife) as soon as possible.[3] I expect that the malaria flagellulae have an *axial* nucleus like the coccidial flagellulae described by Simond.[4] Hence the reason why you cannot make out a nucleus - the whole thing almost is a nucleus (?).

I am in despair about my specimens having gone bad, because now I dare not send you the two slides of pigmented cells in the mosquito, since they also have been mounted in formaline. I suppose it was the Red Sea, because my own specimens of coccidia & octospores are in perfect condition. I cannot understand how bacteria however numerous could have destroyed either of these which are hard resistant bodies. Are you quite sure that you have not overlooked them? The octospores are found *among* the abdominal scales; the coccidia in the stomach. For both use an oil immersion. My coccidia now look like worms eggs, very distinct; but the octospores may be mistaken for fat globules.

You will be dying to know about the new cells. I have had a maddening exasperating week owing to my not finding any more of those infernal brown mosquitoes; and at the end of this week I must go to Bangalore to see my wife & children. Is it not annoying? I have had half a dozen men out hunting grubs & have obtained *scores* of batches - all brindled, or grey. The ones I caught in the ward turn out not to be exactly the right kind, though very closely allied, being whiter & more slender. I cannot find where even these come from, &

those caught by hand won't bite even at night. These kinds constitute evidently a separate family of mosquitoes characterised by having dappled wings & peculiar boat-shaped eggs. I will be on them in time.

I have examined crowds of other kinds for the pigmented cells, without result. I am now going methodically through a grey species with six dark grey bands on back & grey plain wings. Will let you know result up to 4th day tomorrow.

Now to open my heart freely - I really believe the problem is solved, though I don't like to say so. I look at my cells daily; those of the fifth day have grown bigger than those of the fourth day; such bodies are not found normally among the elementary cells of the mosquito's stomach (which are alike in all species of course); they have as yet been found only in malariated mosquitoes; above all, they contain the characteristic pigment peculiar to the malaria bug. What are we to think? What do *you* think? I fancy when you first read the word "pigment" you guessed what it was.

Well now, I daren't send you these specimens for fear they spoil on the way. I will take them to Bangalore & show them all round. John Smyth[5] is there I think & some other men who have got a little knowledge of the malaria bug. I'll make them write descriptions, which I will send with a short note of my own to the B. M. J. Then on returning here I will try & photograph the cells (if I haven't succeeded in finding them again). I think, after deliberation, that the find should be notified as soon as possible, as it may, for one cause & another, be weeks before I get on the cells again, and in the mean time some lucky Italian or American, who has happened to hit off the right species of insect, may polish off the whole business. My note to the B. M. J. will contain description of the mosquito & of the cells & will draw only such cautious inferences as we are as yet entitled to make. In reality - *pigment* - it is almost proof already! What else can the thing be? Mosquito's cells don't contain pigment or anything like it. I am not mistaken - it is *pigment*, absolute, unmistakable *pigment*! I have hardly restrained myself from wiring "pigment" to you, but fear you would think I had gone mad. Well, I know pigment by this time. I *am on it.*

1st Sept. The grey mosquitoes don't contain pigmented cells up to the 4th day. Several more batches of grubs yield only brindled mosquitoes. My crescent cases are nearly exhausted. Hence I must now defer study until I return from leave. I think you will agree with me that I should not risk my two precious specimens until I have shown them & got some photos. Owing to the border war[6] it is quite possible I may be sent on active service. Leslie has not troubled to reply to my letter. Nor have Sir M. Young, Maharajah of Dholpur, Cleghorn and a friend at Simla, to all of whom I wrote months or weeks ago.[7] Funny people out here. I shall look out for brown mosquitoes at Bangalore & am offering large rewards to my hospital servants here for them. There was no gregarine (except perhaps accidentally) in the specimens I sent you. With kind regards, yours truly

R. Ross.

1 Manson (1898a). It was published in April 1898 and sold for 10s. 6d.
2 Letter 90, note 1.
3 Although Ross continued to send his letters handwritten, his writing is much easier to decipher than Manson's.
4 Simond (1897a).
5 John Smyth, (1857-1927), IMS Madras, resident surgeon at Madras General Hospital and Professor of Pathology. He was appointed surgeon to the Maharajah of Mysore in 1897.
6 See Letter 81, note 2.
7 In a draft of a letter dated 20 May 1897, (**RA** 01/097), Ross asked William Mackworth Young to support Donald Robertson's recommendations that he be transferred to the Foreign Department. See Letter 74, note 3, and Letter 85.

Letter 92
02/126

Bangalore
13th Sept. 1897

Dear Dr Manson,

I have packed & posted the two specimens (worth £1000 each) and enclose the registration receipt. The slides are enclosed in three boxes & several layers of wraps & if they don't arrive safely it won't be my fault. The Red Sea will be fairly cool at the end of this month, so that the specimens ought not to be disorganised by heat. They ought to reach you about 2nd or 3rd of October. Before dispatching today, three weeks after being made, the specimens were *perfect* - please remember this. If they go bad on the voyage we shall be fully entitled to utter what imprecations we please on the Fates.

I enclose maps of the two specimens.[1] Please place them on the stage with the label to the right. The tail, ovaries, malpighian tubes, intestine & stomach (in one group) will then be in the right further corner of the cover-glass. A 1-inch lens will enable you to follow the maps. Then begin with a $^1/_6$ inch on the *second* specimen dated 21st August, that of the mosquito at 5 days. You will be able to make out some of the cells with this power in the oesophageal half of the stomach, that is to the *real* left & *apparent* right, and you can even make out the pigment. Begin looking just to apparent left of the first group of air-vessels you meet on travelling away from the oesophagus towards the centre of the stomach. Here, under the oil-immersion there is a field containing seven or more parasites at different depths. In some the pigment is more visible than in the others. I think there are 19 parasites now to be seen in this mosquito. In the earlier one there are only 5 or 6 (I think), the others having disappeared because of the increased opacity of the tissues under formaline. There are two good ones close together at about $^1/_3$ of the length of the stomach left of the oesophagus. You will observe that in this specimen the parasites are more hyaline & smaller (generally) than in the mosquito of the 5th day. I pray fervently that you will be able to find them all, photograph them & demonstrate them publicly. If you think fit you may like to add a note, with photos to my article & Smyth's note, sent by me last mail to the B. M. J.[2] I think that the course of publishing at once is highly desirable as it really *may* be months before I can find the brown mosquito again. When you have examined the cells I believe you will agree with me that there can be little or no doubt that they are the malaria parasite in the mosquito. The formal proof ought to be easy. John Smyth is amusingly grave over the matter. He thinks more than he dare speak. I showed them to Srinivasa Rao, Mysore bacteriologist, & asked him to guess what they were. He said "pigmented leucocytes".

Well, I return to Secunderabad tomorrow & will have crowds of mosquitoes awaiting me. No brown ones here.

As Leslie has not condescended to reply to me I have sent Sir C. Crosthwaites letter to Mr Hewett & asked him if he can do anything.[3] The frontier war ought to be over by Xmas. I hope the theory will be proved by then. I anxiously await your opinion of the cells - will you let me know it by return?

Yours very sincerely
R. Ross

1 Figures 8 and 9.

2 R. Ross, 'On some peculiar pigmented cells found in two mosquitos fed on malarial blood. (With a note by Surgeon-Major Smyth, M.D., I.M.S.)', *BMJ* (18 Dec. 1897), 1786-1788.

3 Letter 83.

Figure 8
Diagram of mosquito showing pigmented cells.

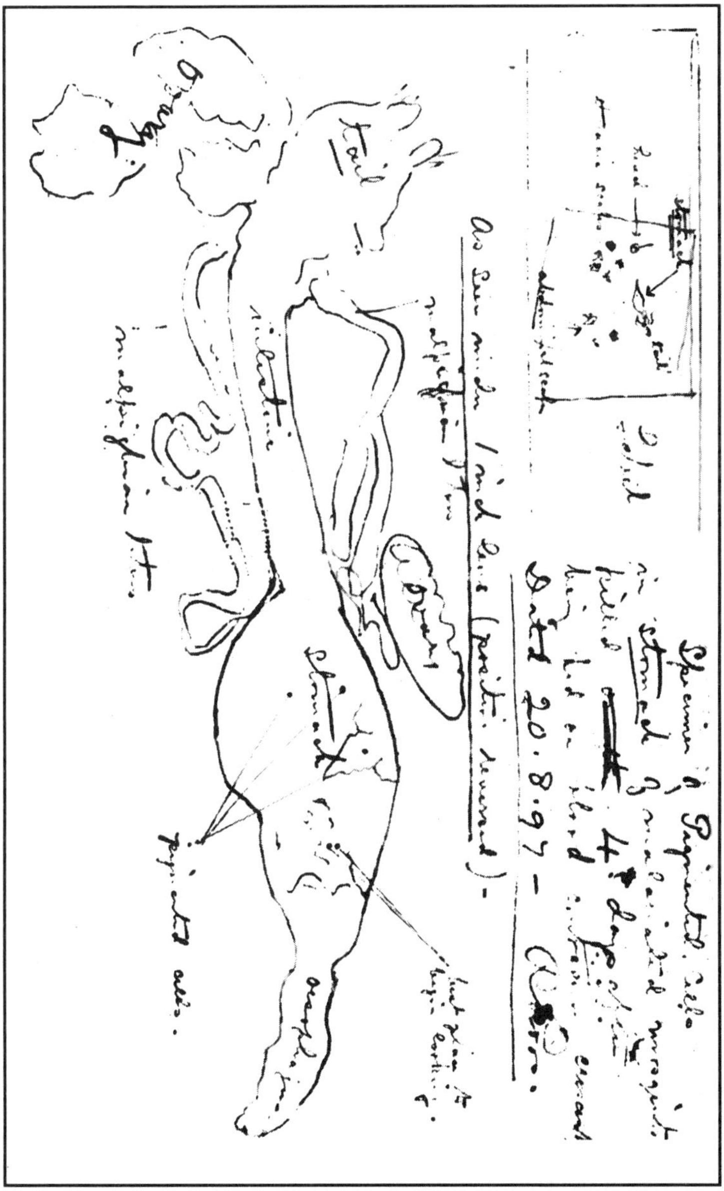

Figure 9
Diagram of mosquito showing pigmented cells.

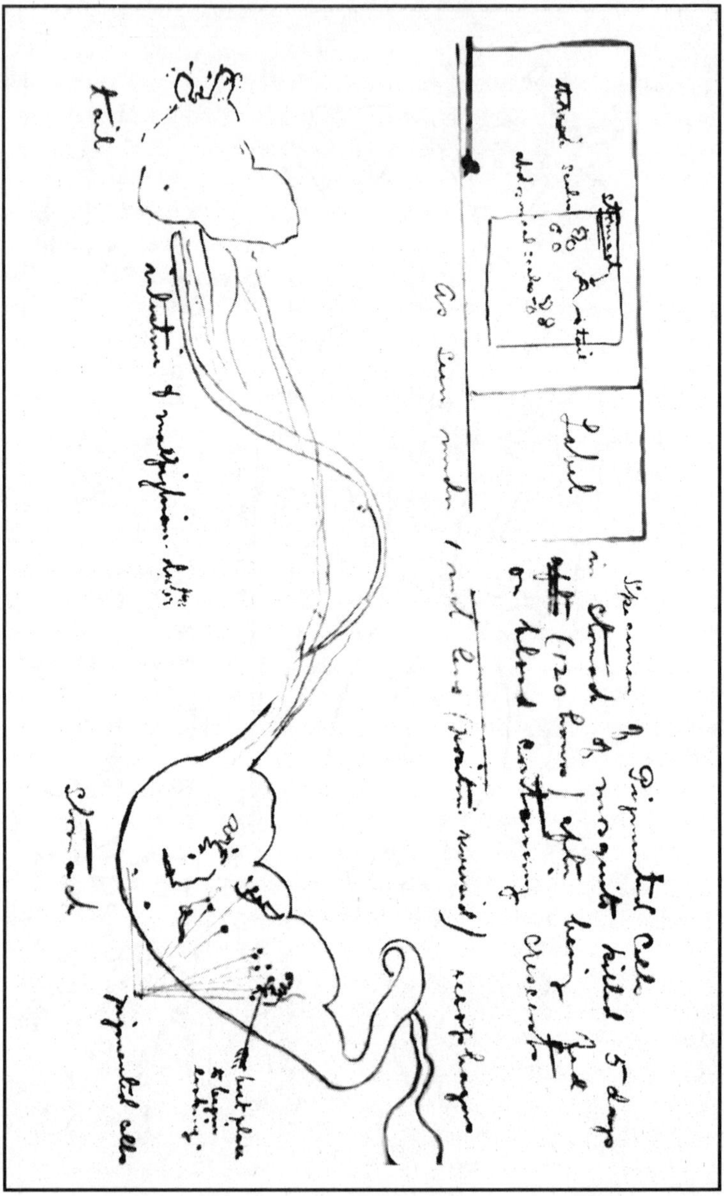

Letter 93
02/128

Secunderabad
21st Sept. 1897

Dear Dr Manson,
The progress is slow, but I think, sure. I am on the pigmented cells again.

On returning here I found about 30 samples of grubs awaiting me; but they were all brindled and grey insects. Several fresh samples a day failed to yield any others, until this morning when I found some brown insects in a rain puddle. I am doubtful whether these are the true kind or the allied species; anyway they quite refuse to bite up to the present.

But often when labour fails fortune strikes in. You remember the grey mosquitoes with plain grey wings, plain legs, white bellies & barred backs, of which before going to Bangalore I had fed a number on crescents with negative results? Well, on the 18th a case of *tertian* (mild), found by microscope, was asleep at 9 a.m. in his corner of the ward & one of these mosquitoes was biting him.[1] I secured her. She was evidently an old lady already, say 3 or 4 days, because the white ovaries were visible through the scales, & she had probably been nipping steadily on the man's blood for some time whenever he fell asleep. Her stomach was crammed with black (old) blood. I kept her up to 11.30 this morning (3 days after feeding last) & then killed. Stomach nearly empty but still some residue of blood. Eggs all fecundated & nearly ripe. Stomach *full of pigmented cells.*

These were much more numerous than in my mosquito of 21st August, were of all sizes from about 5μ to 25μ or more, pigment I think finer, scantier, & browner, and oscillating in the smallest cells. The largest cells appeared to have lost their vacuolated structure & looked more hyaline than the middle-sized ones, while their pigment seemed to be contained in an internal vacuole, but they and also some of the middle- sized cells had a few 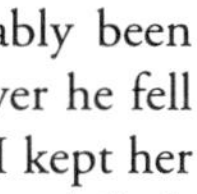 bright, blue, sharp cut bodies  scattered throughout them - like the granules of eosinophile 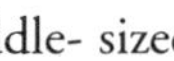 leucocytes, only larger & much fewer. No amoeboid motion (??). Now mark; I have not finished with this mosquito. You remember the swarms of flagellulae which I found in some of the Sigúr mosquitoes & which I thought were derived from free Euglenae in the water. The stomach contained numbers of these, that is, several large sporangia breaking up on access of water into these swarm-spores. You remember also that a man to whom I gave these swarm-spores was attacked with fever five days afterwards.

In this case the flagellulae were almost as large as trypanosomes & took on active movements only as the water pervaded the tissues. The breaking up clusters were lying among the blood-debris in the stomach & the free flagellulae rushed about actively in its cavity. Is it possible that these bodies are the sporulating forms of the pigmented cells? I think it quite possible. We shall see.

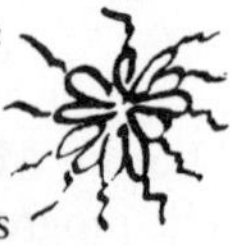

In this mosquito, the pigmented cells are so large & clearly defined as to be found with ease by a 1/6th inch lens. Remember now that I have examined scores of this species either unfed, or fed on crescent blood, without ever having found these bodies, which are however seen at once in an insect fed on tertian blood. From this fact as well as from the marked bulk, definiteness, evidence of growth, it is *evident* that the pigmented cells are *parasites*; they also contain pigment; what is the betting?

It ought to be a question of days only, but yesterday I threw away bottles-ful of barred-back mosquitoes, and my tertian cases are cured. I was a pure fool not to try this species of insect on this kind of fever before. *Both* are very common here; but like all idiots I stuck to my principles, namely to crescents, instead of plunging right and left into chance. You must not be disappointed if I don't work out immediately. The fact is these species of mine, brindled, barred-back, brown mosquitoes are really *families* each comprising many species & it may turn out that each kind of malaria will "take" only in a single one of these species. Hence the hunt may be a long one. Practically however I have only one thing to do now in order to obtain absolute formal proof, and that is to produce the pigmented cells at will from malarial blood. It is, I think, only a question of time, of the exact kind of mosquitoes, & plenty of them. Details of growth & sporulation of the cells will come of themselves. I suspect the swarm-spores like the devil.

If you get a telegram from me it will mean only one thing - absolute proof.

22nd Sept. I have just succeeded with great difficulty in inducing four of the allied dapple winged brown species to bite a case with numerous crescents. These little wretches die if one looks at them; but if they live until the 25th & are then found to contain the pigmented cells the theory will be practically proved, though the experiment must be repeated several times before I telegraph. This evening I hope to get some barred-back grey mosquitoes off a new good tertian case. I shall be much disappointed if I don't get practical proof in a week's time, but all experiments must be verified by frequent repetitions before I announce definitely. This may take a month's work. A telegram to you will mean this definite announcement, & when you get it you may know that I am *absolutely sure*. The only possible source of doubt appears to be that the pigmented cells are some parasite of the mosquito unconnected with the malaria parasite and therefore not depending upon the ingestion of malarial blood. The question will easily be set at rest. It is improbable to say the least of it. The three cases of pigmented cells hitherto found by me were all malariated mosquitoes.

Tomorrow I shall examine some unfed dapple-winged mosquitoes & shall also try to feed some on healthy blood. If these give negative results & those fed today on crescents give positive results the inference will be pretty sure. Remember that I have already examined numbers of this species not malariated with negative results.

23rd Sept. As I feared two of the mosquitoes fed yesterday have died but I fed four more this morning on crescents, and I obtained two barred-back mosquitoes last evening from a tertian case. It is only a question of time.

I don't know what to do with the article I sent to the B. M. J. two mails ago & think I had better leave it to you to publish or not as you think fit. It will always be useful as a basis for a *full* article which I will write after complete proof is obtained; but I don't think I shall be prepared to write such an article for another month or two, and in the meantime I may be sent away on ~~sick leave~~ active service any day. Perhaps it will be best to publish the article already sent, with Smyth's note, and, if you like, one from your description of the cells. I have abstained from theorising in the said article so that it won't do any harm even if by some remote chance the pigmented cells turn out not to be malaria parasites.

Will you kindly let me know where the two articles on flagellate forms of coccidia were *published*.[2]

With kind regards

Yours sincerely

R. Ross.

1 *Memoirs*, 234, identifies it as *Culex fatigans*.

2 Letter 90, note 1.

Letter 94
02/129

Bombay
27th Sept. 1897

Dear Dr Manson,

I fear I must stop my malaria work at this point as I have been ordered to the front on active service. This, so far as my share in the work is concerned is unfortunate as, when I received my orders, I hoped to complete the mosquito theory in a week or so, & now I think it very unlikely that I shall be able to resume investigation for many months, if at all. Perhaps therefore, I should give you a winding-up statement of my studies since I first met with the pigmented cells.

Since the 20th August when I first saw them, I have not been able to find the large, brown dappled-winged mosquitoes again. On the 18th Sept. however I saw a grey mosquito (legs & wings plain, belly nearly white, back of abdomen barred dark brown)[1] feeding on a patient whose blood the microscope had shown to contain the mild tertian parasites. Numbers of similar mosquitoes to these, unfed or fed on blood containing crescents, had been previously examined by me and found not to contain pigmented cells. This one was secured. She was an old insect to judge by her ovaries & had, I thought, often fed on this particular patient who slept in a corner of the ward. I kept her alive for three days more and then examined her. Her stomach contained numerous pigmented cells varying from about 10µ to 25µ in diameter (I have no micrometer), most of them like those formerly found in the brown mosquitoes, except that the pigment appeared to be finer, scantier and browner, while the cells differed much in size & some of them were very large. A few of the largest cells however differed markedly from the others, the substance being apparently free of vacuoles & consisting of a hyaline substance in a capsule. In the centre there was a nucleus (or vacuole?) on the surface(?) of which the pigment was scattered. In the smallest cells the pigment was often oscillating just as in some forms of the haemamoeba; but in none of them did I notice any amoeboid movement.

The discovery of the cells in the mosquito immediately suggested of course that the grey mosquitoes with barred backs, though they appear immune to the summer-autumn parasite, are susceptible to the mild tertian. Proof appeared easy to obtain, by feeding numbers of this species of insect on mild-tertian blood & dissecting them after some days. Unfortunately I was not able to do this until the day before I left Secunderabad, and the insects have all died in the train.

I was however a little more lucky with some of the delicate, brownish-white, dappled winged insects[2] which I have already referred to as being closely allied to those in which I first found the pigmented cells. I obtained the grubs of these with great difficulty (they appear to breed only in rain-puddles) & fed the imagos on crescent-blood. They are wretched little creatures & die at once almost, but I managed to examine two, 24 hours after feeding, and one, 48 hours after. In the former I could find nothing, in the latter there were a number of pigmented cells, all nearly the same size & very small, only about 8µ in the long diameter, containing very marked &, for the size of the cell, copious pigment which sometimes oscillated & was sometimes arranged in the form of a ring. The cells themselves were so hyaline that they were scarcely visible; but there could be no doubt about the pigment which was typical of the malaria-parasite. I had no time to experiment with any more of this species.

This then closes my list of findings of pigmented cells, namely twice in large dappled-winged mosquitoes fed on crescent-blood, once in a small dappled-winged mosquito fed on crescent blood, & once in a barred-back, plain winged & legged insect fed on mild-tertian-blood. Of the small dappled-winged insects, I have examined numbers, fed on healthy blood or unfed, without finding the cells; of the barred backed insects I have dissected as many unfed or fed on crescent blood, without seeing the cells. It would appear then as if these pigmented cells are the direct result of feeding appropriate insects on appropriate kinds of malarial blood. I am not sure of course; but I think so; and I have been studying mosquitoes closely for two and a half years. This supposition taken with the fact (which I think can scarcely be denied any longer) that the cells are parasites, and with the fact that they contain pigment exactly like that of the malaria parasites, lead us, especially when coming on the top of the strong theoretical reasons given by you for the mosquito theory, almost to believe that the pigmented cells must be the long-sought alternative form of the parasite of malaria in the insect. Scientific caution should prevent us giving way at this stage to ~~assertions~~ conclusions, but I must confess (especially as I am writing a "winding up" statement) that I think they are so.

Supposing so, the parasite in the mosquito should be directly derivable from the escaped flagella of the flagellate bodies so called (they *should* be called, after Lankester,[3] flagellula-cysts containing flagellulae, or, simply, cysts containing swarm-spores). The point should be easily proved by feeding the proper kind of insect on the right kind of malarial blood, & comparing with similar insects fed on healthy blood, when the pigmented cells should be found in a certain percentage of the former only. The parasites would then appear to grow to about 8μ in 2 days, 16μ in 4 days & to about 25μ in a week or more, that is towards the close of the insect's life. The young parasites have as many granules of pigment as the older ones. Lastly (this is only a "winding up" hazard) sporulation occurs about the time the insect dies and falls into water.[4]

But there is more than a guess here. In the barred-back mosquito containing pigmented cells (she must have been quite a week old) the stomach contained three large clusters (40 or 50μ) of swarm spores, each cluster breaking up rapidly under the influence of water into a multitude of these swarm-spores or flagellulae, & each flagellulae almost as large as a trypanosome. All the latter then rushed about in the cavity of the stomach with the ordinary movements of flagellulae. I have seen these parasites before in the malarious locality of the Sigur Ghat.[5] The question now arises whether they are not the spores of the pigmented cells, the homologues of the ordinary flagella arising from crescents, etc, but which, in this case, continue the life of the parasite in external nature, or perhaps are deposited on the human skin.

I must now conclude; and shall do so by laying great stress on the presence of the so-called pigment in the cells. This is a substance not found in ordinary physiological cells; or in ordinary protozoa; or in gregarines & coccidia; or even in the gregariniform blood parasites of reptiles: it is seen only in the haemamoeba of men & birds. What is to be said then when we now observe it in mosquitoes actually fed on blood containing haemamoebae?

Yours sincerely

R. Ross.

1 *Memoirs*, 236, identified this as *Culex fatigans*.

2 *Memoirs*, 237, identified this as *Anopheles culicifacies*.

3 Lankester (1875-89) provided the classification of protozoa which Ross used most.

4 Although Ross omitted this paragraph in the letter quoted in his *Memoirs*, it shows that he still entertained the possibility that malaria was spread through drinking contaminated water.

5 Letter 70. Ross did reproduce this portion of the letter in *Memoirs*, admitting in the discussion of it (p.238) that he had been wrong.

Letter 95
02/130

Bombay
28th Sept. 1897

Dear Dr Manson,
I have had a stirring week having been ordered suddenly to Bombay on military duty, which I and everyone else supposed meant active service & six months marching about the Afridi hills.[1] On arriving here definite orders for me had not come, but the P. M. O. told me I should have to go to the front. This meant throwing over the theory for a long time just as I seemed to have the solution in my grasp & it also meant that I should have to apply for pension as soon as the military duty should cease. Hence I was *down* enough I assure you, and wrote you the "winding-up statement" which I enclose. I still send it you, & you will be able to see by it that I was able to find the pigmented cells in yet another mosquito (malariated). If you are contemplating adding a note to my paper on the cells & would like to make use of any of this statement, please do so.

Fortunately when my orders came I was told to go not to the front but to Rajputana where I shall get my Residency Surgeoncy, I believe, at last. My wife & children will follow in a few weeks probably, but I don't know what the place is like. Address in future

Surgeon Major Ross
Meiwar Bhil Corps
Kherwara
Rajputana

Hope to start work again immediately on arrival. Am leaving Bombay tonight & arrive at Kherwara tomorrow.

Believe me
Yours sincerely but in a great hurry
R. Ross.

1 The Afridi tribe inhabited the mountains on the Peshawar border of the North-West Frontier province of India. See Letter 81, note 2.

Letter 96
02/131

Oodeypore
5th Oct. 1897

Dear Dr Manson,
Here I am after nearly a week's travelling at the Venice of India[1] & am doubtful what is going to be done with me. Kherwara is not a Residency Surgeoncy but only military employ of a sort considerably worse than I had in Secunderabad; but I believe they have been forced to send me there in order to avoid dispatching me to the front. They are taking every doctor they can get hold of for the Afridi expedition. On its cessation I expect I shall get something; but I fear it won't be anything good, because on enquiry here I learn that all the good Residency Surgeoncies have been bespoken long ago. On the other hand I hear that I may be sent again to Bangalore, because, since I left, they have been fighting to such an extent that they want me back. Hence I abandon myself to drift on the waves of fortune.

I now write to urge you to exert all your influence to get the Indian Government to take up the malaria question directly the Tirah expedition breaks up (which ought to be by Xmas). Since the subject was last mooted to Govt. the pigmented cells have been found; and it seems to me that it would be insane on the part of the govt. of a large tropical country like this to hesitate any longer in taking up the matter, especially as the thing can be arranged at once free of cost. Of course Govt. will say they have no funds after recent events, but this is no impediment! You remember that the Maharaj Rana of Dholpur & other Indian Princes have come forward with funds for a Health Institute.[2] If the Indian Govt. could see its way to mooting the point to them, I believe they would subscribe at once to pay me while on special malaria duty. This would practically start the Institute immediately on its protozoal side, for which a complex building & laboratory are not essential. Remember that the Maharajah of Patiala proposed in 1895 to do this entirely out of his own pocket. The suggestion emanating from you would I believe bear issue at once if placed in the proper quarter. My own letters to the Maharaj Rana of Dholpur, to Mr Hewett (Home Secretary) and others[3] have as yet received no reply & I don't think I can do anything more; but I believe Surg. Gen. Cleghorn will try; & if you can manage to get the hint sent out from home I believe matters could be arranged by the 1st January.

I have found the dappled-winged brown mosquito in the Residency here (where I am living) but not their grubs. Mrs Ravenshaw the wife of the Resident,[4] whom you know, says she is quite recovered now owing to your advice. Yours sincerely

R. Ross.

1 Oodeypur, 'the beautiful city of lakes and palaces', *Memoirs*, 258.

2 Letter 80, note 1.

3 Letter 91.

4 Major C. W. Ravenshaw, Resident at Oodeypur, formerly Assistant Resident at Bangalore while Ross was there.

Letter 97
02/132

Kherwara
Rajputana
12th. Oct. 1897

Dear Dr Manson,
On examining again today my 3rd mosquito with pigmented cells found three weeks ago I observe that the formaline has made the pigment turn into clusters of black crystals which make it appear different to what it was at first & much more bulky & distinct. Johnston,[1] the doctor here, says the crystals look like haematin ones. I tell you this to warn you that the pigment of the specimens which I sent you may have undergone a similar change; so don't be surprised if their pigment differs from the description of Smyth & myself & from that of the malaria parasite in man. I fancy formaline has some chemical action on pigment. My fourth mosquito does not show this change.

You will be disappointed to hear that there is *no fever* here & I cannot go on with the work at present. I expect to leave the place in a week or so, however, as Johnston whose place I had come to take (a 3 years' service man) is now well enough to continue his duties here. This is only military employ worse than my regiment in Secunderabad. After leaving it I expect to be sent to the front or to some other inferior place. I have however written to Colonel Robertson & asked him to find out if they are going to do anything or not for me.[2] I enclose Mr Hewett's reply to my letter asking when if ever Govt. would take up the malaria subject.[3] You observe the vast amount of interest he takes in the matter; and I can only assure you again that there is scarcely a man in the Govt. or in the department that really cares one button for all the science in the world. Many men who are doing nothing might for instance have been sent on this goose-chase instead of me.

If Col. Robertson's reply to me be unsatisfactory I shall probably apply for furlough from 1st Jan. as my wife and I can't stand any more of this. I shall write more definitely next letter. In the meantime there comes a gleam of hope from Owen of Patiala to whom I wrote.[4] He says he will try to get the Indian Princes to apply for my services for malaria work & pay my salary in anticipation of the Jubilee Health Institute.

Yours sincerely
R. Ross.

Hewett's letter is pure bunkum. In another month there will be hosts of men to spare. Neither he nor anyone else will take any *trouble* about the matter.

1 In *Memoirs* Ross has deleted the name. Probably Dudley Cater Johnston, IMS Bombay (1870-1901) who was murdered by a fanatic Ghazi at Loralai.
2 The Resident at Bangalore. See Letter 75, note 6.
3 **RA** 01/170 (28 Sept. 1897). Hewett says he will bear Ross's request to do malaria research in mind but the present financial position and the need for medical officers make it impossible to take up the matter. He adds that the Public Health Institute will not be established for some time (Gibson, 1983).
4 **RA** 01/109 (6 October 1897). In a letter to Ross, Owen said that the Rana of Dholpur was founding a health institute under Haffkine and suggested that Ross asked for secondment to it; he advised him, however, against leaving the IMS (Gibson, 1983).

Letter 98
02/034

21, Queen Anne Street,
Cavendish Square. W.
1st October, 1897

My dear Ross,

I put off replying to your last two letters hoping that the next mail would bring some fresh news about those most interesting pigmented cells. The B. M. J. sent me your paper asking my opinion about its publication. I told them it should be published at once partly because we want to secure priority for English discovery and partly because it will stimulate others to work on the same lines. It will do you good too by showing that you are not lying on your oars. The thing is really most promising. If you get another opportunity try the chemical tests for the pigment. It is a pity you did not do that at the time; I can quite understand however your disinclination to spoil the specimens. There is just one thought that occurs to me. Is it not possible for a stomach cell to include pigment from pigment in the blood in the contents of the stomach. I fancy some doubting Thomas may raise this point and it would be well for you to notice it so as to show that you are alive to all objections and that you do not fail to weigh them.

You must get more of these mosquitoes and go over and over the ground a dozen times to be sure that the step is a genuine one. If it is genuine the problem seems to be practically solved for the rest is merely a matter of work and detail. You know where to go for your material now.

I spoke again to Hooper[1] about you. It seems that Cunningham[2] of Calcutta is likely to retire soon. His billet would be just the place for you and I fancy that Hooper if he has any say in the matter will say it in your favour. I suppose the emoluments are sufficient. I am sure the work would be to your mind.

I am going off for a week's holiday tonight after an introductory lecture which I have to give at St Georges this afternoon. I am going to speak about the necessity for special education in tropical disease.[3]

Yours sincerely
Patrick Manson

1 Surgeon-General Sir William Hooper, (1837-1921), President of the Medical Board of the India Office, 1895-1903.

2 D. D. Cunningham, (1843-1914). See **Biographical Appendix**.

3 Manson (1897c).

Letter 99
02/035

21, Queen Anne Street,
Cavendish Square. W.
21 October, 1897

My dear Ross,

I have been so oppressed with work lately that I have not found time to answer your last two or three letters which, I need not say, interested me acutely. You seem to be on it at last. The slides arrived a fortnight ago and while I was away in Scotland on my week's holiday. I examined them at once on my return and found them in good condition enough to recognise the cells you describe. But the preservative medium was evaporating and fearing the cells might perish I had them drawn at once by a good artist and I hope they will appear soon in the B. M. J. along with your paper. I showed them to Thin[1] and to Bland Sutton[2] who at once recognised their likeness to the malaria parasite and the importance of your find. Personally I believe you are on the road to a great discovery but first you must be sure of where you are. Two things occur to me. The pigment in the cells may be absorbed by these bodies from free pigment in the mosquito's stomach; second, the pigment may represent an entire malaria parasite which has been bodily incorporated from the blood by the stomach cell. In either case it would not represent a phase in malaria evolution of course. These possibilities you must try to get rid of if you would choke off carpers. I asked the editor of the B. M. J.[3] to request Thin and Bland Sutton to make a brief statement to the effect that they had seen your slides and that they considered your descriptions were correct. A similar statement I have made myself and I suppose these corroborative statements will appear as an appendix to your paper. I told them to hurry up with the publication.

I hope your new appointment will suit you in every respect. I have been urging your claims in all directions and I hope there may be some good come of it. I have suggested that you should get Cunningham's billet.[4] Meanwhile I enclose a letter sent me by Sir Charles Crosthwaite which will show you that you are not being forgotten.[5] If you would only make one step further in malaria you are safe.

Laveran has written a new book.[6] He sent me a copy and I have written Lewis to get one for you as well as one of the Ann. Pasteur with the full paper on the coccidium business by Simond.[7] Both of these I am sure you will be glad to have by you.

I am being worked to death just now with one thing and another. My book will soon be out of hand but then there are a dozen other things coming on which will keep me from original work for I dont know how long. I have vowed a vow to do no more writing except to please myself. I am a perfect slave just now and have hardly time to sleep.

You will have seen from the medical papers that I have been rubbing it in again about medical education re tropical subjects.[8] That has bruised a good many toes and has made me enemies as well as many friends. I have only spoken the truth and they can revile as much as they like. My colleagues, or at least one of them,[9] at the hospital are apparently very wroth about it.

I hope you have got a plentiful supply of mosquitoes and malaria cases and that you are now thoroughly settled down and at work again. I quite expect that ere the winter is over you will have solved the business, at all events in its main features and that it will have been conducted so far by you that a crowd of workers will be on the details. Dont worry over them. Establish the principle and leave details to others; meanwhile move on yourself to some other big subject.

Yours sincerely

Patrick Manson

1 George Thin, (1839-1903). See **Biographical Appendix**.

2 (Sir) John Bland Sutton, (1855-1936), assistant surgeon at the Middlesex Hospital. See **Biographical Appendix**.

3 Dr Dawson Williams, editor of the *BMJ*. Thin and Bland-Sutton's comments are added to Ross's paper (Ross, 1897f).

4 See Letter 98.

5 **RA**02/036 Letter from Crosthwaite to Manson (21 Oct. 97) "Here is the reply about Ross. I am afraid we must wait. Sir Arthur Godley also wrote to Lord Elgin about it I believe."

6 Presumably A. Laveran, *Traité d'Hygiène Militaire* (Paris: G. Masson, 1896); his *Traité de Paludisme* was not published until 1898, though this could have been an advance copy.

7 P.-L. Simond, 'L'évolution des sporozoaires du genre coccidium', *Annales de l'Institut Pasteur*, 11 (1897), 545-581.

8 Presumably his introductory lecture at St. Georges (Manson, 1897c).

9 There was a good deal of vigorous debate about Manson's efforts to establish a school of Tropical Medicine in London. See Letters 164 and 166, note 1.

Letter 100
02/133

Kherwara
Rajputana
10th Nov. 1897

Dear Dr Manson,
I was greatly relieved at getting yours of the 21st Oct. with enclosures and at hearing that the specimens had arrived all right. All I hope is that the pigment in the cells has not undergone crystallisation under formaline as in one of the specimens with me. The pigment ought to be in dots, not in rods; like this

 not like this .

I did not apply tests for pigment because it would not do to destroy my first invaluable specimens. This and staining for nuclei, etc, can easily be carried out afterwards. The crystallisation of the pigment is however a test itself, because I note that the formaline has had precisely the same action on a small residue of blood remaining in the stomach, that is, has converted it into minute black haematin crystals just like those in the cells.

Now for the view that the cells may be ordinary stomach cells which have absorbed and converted haemoglobin or which have incorporated entire parasites. As a matter of fact this is what I thought they might be when I first saw them; but a little reflection showed it to be extremely unlikely. If the cells be such they must be *physiological* cells, that is, *ordinary* cells of the mosquito's stomach capable of such action & should therefore be found in all, or in a large percentage at least, of mosquitoes. Such is distinctly not the case. I have *never* seen them in hundreds of brindled malariated mosquitoes; nor in scores of barred-back mosquitoes fed on crescents or healthy blood; or in numerous small dappled-winged mosquitoes fed on healthy blood. But I have found them in both of two large dappled-winged insects fed on crescents, in one barred-back insect fed on tertian blood, and in one of two *small* dappled-winged mosquitoes fed on crescents. This rarity of the cells precludes their being physiological & the objection is practically dealt with briefly in my paper already when I argue that the cells cannot be physiological for this reason. The thing comes under the obvious law that the constantly-found cell is physiological, the exceptional cell parasitic, or at least pathological. If these cells are as you suggest why are they not found in all fed mosquitoes? Besides, *do* the stomach cells take up solid particles from the stomach? On the second day of digestion the stomach is full of solid yellow particles, but I have never seen any such in the stomach cells. If the stomach cells can incorporate whole malaria parasites, why can't they incorporate whole blood corpuscles or other objects? Lastly, my pigmented cells show distinct evidences of growth in relation to the time after ingestion. They were small in the mosquito at 2 days, much larger in that at 4 days, still larger in that at 5 days, and largest of all and in company with large clusters of flagellulae in the mosquito at one week or so. Stomach phagocytes would not have this history. As a rule the largest physiological cells are phagocytic, so that in the mosquito at the 2nd day large instead of small pigmented cells should have been found. Then, are stomach cells ever known to be phagocytic? If so we should expect to find numbers of them filled with débris of all kinds. No, I don't think the pigmented cells are physiological, but, as I said at first, the point requires formal proof. A month's work would give it. All the same the betting is, even now, thousands to one that the cells are the malaria parasite in the mosquito.

Alas for your hope that I shall have a plentiful supply of mosquitoes and cases here! None of either (or very few); the cold weather is in, & the people here (Bhils)[1] so savage and superstitious that they won't allow experiments to be made on them. I had a very slight case of tertian two days ago, & some small dappled-winged insects. The fool flatly refused experiments. I don't think the insects would have bitten though, it is too cold. People sleep here without mosquito nets.

I was quite knocked over by disappointment anent the theory when I got here, and suffered from sleeplessness & neuralgia for weeks, but am better after a course of fly-fishing. You must confess that it is trying to be snatched away just as one is on the point of proving a theory which one has been thinking of and working at for nearly three years; let alone being sent to a wretched place with two or three Europeans and a few itch cases & febriculae in hospital when one has had every right to expect something fairly good. Fortunately however I think it is only temporary while the war lasts. I asked officially if this were so & mentioned how I had been taken from my research. This was the reply word for word from the P. M. O. Bombay (Churchill)[2] - "I don't understand what this officer means. He was sent to this command by H. E.[3] the Commander in Chief & here he will remain until H. E. orders him away." Sensible and polite, and as you may guess, from an A. M. S.[4] man! However, I expect to be relieved as soon as the troops return from Tirah and think that I was sent here only because they want medical officers at the front.

Wish now that they had sent me there. Some fun at least; and I must say that some better use could have been made of me - plague for example. But medical administration in this country has become too terrible for words. On the other hand, for all I know I may be here for months or till next hot weather. If I see any chance of this I shall write at once to Mr Hewett[5] & complain, & I daresay he can manage to get me back to Secunderabad at least. I commend my own wisdom now for having sent that article on the pigmented cells, as it is really quite possible that I may not be able to get to work again till next rains (May or later).

I had actually written my application for furlough to England (considering the above circumstances and that there was no chance of malaria investigation for the present) when matters began to look brighter in an unexpected manner. I wrote to Surg. Colonel Owen C.M.G., C.I.E. med. adviser to the Maharajah of Patiala to ask whether that potentate would come forward with funds for the investigation.[6] It turns out that he (Owen) is running the Princes' Health Institute idea, and he has come forward promptly. He thinks it very likely that the Maharajah of Dholpoor[7] will apply to Lord Elgin[8] for my services as soon as he (Dholpoor) returns from the war. The Prince will pay my salary. Owen will also try to get me on the projected Health Institute. Failing this, a Residency Surgeoncy is open at Rewa. I may perhaps get it. Failing both I may be able to get back to Sec'bad very shortly & knock off the formal proof about the pigmented cells. So there are plenty of irons in the fire. Many thanks for you efforts *in re* Cunningham's billet.[9] I fear there is not the least chance, as some young chap (Tull Walsh)[10] is I believe sure to get it - in this connection read enclosed: Hewett's letter to Sir. C. Crosthwaite shows that they have not forgotten me certainly, but "financial position" & all that - bunkum. They can put Davies[11] on some foolish bacteriological work (see enclosure).[12] Anyway I *must* get settled soon, or leave. My family now at Bangalore must go either home or to the hills next February. If the former I go with them. Many thanks for Laveran's book. etc. I am anxious to see yours. Your opening lecture was splendid.[13] The cap fits in many quarters. Yours sincerely

R. Ross.

1 The Bhils, a largely tribal ethnic group in Western India, were officially classified by the British as incorrigibly and hereditarily criminal. James (1997), 200.

2 Possibly Alexander Ferrier Churchill, AMS, (1839-1928) or Charles

Fleetwood Churchill, AMS, (1841-c.1920). Ross *Memoirs*, 244, says illegible, but he clearly wrote Churchill.

3 His Excellency.

4 Army Medical Service.

5 See Letter 83, note 2.

6 See Letter 4, note 2.

7 One of the princely states of eastern Rajasthan.

8 Victor Alexander Bruce, 9th Earl of Elgin, (1849-1917), then Viceroy and Governor-General of India.

9 See Letters 98 and 99.

10 John Henry Tull Walsh, (b. 1859), Surgeon-Major, I.M.S. Bengal.

11 Surgeon-Major Arthur Mercer Davies, formerly assistant professor of hygiene at the Army Medical School, Netley, was attached to the Office of the Principal Medical Officer in India to carry out bacteriological and sanitary investigations; reported in *BMJ* (13 Nov. 1897), 1444.

12 Missing.

13 Letter 99, note 8.

Letter 101
02/134

Kherwara
Rajputana
17th Nov. 1897

Dear Dr Manson,

Another reason why the pigmented cells cannot be phagocytes is that they all contain the same number approximately of grains of pigment. If they were phagocytes some would contain a large amount of pigment, others a small amount - compare parasites with pigmented phagocytes in malarial blood.

Many thanks for Laveran's and Simond's books[1] which I have received. Marchoux[2] of Senegal has also sent me his brochure. No, we won't let Laveran assume the honours of the mosquito theory. It is amusing the way in which he thanks you for supporting *his* theory. Some people think that they can claim the full honour of the discovery because they happened to guess that such & such would be the case. Laveran's mosquito theory, like that of others, was founded only on loose epidemiological considerations; yours on the divination of the fact that the so-called flagella are really flagellated spores - a *slightly* more important and substantial foundation for the theory. Until you came up with this explanation, no one had the slightest idea as to what the flagellated bodies were; Laveran once thought the flagella were organs of locomotion! Oh no, *he* shall not have the kudos. But before putting this matter straight let me try to find the formal proof about the pigmented cells; then your triumph shall be complete. Simond thinks his flagella are spermatozoa; they are simply flagellulae like the young of many protozoa - swarm-spores in fact. So are the malarial flagellulae. These parasitic protozoa require to develop in two directions - inside the host & outside; and they therefore require two kinds of spores, amoebulae, not needing to be motile, and flagellulae, which do need it. That is all.[3]

I wrote on the 5th to Leslie applying for Rewa and enclose a copy of his reply,[4] by which it seems that there is very little chance for me. Last June he led me to expect an early appointment (see copy of his telegram).[5] If he had told me before that men in "Foreign Office regiments" have prior claims it would have saved me five months' suspense. But this sort of thing is typical of the Service.

Well, on receipt of this letter of his I wrote (yesterday) again to him applying for Cunningham's post and telling him that it is impossible to work here and that I had been dragged away from Secunderabad just as I hoped to solve the question of the pigmented cells, about which I had already reported fully, officially. I asked him also (with the greatest politeness) to endeavour to let me know as soon as convenient whether there is any chance of my getting Cunningham's place, or any other appointment except regimental employ, because, if not, I would try to get back to Secunderabad as soon as possible (when the troops return from Tirah) in order to finish my research there, or would endeavour to get furlough for six months to England (if I cannot otherwise get out of this place). I hope to get his answer by the 25th if he replies at all.

It is necessary to let you know all this, I think, in case I may never be able to complete the theory & because you have been so kindly trying to get me Cunningham's billet. The fact is of course that I am in such a tight hole here that I really don't know what I may not have to do to get out of it. I *think* I am here only temporarily, but am not sure. I may be posted here for years, and they have expressly refused to give me any information on the point. If I am posted here permanently, good-bye to work, because neither malaria nor dysentery are common enough in the station for research on them. Then, while I am kept in this state of doubt, I cannot bring my wife & children from Bangalore (5 days' journey) because I may perhaps be ordered back to Secunderabad at a moment's notice. I have to keep them meanwhile at an expensive hotel in Bangalore. At the end of next February they *must* go to the hills or to England. If I see no chance of being settled by then I must *take* them to England or else I may not see them for years. As I wrote you last May it does not pay me to remain in regimental employ, more especially as my regiment goes to Burma next year. Hence on the whole it is extremely likely that I shall be forced to try to get ordinary furlough next February. This will not compel me to take my pension next June, but if I can't get it I may have to apply for "furlough in anticipation of retirement" which will finish me so far as the Service is concerned. All this of course would be nothing for a bachelor, but it is very different when one has a family to consider. All this uncertainty for instance is making my wife ill & is not improving my health, and my children must have a cool climate after February. I shall, you may be sure, do my utmost to clear up the "pigmented cells", but I should tell you that it is quite possible I may never be able to tackle them again. Somebody else can do it now, however, and even if I can't get a civil appointment I may, just possibly, be able to get back to Secunderabad in December & put in a few months' work before the hot weather. Then perhaps Owen may get the Princes to take me up (?) or the unexpected may happen. So I don't despair of the Service yet. Another month ought to settle it, & I will let you know what occurs.

With kind regards
Yours sincerely
R. Ross.

P. S. By the way it is sad to see that Laveran still sticks to the folly of the unity of the parasite. Marchoux also adopts it, and Metchnikoff[6] has gone in for it, apparently on Laveran's persuasion. What a curious argument Laveran uses. He admits that different forms of the parasite are found but says that the difference is due to climatic and similar influences. Marchoux says it is due to the resistance of some patients being greater than that of others. Not only is this quite unlikely and about as much as to say that a horse will change into a donkey if fed on thistles & kept in the proper kind of paddock, but won't explain facts I, for instance, have seen. At Begumpett we have tertians & remittents; close by at Hyderabad there are *quartans* & remittents. At Madras there are nearly all quartans; at Bangalore nearly all remittents with a few tertians from one locality. Fresh infections always (with the exception of rare cases of mixed parasites) show one or other of the various species.

The thing is so marked out here that I personally have no doubt of plurality of species. What a lot I scribble to you! Absolutely nothing else to do

R. R.

1 Presumably Laveran (1896) and Simond (1897b).

2 E. Marchoux, (1862-1943), then working in Saint Louis, Senegal. See **Biographical Appendix**.

3 *Memoirs*, 251, admitted that Simond had been correct, though Ross did not reproduce this portion of his letter.

4 **RA** 02/135. Ross's transcription of a letter from Leslie dated Simla 12 Nov. 1897:
"Dear Surgeon Major Ross. In reply to your note of 5th inst. You may be sure that the Director General will not overlook your claims, but it will be necessary for the Foreign Department to provide, in the first instance, for officers who have been serving in Foreign Office regiments in hopes of civil appointments under the Foreign Office.
Yours sincerely
J T W Leslie"

5 **RA** 02/135. Ross's transcription of a telegram from Leslie, dated Simla, 28 June 1897: "You will probably get an appointment under the foreign office soon but cannot say when."

6 Elie Metchnikoff, (1845-1916), bacteriologist at the Pasteur Institute, Paris. See **Biographical Appendix**.

Letter 102
01/176

TELEGRAM

Bombay
2. 12. 97

To Dr Manson
21 Queen Anne Street Cavendish Square London.

Health Institute refuses apply for my services advise you make one last effort on behalf of theory and myself if not almost certainly leave India next March if possible wire result.

R. R.

Letter 103
[Enclosed with Letter 106]
02/136

Kherwara
6th Dec. 1897

Dear Dr Manson,
Just before last mail left I heard from Owen that there is no chance of my becoming attached to the Health Institute.[1] Accordingly I wired off (post-registered from Bombay) acquainting you with the fact.[2] Since then I have heard that the appointment at Rewa, which I was hoping to get after the Director General's telegram of last June, has been given to another.[3] I have also heard from Surgeon General McVittie[4] P. M. O. Madras Command in reply to my letter of six weeks ago asking to be transferred from my regiment the 19th M. I.[5] at Secunderabad to one of two regiments at Bangalore which will be vacant in a few months, & explaining that such a transfer would enable me to remain in India & continue work. The matter is a trifle to arrange and a similar transfer has lately been made in the case of one of the very regiments I have asked for; but my request has been absolutely refused. Lastly, I have received no answer to my letter of a month ago to Leslie, asking him if there was any chance of my getting Cunningham's place or any civil billet.

I wired also asking you whether you could make one last effort on behalf of the theory and myself. This I did with much hesitation since you have already taken so much trouble in the matter; but after long thought I *do* consider it advisable to worry you once more & I sincerely hope for the very last time. But what I will do is simply this - put the present position fully before you & leave you to judge whether it is or is not *possible* for you to do anything, or *advisable* or *necessary*. I leave that to you; but I shall be very grateful to you if you will telegraph to me (I enclose cheque for £2) whether anything can or cannot be done.

My prospects as a medical officer are now as follows:-

If I enter the Foreign Department I can do so only at the tail of the list (since Rewa is given away & since Leslie says that precedence must be given to officers already in regiments in that department), & this order will probably be followed hereafter, so that I must come after men even ten years my juniors, to the end of time. This means there is nothing for me here.

In the Madras Civil Department the same thing holds, so that there is nothing for me there.

In the Madras Military Department I must stick to my own regiment (which goes to Burma next year) and owing to the number of men above me I can perhaps never hope to reach the administrative grade - a simply wretched prospect.

The Health Institute is I fear a dead hope.

Hence all I have now to look forward to in the service is inferior appointments, bad pay, & probably bad stations. The last will certainly necessitate my sending my wife & children home, so that I shall scarcely ever see them for years. My income, small as it will be, will be divided in two in order to keep up two establishments. I see no prospect of ever rising to the top of the tree in any department of my service, nor any prospect of doing interesting & useful sanitary work, or ordinary professional work except on the most limited scale. Research work may not be possible if I am kept in stations like this, and it will never be easy with a "sore back". I shall see men years and years junior to myself drawing double my pay all round me. Thus I picture myself (and I assure you, without the smallest exaggeration) growing old in some small, hot, out-of-the-way station, apart from my wife and children, hard-up, disappointed, with nothing to do, research work possible only a few months in the year, hopeless prospects, and finally indifference to all work - there are scores - hundreds of such men in India at the present moment. And do not believe that *any* work done by me in the future will get me out of such a groove. I saw clearly last May when I first bothered you with all this, that if the work done by me up to then would not help me, no work that I can ever do ever will help me. Work such as mine in Bangalore would in any other branch of public service have pushed me on. In the medical it is of no use, because the medical services have become stagnant ponds full of torpid old carp (so to speak!). The heads of the service don't & won't recognise anything but seniority & red-tape rules. I am afraid this is a little bitter, but is it not absolutely true? Look at the whole state of tropical medicine in this country. I don't believe that 2% of the men know how to find the malaria parasite & I really don't believe that three men *in all* in both the services have ever seen *amoeba coli*. Do you think that these men will push a man for researches? Never. Quite the reverse, if anything.

Well, I draw this picture of my future prospects chiefly in order to justify myself to you in case I have now to give up *the theory*. I feel that it would be impossible for me to acquiesce in such a future - and this future will most certainly be mine unless I can make an effective move at this juncture. It would be *impossible* because I should only become ill & have to leave whether I liked it or not.

If I give up the service now I shall have my small pension of £292 a year which with the little money which we have of our own will enable us at least to live. I shall be independent. I am comparatively young and can work. I shall have my wife & children with me and I shall be spared the discomforts of Indian life.

Which would you choose if you were me?

You will ask, why can't I remain in Secunderabad, clear up the pigmented-cell business, and *then* decide about the future. For many reasons. (1) I may be kept here where investigation is, I assure you, quite impossible, or I may be sent on plague duty. (2) I doubt whether I can completely prove the theory in a short time; I think I could prove the matter to our own satisfaction in a few weeks or months, but then I should have to make numbers of specimens for demonstration, I should have to test various species of mosquito with various kinds of fever, & lastly I should have to find how the germs pass from mosquitoes to human beings - work possibly requiring incubators & laboratory conveniences. It would all take me two years perhaps. I have thought it out well. (3) If I am to leave the service at all, the sooner I leave it the better. I am over forty & can't afford to throw away years as if I were twenty. (4) My family must leave Bangalore in March either for England or for the hills. If the latter I shall scarcely see them at all until about this time next year, & after that my children will be old enough to go home for good. I have seen them for only one week since last June. Lastly, the pigmented cells may turn out a false scent (not at all likely, but possible) in which case all my sacrifice of time & labour will be thrown away.

Next you will exclaim, "but the Government have promised to put you on malaria duty." Yes, but *when*? I fear I know Govt. very well. After this frontier business there will be the plague; after that the "financial condition" will remain. Then someone will pooh-pooh the whole theory. Then they will forget all about it; and lastly, if I remind them of it, they will tell me to mind my own business.

Well, all this may sound pessimistic, but I think it is only right to consider it carefully. The question is, how to get out of the *imbroglio*? There is only one way, and that is to be got at by considering the main point at issue - the theory, and how to get it proved. If I go home without proving it after having reached the stage of the pigmented cells, I shall ever afterwards feel myself a weak kind of ineffectual creature. If I can succeed in proving it I shall not care what happens & can leave the service if necessary with a good conscience. The way to get it proved and at the same time to enable me to prove it without giving up my whole future prospects to it is to *get Government to start the investigation as soon as possible.* Instead of my struggling on with private research, interrupted by other duties & liable to be packed off at a moment's notice to plague duty or cholera duty, I shall have a free hand, full time & perhaps laboratory conveniences & shall be free from the "sore back" which I suffer from at present. At the end of the investigation if they don't choose to give me something in the service, I can leave it with a sense of duty done. I think you will agree with this. In short, I am not prepared to sacrifice, with my present prospects in the service, one or two more years of my life, for the mere *chance* of being able to continue my malaria work; I am prepared to sacrifice them, and with pleasure, for the certainty of continuing it. I would even prefer to take my pension & work in the malarious parts of Italy rather than waste my time here as I have been compelled to do during the last few months.

And in asking to be put on malaria work now I ask in reality nothing at all. It is so easy. As soon as the frontier operations come to a close, quite a hundred doctors will be released and Govt. will have no lack of medical officers, more especially as a number of doctors have been lately sent out from England to manage the plague.[6] Moreover the investigation will not cost Govt. *one penny.* I am willing (and please say so if you think necessary) to undertake the research on reduced pay, namely on the bare salary of my rank, and to give up my regimental allowance to the man who does my work in the regiment. I am also willing to pay my travelling expenses myself. Hence the plea of cost cannot be opposed to the proposal. Nor can the plea of paucity of medical officers be put forward, both because there will be no such paucity in a month or two, and because the doctor in charge of the regiment next to mine in Secunderabad will readily undertake my work, as he does at the present moment, for the R100 a month regimental allowance which I am willing to give up to him. In fact we ask Govt. to do really nothing more that to take the trouble of *drafting an order.*

I think you will agree that we are entitled to ask this little from Government. The work is of the utmost importance to India, the mortality from malaria being from five to ten thousand lives *daily* according to statistics. We have been thinking & worrying over the business for years. I have given up for it leave, leisure and appointments, and with your instructions have now carried the theory to the point nearly of proof, and that without the slightest assistance, active or passive, of Govt. or anyone but yourself - quite the reverse because when on the point of success I have been packed off to a station where it has been impossible to continue work. Surely then we may now venture to ask Govt. to take a little - ever so little - trouble, not expense, for the sake of the work.

You will now ask, why can't I apply direct to the Govt. of India in the above terms? Because I am nearly sure that the application coming from me would receive only the same answer "not practicable at present." Or it would take months in being dealt with - or I should be simply told not to give trouble. I should have to waste months in waiting for a reply and then it would be unsatisfactory.

Lastly, you will ask why, since I am willing to sacrifice pay for the research, do I not ask simply for one year's ordinary leave in India & do it. Because I don't think I would get it; because I should be always liable to recall at a moment's notice; and because I should like to get furlough after the work is done in order to come home & show you everything in order to put the work on a sound footing, and I could never get furlough after a year's leave in India. In fact I feel that I have done my utmost already; & you must remember that I cannot write all this frankly to my superiors as to you. Indeed I am scarcely allowed to write at all.

No, there is only one thing to be done, and that is to get the Secretary of State to interest himself in the matter. If he does, the Govt. of India will I am sure come forward at once; if not there will be delays *ad infinitum* in spite of Mr Hewett's statement to the effect that the Govt. of India are anxious to undertake the work. A word (but a strong one) from the Secretary of State will finish the matter. I don't mean to say that the Govt. of India will not do their best; but they have so many claims upon them that without urging and reminding they are, I feel, very likely to forget our humble investigation. They are also apt, I fear, to forget that their humble servants have exigencies as well as themselves and that sometimes they cannot be kept waiting for ever. The work is deferred, the instrument allowed to rust. When the work is at last taken in hand what wonder if the instrument be sometimes found to be no longer available? I think the facts of the discovery of the "pigmented cells" and of my being now placed in a situation where I cannot continue work will be enough to warrant our going before the Secretary of State again. Unless he acts, the investigation will be almost certainly deferred until the plague ceases - a poor prospect, because the plague will probably last for years yet. By that time I fear that, unless something unforeseen happens, my services will no longer be available.

If the Secretary of State will act, it is important to note that the investigation should last quite one year, that it should be directed entirely to the mosquito theory and that I should be given a pretty free hand. If not I may be put on all sorts of odd jobs & sent to places which are not suitable for research.

I have no *complaints* to make. My poor prospects are a great deal my own fault in my not having got a footing in the Foreign or Madras Civil earlier.[7]

With kind regards

Yours sincerely

R. Ross.

1 Telegram from Owen (1 Dec. 1897) saying no arrangements were practicable at that time. **RA** 02/299, (Gibson, 1983).
2 Letter 102.
3 The person who received the appointment has not been identified.
4 Charles Edwin McVittie, (1842-1916), Surgeon-General (military), Madras.
5 Madras Infantry.
6 For recent accounts of the Indian plague epidemic, see Harrison (1994) and Arnold (1993).
7 Harrison (1994), chapter 1, examines the career structure of the IMS.

Letter 104
[Enclosed with Letter 105]
02/037

21 Queen Anne Street,
Cavendish Square. W.
10th Nov. 1897.

Dear Ross,

The Council of the British Medical Association have determined (wisely I think) to give Tropical Medicine a recognition at the forthcoming meeting at Edinburgh next July and (unwisely I fear) have appointed me President of the Section.

Naturally I am anxious to have the Section a success, and would be very much obliged if you would come to my assistance with a paper on some Tropical Medical or Surgical subject, and, also, with any preparations, microscopical slides, drug, or instrument having a bearing on Tropical Medicine. Please do what you can to let people here and on the Continent know that we are not asleep.

Hoping you are all quite well and with kind regards,

Believe me,

Yours very truly

Patrick Manson

Letter 105
02/038

21, Queen Anne Street,
Cavendish Square. W.
17th November, 1897.

My dear Ross,

I hope you will try to do something in response to the enclosed. I have sent it to a lot of workers in tropical medicine and trust the result will be to get a good practical justification for the B. M. A.'s determining to institute a tropical section at their annual meetings.

Probably this week's Journal will contain your article and you will see from it what I have done to shove the matter on. Your position has been well guarded and there, in future, can be no question in the matter of priority in discovery. I also wrote the leader so as to give the friends you have a handle to work with in attempts on the Indian Government. I have ordered a number of reprints of article and leader. Some of these I will send to you; some I will keep for distribution here. Don't despair. If I can work it I shall not lose an opportunity of doing so.

You will see in last week's Lancet a short notice by MacCallum of Johns Hopkins's[1] Hosp. about a new view on the meaning of exflagellation.[2] It may be correct; but even if correct it does not invalidate the mosquito theory. Perhaps fecundation of the sphere takes place in the mosquito's stomach prior to the formation of the vermicule which is really the penetrating spore carrying the plasmodium into the mosquito cell. Thin is wrong about oil having got into the slides.[3] One, somehow, has gone off very much but the other still shows the pigmented cells very well and I have had them photographed and the photographer is still at work on them trying to get the best results. They are a fact and I dont share with Thin his view that they are simply pigment absorbed by the epithelium. He has his own axe to grind about the influence of pigment on liver cells and he drags in your discovery to strengthen his own position.[4] Does it not occur to you that it is quite possible the plasmodium might be able to manufacture a black pigment from organic material other than haemoglobin. There are many black pigments that do not contain iron. I fancy we are to apt to think that the black pigment is black because it is manufactured from haemoglobin and because this substance contains a notable proportion of iron. I do not know that it has been proved that melanin owes its colour to iron.

I have read Rogers' report on Kala-azar.[5] In many respects it is a goodish report but he is too weak altogether on the subject of the plasmodium. He evidently does not understand the subject thoroughly and it would be well if some one like yourself would go over the ground again entirely from the stand point of the parasite. He says he has never seen crescents in Assam malaria. I, even here, have frequently seen them in Europeans from Assam. He says crescents are very rare in Indian malaria. I have just now no fewer than three patients with malaria contracted in the river at Calcutta with plenty of crescents in their blood. He has written too cock-assuredly altogether and too much from the stand point of infallibility.

I made a curious observation on flagellated body evolution on Monday. I was watching a sphere in the throes of parturition. I saw it shoot out flagella first on one side then on the other but it failed to get the flagella through the cyst wall and *quickly drew them in again* and *tried in another place*. This it went on doing for quite a quarter of an hour; finally it got one through but it was so spent that it had not force to break away and after two or three languid waggles ceased to move. I could see the cyst wall distinctly outside the flagella as they were poked this way and that. The presence of the cyst wall at the base of the flagellum gave it a triangular look - like a very much elongated isosceles triangle.

Thus:

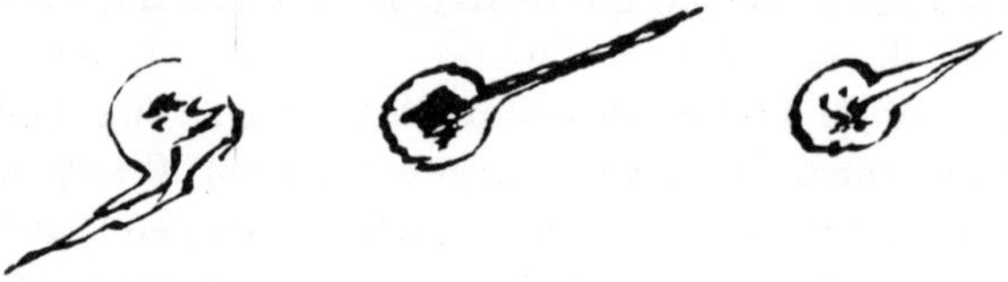

I hope you have got a move to some suitable station for the prosecution of your mission which is, the solution of the problem of the extra-corporeal life history of the malaria parasite.

Yours sincerely
Patrick Manson

I forgot to say that the best article on coccidial flagellation is in Annal. du L'Instit. Pasteur - July 1897.[6]

Your experiments on the tertians are most interesting & I only wish you could follow them up. Yanks, Italians & French are all on the scent now, I fear.

1 As in Letter 38, Manson wrote '**John** Hopkins'.
2 W. G. MacCallum, 'On the flagellated form of the malarial parasite', *Lancet* (13 Nov. 1897), 1240-1241. See **Biographical Appendix**.
3 Thin wrote that before he examined the preparations a second time, some change had taken place which caused the tissues to refract the light more strongly and that this was probably caused by the introduction of cedar oil under the edge, (Ross, 1897f).
4 In discussing the pigment in Ross's preparations, Thin remarked that liver cells have a peculiar capacity to take up pigment.
5 Rogers (1897b). See also Helen J. Power, 'Sir Leonard Rogers FRS (1868-1962): Tropical medicine in the Indian Medical Service' (PhD thesis: University of London, 1993).
6 Simond (1897b).

Letter 106
02/137

Kherwara
9th Dec. 1897

Dear Dr Manson,
I wrote you the enclosed lugubrious letter the other day when I felt rather down at having all my applications refused. Since then I have been much heartened by yours of the 17th Nov. but on reading over my letter find it sound enough still to send you. I think the only way out of the wood is to try to get the Sec. of State to act. It is perfectly useless my writing to Leslie or to anyone else in this country, and I can't form a conception as to what they are going to do with me or how long they will keep me here. We are now fully justified in going up to the Secretary of State again. If we let the investigation slip through our fingers now we shall probably never catch it again. At least, if the S. of S. does not see his way to hurrying up the investigation he may tip them the word to put me somewhere where I can work, or even to send me back sharp to my regiment. I think however by your letter that you are already taking action.

Will you do me one more favour? That is to wire to me if you *ascertain* that any *strong action* is going to be taken. It would be a boon and may save me applying for furlough. If nothing can be done, or nothing at all certain to be effective, please don't wire. On the other hand, if I hear anything which will obviate action on your part, I will wire it to "Finically, London".

I fear there is no chance of Cunningham's place, but it would enable me to do really good work & is worth trying for. They have made Grant[1] Bacteriologist in Madras. The Madras men say he knows nothing. That is the way things are done. Owen's refusal to put me on the H[ealth] Institute appears now to be temporary (?). His letter[2] is very kind and polite but through it evidently runs an entire distrust of the theory. I can scarcely send it to you. He is afraid that if the Institute takes me on and then the theory fails, the Institute's reputation will suffer! He also seems to think that I have been theorising too much & talking too much. Haffkine[3] who is to be the head of the Institute advises "quiet pursuance of your studies without stirring up exaggerated expectations & artificially exciting attention". I am replying suitably & reminding him very gently of the cholera inoculation business![4] In this world it is necessary to excite attention, I fear. Well, if this is the spirit in which men like Haffkine & Owen take the theory, you can imagine that Cleghorn, Sibthorpe & McVittie look upon it as either an amusing scientific bagatelle or else a kind of charlatanism to attract notoriety. They won't lift a finger to assist, I assure you, as has now become quite clear to me. In fact I saw in May last that if the affair is to be carried through the impetus must come from England and must be pushed even against the resistance of the medical services. Well, it is worth trying, but no help in India is to be expected, I warn you.

I am delighted to hear of the tropical disease section with you as President. If I can only get to work again I will promise you something worth reading. The B. M. J. of Nov. 20th does not contain the article on the cells, so I will wait until I see the same before discussing the cells further.

Yours sincerely

R. Ross.

Make use of my letter of the 6th enclosed as you like.

1 Letter 78, note 3.

2 Letter from Owen (3 Dec. 1897). **RA** 01/113. See Letter 107.

3 Waldemar M. W. Haffkine, (1860-1930), Bacteriologist in Calcutta. The quotation is from Owen's telegram, Letter 103, note 1. See **Biographical Appendix.**

4 Haffkine had arrived in India in 1893 from the Pasteur Institute with his anti-cholera vaccine. See Ilana Löwy, 'From guinea pigs to man: the development of Haffkine's anticholera vaccine', *Journal of the History of Medicine and Allied Sciences*, 47 (1992), 270-309.

Letter 107
02/138

Kherwara
14th Dec.
1897

Dear Dr Manson,
I have of course been making every effort to get to work here. I fear that this is the most impossible place in India for it. I get only a very few cases of fever which turn out to be the mildest possible quartans with one or two parasites found with great difficulty in a whole specimen, & temperature reaching only about 101°F, and generally no second attack. Next, it is so cold that there is great difficulty in breeding mosquitoes at all, and, when hatched, they die as soon as they are let out of the bottle, & absolutely refuse to bite under the net - I have tried them on myself. Lastly the people here who are very ignorant & superstitious jungle folk (Bhils) won't have the experiments at any price. It is no go, in fact. I have however been examining bloods of frogs, toads, fish & numerous birds without result, until today, when I got Halteridium in a blue-rock pigeon (dead three hours). No flagellate forms & no fleas - but I will examine more of these birds. The forms were

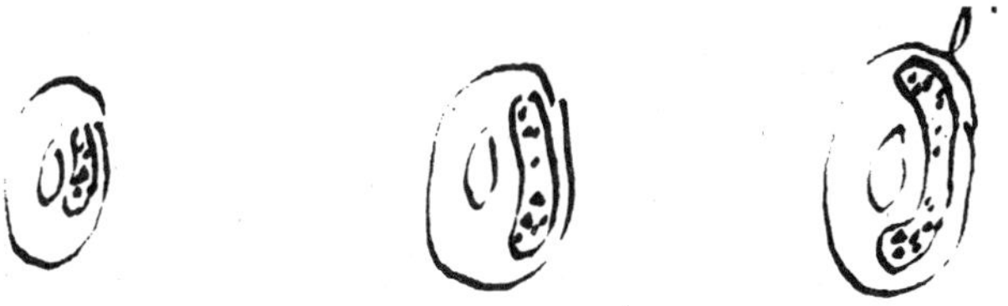

They became spherical on addition of water & the corpuscle lost the haemoglobin.

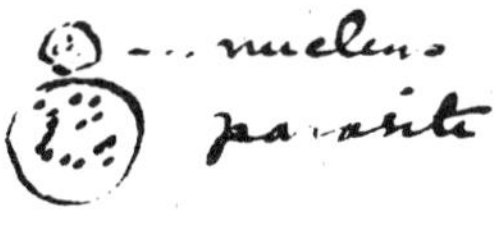

The figure then presented was closely similar to that shown by a crescent-sphere 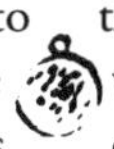 with the familiar little ball on its edge. Hence I think that this little ball may be the *remains of the nucleus* of the human red blood corpuscle. If I could examine fleas from pigeons containing halteridium I might do some work.

The more I look at my two specimens of pigmented cells the more difficult it appears to consider these bodies as anything but parasites. They *can't* be physiological cells, phagocytes, etc. They are too exceptional altogether. They don't *look* like phagocytes, all of them having almost exactly the same amount of pigment. Then they certainly appear to grow in size in proportion to the time after ingestion.

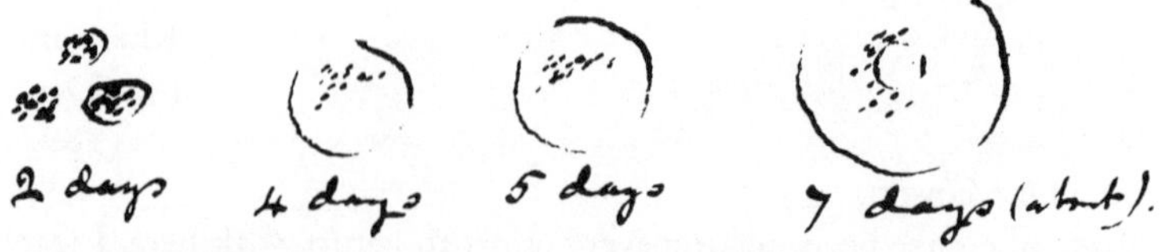

You say in yours of the 17th. Nov. that the cells are not to be made out very clearly in one of your specimens; that was the one at 4 days. I told you it was difficult, in my letters.

It makes me gnash my teeth being here! Just like a prison. One family of Europeans, one sick Lieutenant, two case of itch, one of ulcer & one bruise case in hospital. Absolutely nothing to do from morning to night & no work possible. It takes 5 days to get an answer by *telegram* from my family at Bangalore & 11 days by post! Luckily they are well at present. I will try my best with the blue-rock pigeons.

Owen's letter is a very funny one.[1] I wish I could send it to you, but he seems to want the matter kept private. However, I think I may give you the heads of his discourse. He, Dholpur[2] and Haffkine seem to have had a committee meeting over my application. They won't apply for me because they think Govt. will put me on malaria duty. That is all well, but then Owen goes on to remark "how fatal it is for any investigator to attract undue attention to his work at a time when the results he has to show are full of doubt & uncertainty." It would ruin the Health Institute if such an investigator should be brought on its strength & then fail. Then the solution of the malaria problem may lie in another direction to that in which I seem to believe, and (he thinks) I even have an inkling of this! "You can estimate (he says) what might be your position if such should be the case." My ideas may possibly change when I commence real laboratory work as they did when you first showed me the malaria parasite. Then he advises me to read the "vast literature of the subject" & above all to go and see Haffkine, if I can do so "quietly & without attracting attention", and he will be able to clear up many "doubtful points." I replied thanking him & saying that if the theory were disproved tomorrow I should have nothing to lose, but that, on the contrary, the negative result would be important. I might have added that the more attention is attracted to the subject the better, even if the theory prove wrong in the end, especially in a country where every scientific problem is grossly neglected. But what was the use of arguing? This is the common view in this country. If a man is enthusiastic he is advertising himself; if he takes up a subject, he is a faddist and a crank; if he does not belong to some Institute or other, he is a mere amateur!

The Pioneer published your lecture[3] and shortly afterwards an absurd letter from B. Sc. appeared controverting your views.[4] I am sending this letter to the Editor B. M. J. as a curiosity and as a convincing proof of your strictures on education in tropical disease. It really ought to be reprinted *in extenso*; the writer is an unconscious humourist of the finest water. I don't know who he is. *Not* Lawrie *certainly*, because a letter from him appeared formerly in the same number of the Pioneer as one from Lawrie; but of the tribe.

Has anyone ever been convinced by argument even to demonstration? Seldom, I believe. Men stick to their prejudices like limpets to rocks - the tighter the more one tries to pull them off.

What alarms me about Owen's telegram and letter is the fact that he and Haffkine have great influence with the Indian Govt. & as they don't seem to think much of the theory and hold that it has been too much written up, Govt. is very likely to be of the same opinion and may *very probably* abandon the malaria investigation entirely on reconsideration. I felt this strongly as soon as I got Owen's telegram; and it was this which decided me to ask you to attempt one last effort. Thin's opinions about the pigmented cells will be sure to be jumped at by all of them, so that I should not wonder if the discovery of those cells, so far from making Govt. take the matter up, will cause them to drop it *ad infinitum*. It astonished me that Govt. entertained the idea of the investigation so readily as they did; and I feel that if they are allowed to cool on it, they won't touch it so quickly again. You should not put much reliance on Hewett's letter (which I return with thanks); it is diplomatic, nothing more. No; unless pretty strong pressure can be brought to bear from Home, nothing will be done I fear.

On second thoughts, if you find that Sir C. Crosthwaite & the Sec. of State won't move any more in the matter (as I believe likely) and if nothing pretty likely to be effective can be done, will you telegraph the fact to me? My address should be Ronald Ross, Kherwara, Rajputana, India. Some message like "Secretary State acting", or "Strong action taken" or "No action possible" will give me definite information to go upon. This letter ought to reach you about the 5th January. As my children must leave Bangalore at the end of February either for the hills or for England, I should if we decide to come home, send in my application for furlough by the 15th January at the latest.

If you wire that you can do nothing, I shall be forced to depend on events as they occur here & shall not, therefore, make up my mind to do anything until the very last moment. If I see any likelihood of being able to get work again shortly, you may depend on it I will try to remain in the hope of being able to obtain proof at least of the cells being present only in insects fed on malarial blood. But if I see no such likelihood I think it will be wisest to try to come home on ordinary furlough. I may perhaps be able with your assistance to work matters when at home. I *may try* to get six months' leave in India to carry on the work, instead of six months' furlough to England; but I am pretty sure they will refuse it so long as plague is about. Furlough to England is a kind of right of ours; leave in India for more that 2 months is not.

The B. M. J. for Nov. 27th. (In which I suppose the *article*[5] will be) will not reach me until after this letter is posted. I am looking forward to seeing all your remarks anent the cells. Whether your article[6] (for which, thanks in advance) will affect the Indian Medical *Carp*, except to wrath, remains to be seen. I suppose they will talk about "artificially attracting attention" and so on.

My pay if I remain in India in military employment as seems inevitable will be £500 a year, or a very little over. Out of this we shall have to save quite £100 a year to pay the outrageous price of passages home and the rest will have to be divided into two parts to provide for two establishments one in India & one at home. Thus we shall be actually better off if we take our pension of £292 a year. By my pay of £500 I mean *net* pay after deducting subscriptions to Family Fund, mess, etc which are compulsory & very heavy. Hence it would be absurd for me to remain in India with all its discomforts & separations. My pension will increase only by £70 a year after three years more service. Again my wife, who is not strong & dreads separations, *must* be parted either from me or our children in a year or so. I tell you this to make it quite clear to you that it is almost impossible for me to stay in India in regimental employment. In good civil employment of course, the pay is practically doubled.

I found trypanosomes in a fish today. They were flatter & broader & more scarce than in the rat.

I enclose Col. Robertson's orders on my work in Bangalore,[7] as they may be useful in case you decide on making another effort. I believe something must have gone wrong with the Sec. State's former letter. Don't make any *complaints* on my behalf - it only riles them; and don't trouble *much* any way.

Yours sincerely

R. Ross.

1 Letter 106, note 2.

2 i.e. the Maharaja of Dholpur.

3 Probably Manson (1897c).
4 Not traced.
5 Ross (1897f).
6 Manson's leader 'A malaria problem', *BMJ* (18 Dec. 1897), 1805-1806.
7 Ross had sent a copy of these orders in Letter 76, enclosure 11.

Letter 108
(Telegram)[1]
02/298

21 Queen Anne Street,
Cavendish Square. W.

[27 Dec. 1897?]

Ross, Kherwara Rajpootana[2]
Fayrer Manson have written Cleghorn

1 This letter is in Manson's hand and may have been a rough note for Letter 109.
2 Note spelling (Rajputana).

Letter 109
01/177
Indian Telegraph

From
Station London P.O.

To Station Rajpootana
To Ross
Kherwara
Rajpootana
India

official pressure
injudicious
fayrer written
cleghorn

7 JA 98

Letter 110
02/139

Kherwara
13th Jan 1897 [sic]

Dear Dr Manson,
You can imagine my delight at getting your telegram[1] & also the pigmented-cell article[2] on the same day, the 8th. As it "pans out" it is just as well that official pressure cannot be brought to bear at present, because owing to the continuance of the Afridi business & the consequent closing of all leave it will be quite impossible for me to get away by March. I shall certainly not be able to leave India until May I think, and if leave is not open then, as I doubt it will be, not until June 23rd when my pension is due. I trust Sir W. Fayrer's[3] letter will be able to effect something, but have my doubts as I have twice informed Leslie that I cannot work here. However, as I cannot apply for leave now I must "willy-nilly" await events. If only I could get back to Secunderabad I might almost promise you something really good for the tropical section. I have taken rooms for my family in the Neilgherries from the middle of March. Of course the stoppage of leave prevents me from applying for leave to carry on malaria research, so that, unless the authorities can be moved I shall probably be boxed here indefinitely. Work still quite impossible of course, and not likely to be possible until the rains in June. I have done a small research, interesting but negative, on horse-flies feeding on pigeons with halteridium, and will tell you about it in my next. No pigmented cells in the flies. The notes on the specimens are most interesting to me, & Dr Thin's remarks respecting my work flattering indeed.[4] The editorial[5] is an honour & the illustrations excellent. So I am in a happy frame of mind in spite of suppressed rage at not being able to get on with the work. Dr Thin has fallen into a horrible pit. His needle-shaped pigment & so on in the epithelial cells are the *effect of formaline*! Now I feel that this error ought to be corrected & the two other cases of pigmented cells given. So I have written a letter to the Editor B.M.J. which they may have room for.[6] At the same time as I am correcting Dr Thin's views I have written the enclosed letter to him.[7] Would you mind addressing it?

I see quite clearly that the pigmented cells *cannot* be physiological cells at all. This view is incompatible with the 3rd & 4th mosquitoes. So I have given the reasons as briefly as possible in my letter to the B.M.J.

Next mail I am going to bother you more on this subject; but must leave off now. With many thanks for all your trouble.

Believe me

Yours sincerely

R. Ross.

1 Letter 109.

2 Ross (1897f).

3 Ross meant Sir J Fayrer. See **Biographical Appendix**.

4 Thin's comments at the end of Ross's paper (note 2). Thin concluded his comments by urging the Indian Government to provide Ross with 'support, assistance if required, and every facility,' in order that he could continue his researches.

5 i.e. Manson (1897f).

6 R. Ross, 'Pigmented cells in mosquitos', *BMJ* (26 Feb. 1898), 550-551, but see Letter 111.

7 Not located.

Letter 111
02/141

Kherwara

19th Jan. [1898]

Dear Dr Manson,

Today is mail-day but I have had to go 14 miles into the country to see the Maharawal of Dungapore[1] & so cannot write all I wanted to say about the "cells". I sent the Editor B. M. J. a letter on them last mail, and this mail I am sending him a better written one which I have asked him to substitute for the former one. I think it may be useful to correct the error due to the formaline, to give an account of the two new observations & to put views straight in regard to one or two points as illuminated by these new observations. Perhaps however you may think we have had enough talk on the subject for the present; in which case don't hesitate to suppress my letter, which I suppose will be sent to you for approval.

I have considered very carefully & with great interest all the remarks on the cells. They are very much to the point & Thin's views are intelligible enough considering the unfortunate effect of the formaline. I see however that they are really out of the question after the two new cases. I wish I had sent you the specimens; but I am glad you did not refer to these new cases in your remarks. The cells cannot be any physiological cells; they must be pathological. Looked at from every side they cannot really be pigment *producing* normal cells & how can they be exceptional pigment-producing cells? As for cells absorbing pigment from the stomach cavity - the stomach cells don't do such a thing. They would always be stuffed full of all kinds of debris if they were capable of such action. And why of all things should they take the trouble to absorb dead pigment? Is it likely? Then case 4 is a crushing reply to Thin's hypothesis. No - it won't work. The cells are pathological. What then? - they are the malaria parasite in the mosquito simply because they *can't* be anything else.

I will tell you about my halteridium research in my next. I hope Sir J. Fayrer's letter will do good,[2] but believe that I am likely to be here till June. The P. M. O. has been here & seen the specimens; he says he will try to get me out of the place (?).

With kind regards

Yours sincerely

R. Ross.

1 Dungarpur is an administrative district and town in Rajasthan.

2 Not located.

Letter 112
02/039

21 Queen Anne Street,
Cavendish Square. W.
27th December, 1897.

My dear Ross,

Before proceeding to business let me express the hope that you have had a happy Christmas and that you are going to have a happy and prosperous new year. Presentiment points to the latter.

I duly received your telegram[1] of 3rd inst and letters of 6th and 9th December and also the cheque for two pounds. The telegram came first and I at once set to work to find out what could be done. I wrote to Sir Charles Crosthwaite enclosing your article in the B. M. J. and the leading article thereon. I enclose his reply.[2] Of course the latter is very private and confidential and not to be used. I also went to Sir Joseph Fayrer and had a long talk with him. I also consulted the B. M. J.

It is evident from Crosthwaite's letter that he does not think it advisable to force the hand of the Indian Government and Fayrer is of exactly the same opinion. They both, especially Fayrer, think that to attempt this would set the backs of the Indian officials up and do no good. They say that the Indian Medical Service must be directed from India. Fayrer was very decided about this. By Fayrer's advice I have written Cleghorn, who is an old friend of mine, and have asked him plump to lend you a hand. Fayrer has done the same. Fayrer was dead against going to Lord George Hamilton[3] or to the Viceroy.[4] There the matter rests at present. The article in the B. M. J. was a very strong one and if Cleghorn is to be influenced by public opinion it should do the trick for you. The notes by Thin, Bland Sutton and myself appended to your article will show Cleghorn what people here think of your work.

However things go yet awhile don't throw up the sponge. Of course the hardship you are called on to endure is very galling and almost insupportable; but such is the fate of nearly every one who makes a new departure and much of the merit of the discoverer lies in his faith and perseverance under difficulty. There are very few things worth having that are easily got. You should have heard Fayrer on the treatment that had been meted out to Vandyke Carter.[5] I feel that if you carry this mosquito business one step further that the battle is won and that your future is assured. I feel that if you chicked[6] it now you would regret the step ever afterwards for some one else would enter in and reap the harvest you have prepared with so much labour. If you succeed in proving the mosquito theory and if then the Indian Government will do nothing for you such a howl will go up from this side that they will shake in their shoes and have to mend their ways sharp. All you would have to do then would be to send in your proofs and demand opportunity to go on with the work. If still they refuse you might then apply to the home government and if they refuse there is America which wont.

Wait therefore till Cleghorn has got Fayrer's letter and mine. I think he will do his best for you. If you get a suitable place then work as hard as you can so as to justify his action, prove the theory and you will establish claims which will be irresistible. I think that you will find Cleghorn will befriend you.

I shall not cash your cheque unless I think there is urgency and need for telegraphing.

I hope that your next letter will tell me that you have had a transfer to some suitable spot and that work is in full swing again. The interruption was most unfortunate coming as it did when you seemed just on the point of laying your hand on the prize. No harm can come of it just at present as the Yanks and Italians dont have the chance of working on the mosquito during the winter and by the time their aestivo-autumnals are in full swing you, I hope, will have rounded up and completed the story. Much detail will have to be filled in afterwards, particularly the study of the various malaria bearing mosquitoes and the relationship of particular species to particular parasites. I fancy some of this might be better done in countries where special types of parasite are exclusively present. It would be easy to find out if there is a special mosquito in quartan lands, in tertian lands and so on. The mosquito species have all to be collected, classified and separately studied in relation to the parasite.

Wishing you patience, a fixed purpose and good luck,

I remain

Yours very sincerely

Patrick Manson

1 Presumably Letter 102 arriving a day later.
2 Letter untraced.
3 Lord George Francis Hamilton, (1845-1927), Secretary of State for India, 1895-1903.
4 Lord Elgin, see Letter 100, note 8.
5 Vandyke Carter, (1831-1897). See **Biographical Appendix**.
6 Slang: to show fear or indecision.

Letter 113
02/142

Kherwara

21st Jan. 1898

Dear Dr Manson,

Just after I dispatched my last letter I received your very kind one of the 27th Dec. Before thanking you for it let me finish my say about the "cells".

I told you that I had found Halteridium in a wild pigeon. Well I shot several more of these birds, together with doves, finches, etc, and found Halteridium in some of the first only. But none of the birds had any kind of ectoparasites - ticks, fleas, etc, though I searched them very carefully with a lens. Then I bethought me of Major Cole's tame pigeons.[1] These are persecuted by a horrible kind of black horse-flies which live among their feathers, flying out when disturbed but always returning even when the pigeon is held in the hand. They suck large quantities of blood from the poor birds; but *wild* pigeons do not have them - so that it appeared scarcely likely *a priori* that the Tabanus (horse-flies) could be the carrier of the Halteridium. But I set to work & examined 30 of the flies. The blood in the stomach when fresh contained numbers of Halteridium, showing that the tame pigeons are also infected; but there were no pigmented cells in the stomach or other tissues of the flies. The histology of Tabanus is just like that of Culex, so that here is another argument against Thin's theory.[2] I have also examined numbers of other Diptera - fleas, dung flies, horse flies & a few mosquitoes - but no pigmented cells.

The upshot of all this is that the cells cannot be any kind of physiological cell. At first I thought they might be epithelial cells capable of absorbing haemoglobin from the cavity & of converting it into pigment - a much more likely idea, I think, than that they are epithelial cells taking up dead malarial pigment, which is quite a gratuitous idea without *a priori* likelihood (confess it) or any evidence of facts. But if they are the *first*, we should find similar cells in most blood-feeding Diptera & certainly in most blood-fed insects of the same species. I admit that we may exceptionally find cells differing *slightly* from normal cells, without concluding that the former are pathological because they are exceptional. But the pigmented cells differ from the other stomach cells so markedly that we could not venture to think them normal but *slightly altered* cells, unless they were to be found very commonly. They are much too rare, in fact, to be anything but pathological cells. Cases 3 & 4 are simply conclusive of this, I think. No; look at it how you will, the cells are disease-cells of some kind. Of course it is just possible that they may be disease cells which have no connection with malaria; but if so it is very odd that they should have been found only in 4 insects all of which had been fed on malarial blood. I have really examined just as many if not more non-malaria-fed as malaria-fed insects. Lastly it would indeed be a strange discovery to find that mosquitoes are capable of harbouring pigment-bearing parasites which *du reste* have been only found in men and birds hitherto. On the other hand, *all* the known facts combine in favour of the cells being malaria parasites, and one of them alone - the presence of the pigment, otherwise so hard to explain - gives an extremely cogent reason for this view. You say there are many kinds of pigment; but I think that of the cells is related to haemoglobin, because formaline converts both into the same kind of small crystals. Now look at it all round & say what you think. Personally I believe I am *convinced* that the cells are malaria parasites.

More than this, I think the swarm spores are the spores of the pigmented cells; not because they were present in the Sigur mosquitoes or because they seemed to give a man fever, but because out of innumerable insects examined at Secunderabad the *only one* that contained them contained also large pigmented cells. Is this a mere coincidence? Perhaps; but the chances are heavy against it being so. What happens to the swarm spores? This will be the third part of the story. Are they discharged on the human skin from which they enter the blood through the puncture made by the mosquito; or are they discharged into water or on to damp surfaces where they can develop into Euglenae, mycetozoa or other protozoa?

Well, I will bet heavily on the pigmented cells & will lay odds on the swarm spores. The more I think of it the more I believe that the whole subject is already blocked out in the rough & requires only the filling in of detail, which is a mere question of time & opportunity.

If the swarmspores are zoospores of the pigmented cells, similar cells, without pigment of course, should be found in mosquitoes of malarious localities - in the *larva*, I think, because I found the swarmspores only in the newly-hatched adults of the Sigur Ghat. I can't find these swarmspores here.

A few more observations of the cells will, I think, clear up the matter. To connect them with malaria we have only to compare malaria-fed mosquitoes with insects fed on healthy blood; and to prove parasitism we have only to find sporulation. If I can detect pigment amongst the clusters of swarm spores we have it all. Finally we must produce fever in a few cases. I suppose the cells will be found in a percentage only, even of the right kind of mosquito fed on the right kind of malaria blood.

Well, these are my sentiments after carefully considering the various points raised in the B. M. J. It is excellent of course that the points should have been raised, as they serve to define our ideas. Exactly as you say, the question "now comes to be" what is the melanin? But I don't think it can possibly be the second alternative you suggest for it. There appears to me to be only one possible explanation of the cells other than the theory that they are malaria parasites, and that is that they are pigmented protozoal parasites of the mosquito distinct from malaria - but even this is very unlikely.

All remarks in the B.M.J. were greatly to the point. Your brief statement followed by the excellent and, I think, almost convincing drawings, was better than a longer review would have been.[3] The flattering notice of my work (in excess of its merits) would encourage Sisyphus himself to roll the stone to the top of the hill.

And now I must thank you for all your trouble on my behalf. I quite agree that it was better to go to Cleghorn. I did not know that he was a friend of yours, and fear I have *talked* about him to you in my peevish moments, frequent enough in my solitary confinement here; where for the last two months I have had my meals alone & where I have nothing to do after my ten minutes work in the morning but growl & pace the verandah like an animal in a cage! I hope and believe he will be able to get me to work again - that is all I ask now. But remember that I reported my Sigur work & also about the pigmented cells directly to him four months ago, & have twice told Leslie that I cannot work here. The letters from you & Sir J. Fayrer must have reached him not later than the 17th instant. If they, together with the B. M. J. articles, do not suffice, nothing, I fear, will, unless Lord Hamilton will take it up. I think therefore I should forewarn you of replies you *may* receive from Cleghorn. He may say (a) that as I am in the military department, he can do nothing for me - which will mean of course that he is not willing; or (b) that I was sent here in response to my wish to be posted in the Foreign Department (this place was under that department a year ago & was then the lowest rung of the ladder of promotion in it - it is not now, as he may not have remembered); or (c) that I was sent here temporarily under stress of the frontier operations. You will probably have received his reply before this reaches you, and, if it is unsatisfactory and yet permits another letter from you, you may perhaps try to get him to send me back to my regiment at Secunderabad where I can do excellent work, & where I will stop at least until June 23rd & endeavour to solve the problem. This is asking absolutely nothing; but tell him that the P. M. O. Bombay Command[4] has refused to forward my official request to be permitted to return to my regiment, & has also refused to grant me a month's leave to go to Calcutta & see him (Cleghorn), though I asked for it expressly on the ground that I cannot do malaria work here. Hence I am as helpless as if locked in jail. The P. M. O.'s refusal was sent a week after the B. M. J.'s article was received in India, so that he must have known all about my work. The leave was recommended by my immediate superiors, and I can't understand why he refused it.

I think it best to tell you this, because it is all important now that

I should get back to work as soon as possible. If I can do so shortly I hope I shall be able to send you a really good paper for the Tropical Section. If not, I can do no work here except perhaps with quartan or halteridium later. I haven't had a case of fever *for six weeks*, & there is no dysentery at all. It is the least that Cleghorn can do, to get me back to Secunderabad & to work. Beyond this, I have now no wish at all (though of course a better appointment in another place where I can work will be better). I follow your advice & scatter all ideas of advancement, promotion, etc, to the winds. But I must get back to work. My wife & I have decided that it is a matter of indifference to us whether we leave India - we had just as soon go; but we cannot go now until June. In the meantime & after I have finally made up my mind to stick to the theory, even though we abandon the service (which I shan't do unless forced to it). Hence I no longer trouble about appointments; but try to get me back to work. Have no doubt I shall work hard if you do. If Cleghorn does not come forward, we have already advanced enough in the theory to demand from a higher authority further opportunity for work, such as my being sent back to my regiment. Yours very sincerely

R. Ross.

I return Sir C. C's letter with thanks.[5]

P.S. Jan. 26th - There are times when I think I may have been sent here as a warning not to preach "Laveranity" so eagerly. It sounds absurd, but is quite possible. When the District Principal Med. Off. came here the other day he evidently thought something was going on behind the scenes & said it was very odd that I should have been sent here. If this is the case you will probably receive an unsatisfactory answer from Surg-Gen Cleghorn; and if you do I would advise the strongest possible action. Fact is I believe my health won't stand many more months of this kind of thing, unless I can manage to get to work here.

However, I hope I may be able to do so. A mosquito bit me yesterday, and it is becoming much warmer. I am paying *touts* to get me malaria cases if possible in the neighbouring villages. I fear, when I get them, they will run away at the mere mention of being made food for mosquitoes. But large rewards are offered, & great is the power of the rupee. I find by statistics that this is the healthiest season for the last ten years, doubtless owing to the scarcity of water. I am practising staining mosquitos' stomachs. Am also searching for coccidia. Trypanosomes exist in the fish here; but I cannot find haemogregarines anywhere. If I cannot get to work with quartan, I will try mosquitoes on halteridium.

I will write directly I get orders to leave this place, if I do get them. War promises to be over, but numbers of doctors who have been on active service will then get leave, so that there is but little chance for me. Think I will write to Mr Hewett[6] if nothing happens within a month or so.

R. R.

1 Major R. A. Cole, commandant at Kherwara.
2 Thin suggested that the epithelial cells of the mosquito's stomach might be capable of absorbing pigment, and that these were what Ross had observed.
3 Manson's remarks at the end of Ross's paper. Ross (1897f).
4 See Letter 100, note 2.
5 Letter not traced.
6 John Prescott Hewett, (1854-1941), Home Secretary between 1895 and 1902, with an interval as member of the plague commission in 1898-99.

Letter 114
02/143

Kherwara
1st Feb. 1898

Dear Dr Manson,

You will be glad to hear that I have received the following telegram from Surg. General Cleghorn.

"Government India sanctions your appointment on special duty under Director General for six months. Rupees one thousand per mensem. Your transfer may be delayed."

This was dated 27th Jan. only ten days after Surg. Gen. Cleghorn could have received your letter, and as the Govt. India rarely does anything in so short a time, I fancy the sanction must have been obtained before, probably as a result of your & Dr Thin's remarks in the B. M. J. Anyway it is most welcome & the telegram, which is very business-like, relieves me from all anxiety, thanks to you. You will be further pleased to hear that I am getting to work again here, though only with brindled mosquitoes. It became suddenly quite warm a few days ago & mosquito grubs appeared in the pots of water which I have arranged for them for the last two months. I obtained some batches of brindled insects on the 29th. I suppose the eggs lie inert during the cold weather. At the same time my touts brought me in a number of sick all round. Only two of these contained haemamoeba (or coccidia) - a baby with a very few crescents, and a man with splendid triple quartan, one parasite to 150 corpuscles. I thought the brindled mosquitoes might carry quartan. Up to date I have examined 3 fed on crescents, & 5 on the quartan. No pigmented cells. I feed on the quartan both before and after the access, for comparison. A number more fed insects awaiting study. It is too cold for them to bite well.

I am looking everywhere for barred back & dapple-winged fellows. They are in the station for I find one occasionally in my warm bath room. I fancy the brindled insects will be a complete failure as regards malaria - as with filariae. The secret appears to be this. The brindled species breed in *pots* of water round houses; the other species in wells & rain puddles. I shall exhaust the question of the brindled mosquitoes on quartan in a few days, & hope to get on with some other species too.

2nd Feb Three more brindled mosquitos, one at 4 days & 2 at three days, all fed on the quartan, examined. No pigmented cells. I shall feed a number at 9 p.m. tonight. A few grubs have been obtained from an old well. Some of them may be malaria-bearing species.

I believe that as soon as I get the proper kind of insects the problem will be solved; but there is the difficulty. Everything is quite dried up. I shall strain every nerve to get *proof* together before the official enquiry commences.

You would have been amused at my shifts to persuade the quartan case to let me feed mosquitos on him. I had to lecture on the malaria parasite to the native officers of the regiment & to other natives. I showed them quartans, sporulating forms & phagocytosis, explained how the mosquito carries malaria & finally told the patient that mosquito bites were good for him as the insects take the parasites out of his blood! He is rather grumpy today, & no wonder as he had a sharp go of fever yesterday. But 2 annas for every fed insect is a pretty good reward for him. He will leave hospital with about two months' pay in addition to his usual income.

The article about the new filariae was grand.[1] I shall be on the look out for them.

Let me know if you paid more than £2 for the telegram, you were kind enough to send me.[2] Will you also kindly thank Sir J. Fayrer on my behalf. I hope to justify your action & his.

Yours very sincerely
R. Ross.

1 Manson (1897d).
2 Letter 109.

Letter 115
02/144

Kherwara
8th February 1898

Dear Dr Manson,
To continue my report:- I have completed the research on brindled mosquitoes fed on quartan - negative. Since 29th Jan. I have exhaustively examined 34 brindled insects fed on the case of triple quartan either before, or after the access or at 9 p.m. They have been examined from 2 to 6 days after feeding. No pigmented cells at all & no signs of pigment being absorbed by the stomach cells or anything like it. I think this proves that brindled mosquitos are useless as regards quartan & crescents - as they are as regards filariae. Moreover each of these negative results is a nail in the coffin of Dr Thin's theory. Stomach cells don't absorb solid particles from the cavity; &, if they did, there is no reason why they should absorb spent pigment to the exclusion of other particles.

As I suspected, my pots of water all yield brindled insects, whereas three old unused wells have yielded exclusively a scanty crop of grey or barred-back mosquitos. These while very like brindled mosquitos differ from them in the shape of the egg which is cartridge-shaped & not oval, and in the larva which has a much longer spiracle & other peculiarities. I have a fair stock of these grey fellows & my quartan subject is still going at the rate of 1 parasite to 1000 corpuscles (no quinine & little fever now owing to systemic toleration); but I *cannot* get the creatures to bite. They "simply won't" as Punch says of Mr Balfour. They sit stupidly on the net & won't touch the patient. I have bathed him, put him in the sun to bring his flavour out, & have kept him in the net for hours during the day & also all night. No use. Imagine my exasperation. It is too cold or too dry or something. But I have fed two insects of a closely allied species caught by hand. One contained no pigmented cells on the 5th day, the other will be examined tomorrow perhaps.

9 p.m. All's well that ends well. Have just received orders to be off to Calcutta at once & report myself to the D. G. - thanks to your action. I expected to be kept here for another two months until the war is over. Have just come from trying to find those grey fellows.

Apparently useless; but have bred a larger variety in earthenware vessels kept by me on the roof of the hospital. Will try them tomorrow.

Now comes the great time. Will prove the theory if I can. Always remember that I consider myself only your instrument in this work. You have directed the telescope: it is my part only to look through it & find the new planet.[1]

9th Feb. No pigmented cells in the 2nd grey mosquito. Will write as soon as I reach Calcutta. Am trying *large* grey mosquitos. Wish me luck.

Yours very sincerely
R. Ross.

1 *Memoirs*, 358, comments: 'I hope this proves me to have been a duly grateful disciple.' Ross's final analysis of Manson's role in the malaria transmission cycle was less generous. See Ross, *Memories of Sir Patrick Manson* (London: Harrison, 1930), and **Introduction**.

Letter 116
02/146

8 Harrington Str.
Calcutta
2nd March 1898

Dear Dr Manson,

I missed last mail by accident & so have a great deal to tell you by this one. I arrived on the 17th, after dining with Hankin[1] at Agra on the 15th. On calling on Surg. Gen. Cleghorn I was told that Cunningham's laboratory[2] has been placed at my disposal; that I am to be on special duty for six months for certain and that if necessary I am to apply for an extension; also that I am to go & work at Kala-azar later on. He asked me what my plans are. I replied that it would be best for me at first to try and get on to the pigmented cells again here & that my further movements should depend on developments. I thought that Kala-azar should be left until the rains, but am writing Giles about it.[3] I think you will agree with this programme. Surg. Gen. Cleghorn has gone home & Surg. Gen. Harvey[4] acts for him. I have *carte blanche*, but wish only one thing, that I had been sent back to Secunderabad for two months before the rains begin. However, this is a trifle.

Cunningham's laboratory is an isolated building close to a large European hospital, a native hospital and two jails. It has all necessary appliances. For several reasons hospital patients (in other men's hospitals) are not convenient to work with. They expect treatment & the papers might talk. Hence I am starting my touting system with a constant flow of backshish, & have been at work for a week.

Before I left Kherwara I found proteosoma & filaria sanguinis in two sparrows. The large grey mosquitos would not bite the quartan case, so I brought two bottles of grubs with me. They lived all right. Much to my surprise however I find that the grey mosquitos are the commonest insects here. All except one out of 19 samples have yielded this species. Brindled mosqs. are rare and mixed with the grey mosquitos there are a very few *black or grey dapple-winged* insects. Close to the laboratory there is an old drain swarming with greys & a few dapple-winged fellows. The laboratory itself contains both species in swarms in dusty corners. The greys bite well here but only at night & I hope to feed some dapple-wings tonight. I have to isolate the latter from the former by releasing all together into a mosquito net & then catching the dapple wings in test-tubes, which, stopped with cotton are the best homes for mosquitos. I have fed a number of greys on crescents in order to repeat my former (negative) research on them; but I trust the dapple wings will yield pigmented cells.

There is considerable difficulty in finding cases. I have obtained only four poor crescent cases & I want rich ones. Tertian is also present (2 cases found) & is suitable for greys but one case was a European who wouldn't hear of mosquitos & the other man ran away. I hunt in the native hospital every morning before 9 a.m. After 10 a.m. I see cases my touts bring me & work till 2 or 3 p.m. At 7 p.m. or 9 p.m. I go back to laboratory to feed my nocturnal insects. There is comparatively very little fever here, the cases being evidently remittents of a mild type, leading to a few crescents. They say tertian begins with the first rains. Naturally there is at first some difficulty in finding cases but I shall have plenty shortly. I have also bought some sparrows & will examine their blood tomorrow. Will try mosquitos on them. Crombie has been very kind.[5] Maynard has just returned from leave & will help, I think.[6] Other men are beginning to come to the laboratory. In some quarters there is great scepticism & ignorance not only regarding malaria but other germs.

I have boys out to get me grubs from distant parts & poke about myself after them. Am flooding some ground at the laboratory to imitate a rain puddle. Weather hot & damp.

If I am not on the pigmented cells again in a week or two my language will be dreadful. Perhaps certain meteorological conditions are required before the flagellulae can take hold in the mosquito's cells.

Directly I arrived here, I wired for my wife & children & they arrived a few days ago. They will have to go to Darjeeling in a few weeks as it is getting hot here already.[7]

Surg. Gen. Cleghorn was very brusque with me (as they say he always is); but I owed this partly to the P. M. O. at Kherwara an A. M. S. man.[8] He was good enough to accuse Johnson [sic],[9] the man I relieved at Kherwara, of malingering in order to avoid active service, and me of refusing to give Johnson a sick certificate in order to escape from Kherwara! I certainly wanted to do the latter but scarcely at the expense of another man's health, & besides if I had succeeded I should only have been sent on active service. This story reached Cleghorn's ears, but what he did not hear was that the P. M. O. after going into the matter had *apologised to me* for entertaining the idea! However, it was not difficult to put him right & he refused to hear me further about it because he said the matter had already been dismissed. Can you imagine a more monstrous & idiotic accusation to bring against two men? No wonder men won't go into the A. M. S.

There is so much to be done here that I feel like Aladdin in the cave of the "lamp" - I can't carry away all I can lay hands on. I should like to make a methodical study of all fever cases; also to examine "eye-forms"; also study amoeba coli, etc. not to mention animal parasites of animals. I think however I must resolutely set my face against wandering from the pigmented cells at present.

Imagine my disgust on arriving here to find that there is no reference medical library. I don't know what to do for some literature I want. I am writing to H. K. Lewis for Councilman & Lafleur on Amoeba Coli.[10]

3rd March. Examined two dappled-winged insects to day, between 3rd & 4th day. One had certainly been fed on crescent blood but only a little. The other was doubtful. Neither contained pigmented cells.

Only one out of eight dapple-wings bit the patient last night. I have found a child with a few tertians today. Several men are interesting themselves in getting me cases, but getting under weigh is difficult here. Hope to have good news by next mail. With kind regards

Yours sincerely

R. Ross.

Have had letters from Dr Thin, & Thornhill of Ceylon.[11] One of my sparrows has no proteosoma.

1 Ernest Hanbury Hankin, (1865-1939). See Letter 38, note 4 and **Biographical Appendix.**

2 Lieut.-Col. D. D. Cunningham was about to retire; his laboratory was 'a small isolated building containing only two rooms, offices and a veranda, and was situated in a considerable compound full of trees and bushes', Ross, *Memoirs*, 262 and plate vi, and **Biographical Appendix.**

3 Letter untraced. Surgeon-Major George Michael James Giles, (1853-1916), had reported on Kala-azar in 1890. See **Biographical Appendix.**

4 Surgeon-General Robert Harvey, (1842-1901), took over the office of Director-General of the I.M.S. from Surgeon-General Cleghorn in October 1898. See **Biographical Appendix.**

5 Alexander Crombie, (1845-1906), I.M.S. (Bengal). A District Surgeon in Calcutta. He was one of the first 'students of the *Plasmodia* in India' (*Memoirs,* 263) and known for his classification of Indian fevers. See **Biographical Appendix.**

6 For Maynard, see **Biographical Appendix.**

7 Hill station in the Eastern Himalayas, see Kennedy (1996).

8 Charles Albert Maunsell, (1840-1931), then Surgeon Colonel, AMS.

9 D. C. Johnston, see Letter 97, note 1.

10 W. T. Councilman and H. A. Lafleur, 'Amoebic dysentery', *The Johns Hopkins Hospital Reports*, 2 (1890-91), 395-548.

11 Letter from George Thin to Ross, 3 Feb. 1898, giving advice on preserving mosquitoes in alcohol, **RA** 06/055; letter from Hayman Thornhill to Ross, 24 Jan 1898, saying he was interested in Ross's publications and was arranging to send Ross some mosquitoes from Ceylon, **RA** 06/048, (Gibson, 1983).

Letter 117
02/040

21, Queen Anne Street,
Cavendish Square. W.
7th February, 1898.

My dear Ross,

Yours of 19th Jan. by last mail. I had also a letter from Cleghorn. From the latter I judge that Cleghorn is doing all he can for you. He writes:- "Ross sends me a copy of all his papers and I have read them with great interest. Some time ago I strongly recommended that he be placed under my orders, with a good salary, so that he might be enabled to carry out his investigations without let or hindrance. The proposal would have been agreed to under different circumstances, but financial difficulties and the paucity of medical officers prevented its being carried out. Ross is in military employment and is on the Madras cadre. All available officers have been transferred to military and plague duties and the P.M.O. absolutely declines to give up a man at present. I have no authority over Ross and the Gov of India cannot, even if his services were available, order the Madras Gov. to give Ross a civil appointment. When the medical officers are returned from military duty on the frontier and the present strain is relaxed, something can then be done and I have told Ross this over and over again. Your letter to Sir C. Crosthwaite was submitted to G. of I. and they were quite prepared to do what they can, but it is impossible to do anything now".[1]

It is evident from the foregoing that you have a friend in Cleghorn and that when the war is over and the plague subsides that your turn will come. It is not nice to have to preach patience but it is the only sermon which, in the face of Cleghorn's very frank letter can be preached. I feel sure that you are not being ignored and that when the time comes you will shoot ahead. Meanwhile do the best you can with the poor opportunities at your command. If you cannot get malaria you can get crows and pigeons and frogs and other coccidium afflicted creatures to work on. Much can be learned from analogy and comparative pathology and I am not sure that you could not do a very great deal, especially in the experimental line, by working on the lower animals. Dont forget that mosquitoes bite birds and that the plasmodia of birds are just as likely to be conveyed through mosquitoes as are the plasmodia of man. You should go over MacCallums observation on halteridium[2] and see if it is correct, for, if correct, it is of the very greatest importance. If the polymitus[3] is a fertilising factor in the halteridium cycle then the flagellated body of malaria is also a fertilising factor in the plasmodium cycle. And if this is the case and the fertilised crescent-derived sphere becomes transmuted into a travelling cell-piercing vermicule in the stomach of the mosquito we have the explanation of the pigment in your mosquito stomach cells; they are carried into the cell by the vermicule. I assume you have read MacCallums paper in the Lancet. This is a way of reconciling your observations and his; the one set of facts explains the other.

I have been doing a little lately with the lymphocytes having observed that from 20 to 50 per cent of them in healthy as well as in malarial blood carried from one to three or even more dots of black pigment exactly like that of malaria so far as intensity of colour is concerned. Lately Vincent in an article on phagocytosis in malaria in

Pasteur's Annales said that the lymphocytes took up the pigment. He is wrong; the lymphocytes are normally pigmented. Have a look and you will soon make out what I mean. I have written a short note on the subject and may publish it in one of the journals soon.[4]

Daniels has found the parental form of one of my new blood worms in Demerara.[5] It is about three inches long and very slender - not half the thickness of filaria bancrofti. I have got some magnificent sections of filariated mosquitoes from the specimens Sturmer was so kind as to bring home for me.[6] If you get a good chance I wish you would bottle a lot of filariated mosquitoes for me. Put them up in glycerine pure and simple.

The B.M.J. has not sent me your letter yet. Perhaps they will publish without reference to me on the point. It does no harm to keep the pot boiling. Thin I am sure is quite wrong. I believe with you that you have found the mosquito phase in these cells but, to prove it; there's the rub. Think of the pigment in connection with MacCallums vermicule and try if you can find in the stomach of the mosquito a vermicule phase. I have never seen flagella enter crescent spheres, but such things are easily overlooked if not specially sought for.

Yours very sincerely

Patrick Manson

1 On 14 Feb. Crosthwaite wrote to Manson, confirming that Ross was to be put on malaria duty for a period of six months. **RA** 02/145.

2 MacCallum (1897).

3 A name coined by Danilewsky to describe what he thought was a distinct species of bird parasite. See E. L. Opie. 'On the haemocytozoa of birds', *Journal of Experimental Medicine*, 3 (1898), 79-101, 80.

4 M. H. Vincent, 'Contribution à l'étude du processus leucocytaire dans la malaria', *Annales de l'Institut Pasteur*, 11 (1897), 891-908; P. Manson, 'Appearance of pigmentation in lymphocytes', *BMJ* (24 Sept. 1898), 881.

5 C. W. Daniels 'Discovery of the parental form of a British Guiana blood worm', *BMJ* (16 Apr. 1898), 1011-1012.

6 See Letter 58, note 7.

Letter 118
02/147

8 Harrington Street
Calcutta
9th March 1898

Dear Dr Manson,
I have had rather a disappointing week. Six barred-back mosquitos fed on tertian, & five greenish dappled-winged ones fed on crescents, contained no pigmented cells after from 2 to 5 days. The former experiments are open to question, because the subject, a child with tertian, was in the anaemic stage & possessed on the afternoon before the insects were fed only medium sized parasites. She was so ill & was otherwise such a bad subject that I sent her away next day. The mosquitos were fed at night & I am not sure that the child's father did not substitute himself for her. But the five dapple-wings were certainly fed on the crescent case, though only slightly. They are of the family of those in which I first found pigmented cells, but of a greenish colour.

I am having all sorts of petty difficulties at first. Cases can scarcely be obtained though I hunt the hospitals every morning. It is of course the healthy season. The laboratory assistants are useless & I am training men I have hired. Dapple-wings are very scarce & have to be picked out from among thousands of greys, & then bite very badly. All fed mosquitoes die in large numbers for some unknown reason. The truth is, I think, that since writing to you the temperature has fallen in a wonderful manner quite ten degrees. I have two blankets at night, which is wonderful for Calcutta in March. It will however be warm again in a few days. Perhaps the pigmented cells require a certain temperature - or rather the flagella do - before they grow in the mosquito; this may explain why they have not been found in the eleven mosquitos here.

The question of mosquitos biting birds is certainly settled. Three days ago I put a cage full of sparrows within a mosquito-net full of mosquitos. Next morning a number of mosquitos were found to be fed, & on examination, the blood in them contained all nucleated corpuscles, but no halteridium or proteosoma. This has been twice successfully repeated. Tonight I have six new sparrows some of which I hope have halteridium. I am also getting other birds.

Samples of grubs continue to yield greys, large & small. I think I have made out a sound classification for Indian mosquitos, based chiefly on the shape of the eggs, namely brindled, with round or oval eggs; grey or barred-back, with cartridge-shaped eggs; dapple-wings, with boat-shaped eggs. There are other notable differences of course.

Many thanks for yours of the 7th Feb., just received. There are many facts in favour of MacCallum's theory. Perhaps you may remember, I thought that the flagella may be of the nature of spermatozoa long ago. Certainly a large number of crescents develop into spheres which do not appear to give rise to flagella. Then you may remember the observation which I mentioned to you last September when I saw several flagella attacking one leucocyte.[1] As you say his theory does not affect the mosquito theory. I am thinking it out, & also a method for testing it.

My failure to find pigmented cells in the mosquitos referred to is annoying as it pushes back indefinitely our prospects of obtaining complete proof shortly. It may however be due to coldness of weather; & I shall employ an incubator shortly if necessary. My great trouble is to get tertian cases, & I have to spend hours every day in the search for them. The greenish dapple-wings, moreover, bite very charily & have to be put to the patient over & over again. Many of them die every day.

It *was* unfortunate my being moved from Secunderabad last September. It may be months before I get on the pigmented cells again.

I shall worry on here for another week or so, & then, if prospects don't improve, shall go to Jessore, six hours journey, where there is lots of malaria. If necessary, I shall go back to Secunderabad. The pigmented cells must be found somehow.

I have no doubt Surg. Gen. Cleghorn did his best for me, & am duly grateful to him & to Govt. But the organisation is rotten. I don't remember Surg. Gen. C. telling me "over & over again" that something would be done shortly. I remember only a single sentence to that effect eight months ago. I have got all his Secretary's letters.[2] No use talking more about it, save to thank you. Lucky leave was not open, or I should probably have been in England by now.

Excuse smudged letter.

Yours sincerely

R. Ross.

Congratulations about the parent of the new filariae.[3]

1 Letter 85, in fact August.

2 Several telegrams and letters from Leslie to Ross survive in the Ross Archives (15 April 1897, **RA** 01/090; 19 April 1897, **RA** 01/091; 25 June 1897, **RA** 01/103; 20 July 1897 **RA** 03/064; 12 Oct. 1897, **RA**

03/070; 12 Nov. 1897, **RA** 02/135), (Gibson 1983). See Letter 84, note 5 for the letter of 20 July.

3 Manson (1897d) described a new species of filaria, which he called *Filaria ozzardi*, in honour of Dr Ozzard, the British Guiana doctor who had supplied him with the blood films.

Letter 119
02/148

8 Harrington Street
Calcutta
15th[1] March 1898

Dear Dr Manson,
On the pigmented cells again today (in one mosquito), and have found active vermicules in mosquito recently fed on a crow.

Work as follows:- one tertian case found (a European), who failed in getting mosquitos off himself. Difficulties as to dapple-wings with crescent case remaining. Three more dapple-wings, however, fed on it, and did not contain pigmented cells. Tertian case almost impracticable - quinine.

Seeing these difficulties I set hard to work on birds. Numerous sparrows & larks contained no parasites. Got a new lot; also two pigeons & a crow. Had no time to examine them, so, on the 11th put them all in their cages in a net with a swarm of greys. Next day obtained about 100 fed insects which were put by to incubate; at the same time scanty halteridium was found in crow by puncture & very numerous halteridium of all stages in pigeons. The new sparrows & larks negative. Am consequently working with crow & pigeons. The former has also filariae.

On 12th also, at noon, fed a few greys who were hungry enough to be awake, on the crow. Blood in stomach examined within an hour. Moving vermicules found at once - about six of them - also some spent pigment. The vermicules were exactly as described by MacCallum,

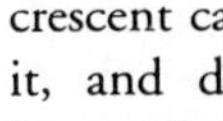

moving sharp end foremost. Other mosquitos examined up to several hours after feeding showed also a few vermicules whose movement ceased apparently two hours approximately after feeding. Experiments repeated not so successfully next day. Parasites too few for such demonstrations. Obtained about 40 fed mosquitos off crow & pigeons on night of 12-13th March. They will be examined tomorrow.

Yesterday (14th) I examined a large number of greys fed on

crescent case & birds (night of 11th to 12th). All were negative. I forgot to tell you in my last that a number of greys fed on crescent case have been negative, according with former results in Secunderabad.

Today (15th) I continued examination of mosquitos fed on all the birds three days ago. All except one were negative. That one contained two pigmented cells. Of course I don't know which of the birds it bit, but fancy it was the crow. The pigmented cells were in the stomach (I glance at all the tissues formally). One was about 15μ & the other about 9μ, each containing about 10 granules of pigment.

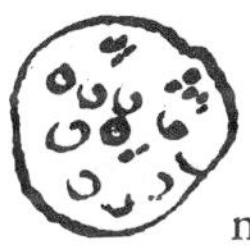

They were just like those formerly obtaining except that the large one had a more definite outline than those found in the 4 days' mosquito fed on crescents. The body of the smaller cell was almost indistinguishable but could be made out by the arrangement of the pigment. The mosquito was of course grey or barred-back, of exactly the same lot as has yielded negative results so persistently with crescents, and lately with the tertian child, but which contained large cells & swarm spores when fed on the tertian in Secunderabad.

The mere fact that only two pigmented cells were to be found in the whole stomach goes against their being physiological.

I think I am doing something wrong with my mosquitos because 80% of them die between 2nd & 3rd day, though I keep them in a large jar with a saucer of water at the bottom, dead leaves, etc. Dead insects don't seem to contain filariae or pigmented cells to account for their death.

16th. Examined 18 (eighteen) mosquitos fed on crow & two pigeons with halteridium three days ago. None contained pigmented cells. Examined also 5 greys fed on crescents - negative; four white pigeons, 2 jays, 2 dead blackbirds, I fever case - all negative. One of my infected pigeons contains one infected corpuscle in six; flagellates seen in it, but no vermicules. Am pretty well dead beat.

There is probably some condition, possibly climatic, which is necessary to the successful infection of mosquitos. It will doubtless be found soon. Am trying different ways of keeping mosquitos. Find that these grey mosquitos lay their eggs just about 72 hours after feeding - a floating raft of eggs as frequently described - but they should live after that & be ready for another feed, because their ovaries still contain numbers of ova. Perhaps to keep them alive easily for more than three days it will be best to exclude males.

Labbé is poor as regards vermicules.[2] He thinks that nothing exists which he has not seen. Now I find that Kruse, Danilewsky, MacCallum & others agree as to vermicules in crows, and Labbé does not appear to have examined crows. Anyway they existed in my crow a day or two ago.

Tomorrow I expect fresh crows, with, I hope, more parasites.

Oddly enough I have not been able to get any fed mosquitos off the birds the last few nights - why?

I think it likely by the scarcity of its pigmented cells, that the mosquito which contained them yesterday bit the crow & not the pigeons. It was foolish to put the birds together into the same net. Tomorrow however I shall have a number of insects fed off the crow alone to examine.

The specimen today shows the outline of the smaller pigmented cell quite clearly 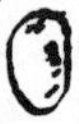 with the assistance of formaline.

17. Two greys fed on crow three days ago had no pigmented cells. Shall examine a large number more today but must stop this letter to catch post.

Owing to paucity of cases have asked Surg. Gen. Harvey for permission to travel to more malarious places. He says sanction of Govt India must be obtained! Just fancy! - that will take some weeks.

Just heard from Civil Surgeon Jessore that there is no fever there at present.[3]

Please give me advice as to the study of Kala-azar. Advice as to other work will also be acceptable. I wish I had followed your suggestion regarding halteridium before, but was put off by failure to find it in Bangalore birds in 1896 - very stupid on my part. Can you possibly send me (or tell Lewis to do so) MacCallum & Opie's full paper (referred to by Osler in Lancet Nov 13th 1897 page 1241) on birds' parasites in the Journal of Experimental Medicine.[4] I also want most particularly Councilman & Lafleur's article or book on dysentery & amoeba coli (Johns Hopkins, I believe).[5] Lewis was written to, but did not send it.

With kind regards

Yours truly

R. Ross.

1 Ross writes 10th in *Memoirs.* 15th is correct.

2 Probably Labbé (1894), but Labbé also published a lengthy summary of his researches in 'Recherches zoologiques, cytologiques et biologiques sur les coccidies', *Archives de Zoologie Expérimentale et Générale*, 3rd series, 4 (1896), 517-654.

3 Letter from D. Basie to Ross, 15 March 1898, **RA** 03/089.
4 W. G. MacCallum, 'Notes on the pathological changes in the organs of birds infected with haemocytozoa', *Journal of Experimental Medicine*, 3 (1898), 103-116; 'On the haematozoan infections of birds' *ibid*, 117-136; Opie (1898).
5 Councilman and Lafleur (1890-91).

Letter 120
02/149

Calcutta
21st March 1898

Dear Dr Manson,
My one wish is that you were here to share with me the pleasure which I have experienced yesterday and today in seeing your induction being verified step by step. Such pleasure comes but to few men, I fancy, though you must have felt it in regard to filaria. I am producing pigmented cells *ad libitum* by feeding grey mosquitos on larks infected with proteosoma. This, of course, means the solution of the malaria problem.

You remember that on the 12th I obtained a number of greys fed on a crow, two pigeons & several larks & sparrows. Out of nine of these I found pigmented cells in one only. Then I fed mosquitos on the crow & pigeons & lastly on the crow alone & a few on the pigeons alone. Of these 35 in all were carefully examined - no pigmented cells. Where then did the pigmented-cell fellow come from in the first series? Probably from the larks & sparrows. Hitherto I had time to examine only a few of these, in which I found nothing; but now, on the 17th, I went through them more carefully, & found *proteosoma*, Labbé, in three larks & one sparrow. What then if the pigmented-cell mosquito had come from one of these? It was easy to find out. On the night of the 17th-18th March 10 grey or barred-back mosquitos were fed on the three larks. Excitement now rose to a high pitch. On the morning of the 20th I judged these mosquitos to be ready. All except one were alive. I was so excited that at 8 a.m. I could hardly dissect the first one.

It contained pigmented cells. I now had to come home for breakfast and could scarcely sit it through. When I returned at 10 a.m. I set to work on the rest of the mosquitos. The second & third of them contained no pigmented cells, but certain peculiar pigment *clumps*. Of the remaining six four contained more or less numerous pigmented cells - that is, pigmented cells were present in five out of the nine greys fed on proteosoma, and the rest all contained pigment clumps. This, compared with the past negative results could be interpreted in only one way. I felt that the theory was proved.

Since the night of the 17th-18th I have been feeding greys on the larks & the sparrow regularly. The insects have been obtained from different sources. Three out of four of those fed on 18th-19th, and two out of two of those fed 19th-20th have had pigmented cells. Control insects out of the same bottles fed on crescents have been *quite* negative both as to cells and pigment clumps. Pigment clumps have been found in *all* the mosquitos fed on proteosoma, in *none* of the others. What are they? - we shall see very soon.

The cells are very like those derived from malaria. I will describe them exactly later. Those obtained from mosquitos after about 36 hours are much smaller than those derived from insects after about 60 hours. Today I found a different kind of cells in a mosquito which may have bitten the sparrow. I also found ***two swarm spores*** in one of the insects. Let us see what I get tomorrow!

23rd March. I[1] have not yet arrived at sporulation but have reached a growth of 40µ after 85 hours. I find that I exist constantly in three out of four mosquitoes fed on proteosoma & that I increase regularly in size from about 4µ after about 30 hours to about 40µ after about 85 hours. I find myself in large numbers in about 50% of the mosquitos and also in small numbers in about one in two mosquitos fed on two crows with blood parasites. I can't get mosquitoes to bite the pigeons in large numbers.

After about 48 hours many of the cells are found to be quite hyaline, that is, free from vacuoles. After 72 hours almost all the cells look like spherical, almost clear bubbles & are easily seen by low powers. The pigment appears to get less & less the older the cells are, until it is entirely absent sometimes after 72 hours. In most of the cells the pigment is contained in or upon a small internal sphere.

Today I watched a curious phenomenon. A specimen after 72 hours contained numerous hyaline cells; in 20 minutes they had all become vacuolated. I was beginning to think that the hyaline cells were dead & degenerate ones; or that there were two kinds, hyaline and vacuolated cells. I now find that the latter are the former *post-mortem*, at least with the older cells.

Of course I have only to find sporulation to complete the life history. Then I shall wire to you. I must also feed greys on healthy larks for a formality, & much miscellaneous work must follow. The difficulty as regards sporulation is to keep the insects alive. Now, they all die after 80 hours with the exception of one or two, though the test tubes are changed daily; but last night I fed three over again - the rest refused to bite. I am starting staining to get at the nucleus but haven't succeeded yet. Most of the insects are being mounted in formaline, as before, in series to send you & to Laveran. I forgot to tell you that I wrote to him & had a very nice reply a few days ago.[2] He wants specimens of pigmented cells.

Though I am working up to 8 p.m., I haven't had time to elaborate the best method of mounting, etc, as yet. That must follow the discovery of sporulation. I want to keep my specimens this week (to look over them again) & will dispatch by next mail. I shall also send crowds of mosquitos in glycerine

I am endeavouring to work *backward* to the earliest forms of the parasite in the mosquito. This presents difficulties before 36 hours, owing to blood in the stomach. All the questions regarding flagella, vermicules, etc, ought to unroll themselves now with ease. Before this the difficulty lay in finding the proper species of mosquito, because *a priori*, the flagella, or vermicules, may be expected to die in the stomach cavity in the wrong kind.

What an ass I have been not to follow your advice before & work with birds. Technique *much* easier. Was put off by finding nothing in Bangalore.

Illustrations, microphotographs, will be begun shortly. Healthy birds must be infected.

24th. One mosquito lived to 102 hours & was examined just now (7 a.m.) Cells not much if at all larger but showing tendency to burst. Pigment absent from most of them. Many appearing to protrude from the outer wall of the stomach into the coelom. I think I saw signs of

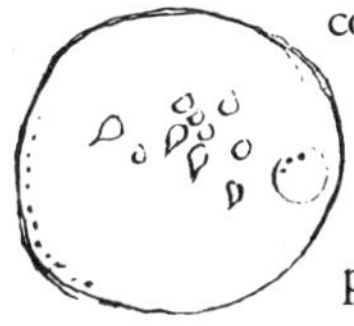

commencing sporulation in one or two - little oat-shaped bodies.

That beastly formaline has ruined many of my specimens. Hope to have time to work with other preservatives today. A number of infected mosquitos were fed again to day & will I hope last up to sporulation. Must be off to work & therefore close this letter for the post with congratulations to you.

Yours very sincerely

Ronald Ross.

1. *Memoirs*, 270, remarks on Ross's turning himself into a pigmented cell, in his excitement, further confirmed by his full signature.
2 Ross referred Laveran to his article on pigmented cells (23 Jan. 1898, **RA** 02/208); Laveran replied that he was interested in Ross's research

and would be pleased to examine specimens of pigmented cells if he would send him some (23 Feb. 1898, **RA** 02/182), (Gibson, 1983).

Letter 121
02/150

UNITED SERVICE CLUB
CALCUTTA
30th March 1898

Dear Dr Manson,

I have not wired to you only because I have not yet found sporulation; but all doubts as to the fact that we have at last succeeded in cultivating the gymnosporidia in the mosquito have vanished. I have been too fagged to write to you daily; but here is the summary of my week's work.

1. The cells continue to be found in three out of four grey mosquitos fed on larks & sparrows with proteosoma, and on crows with blood parasites ((?) proteosoma).

2. The cells begin to be noted certainly after one day (between 24 & 48 hours after feeding) as small bodies from 4μ to 10μ or so, profusely pigmented, lying in the stomach wall, sometimes in the external muscular coat, & apparently *not* intracellular. They increase steadily in size. On about the fourth day they generally lose all traces of pigment reaching at that time a size of about 30μ to 40μ. They then begin to protrude from the external wall of the stomach into the body cavity. On the sixth day this protrusion is generally complete, the stomach having this appearance:-

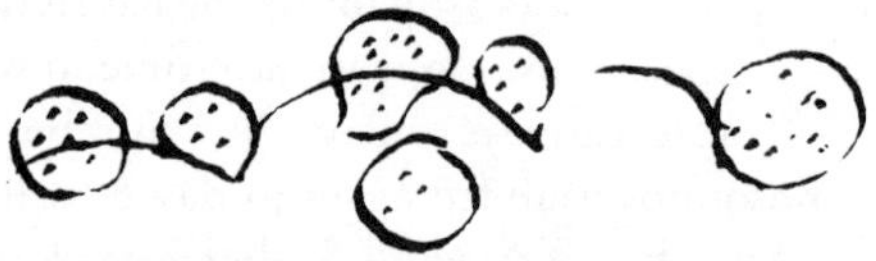

At this stage the bodies may reach 60μ when uncompressed by a cover glass; they are full of a clear fluid containing a few large vacuoles & numerous bright refractive granules, or rather globules, 1μ in diameter; and their capsule is so delicate that it easily bursts before the coverglass is imposed - which can be prevented by adding a little formaline to the water. The contents are poured out slowly *outside* the stomach. The cells, though distinct from the stomach wall, still remain attached to it by some invisible tie.

At this stage I thought sporulation would commence; on the

contrary it seems to me that the cells now burst or disappear; because in mosquitos kept after 6 or 7 days (I have examined them up to nearly 10 days, 240 hours after feeding) the largest sized cells are rarely to be found, while a few wrinkled empty capsules may often be seen still attached to the stomach wall. I have not yet determined whether these capsules are natural, or are artifacts caused by the making of the specimen. It seems likely then that some trick of nature takes place at this point. The cells, either bodily or their contents only, should be found in the surrounding tissues - cellular tissues or perhaps attached to the egg. I have not found any certain sign of them yet owing to difficulties of distinguishing normal cells; but have my eye on some suspicious fellows.

3. The size and appearance of the cells therefore corresponds exactly with the *time after feeding*; & it has been invariably found that medium & full-sized cells *never* occur a short time after feeding, or at any time previous to the natural time for their appearance. Hence it follows *that the growth of the cells begins at the moment of feeding* & at no time previously. Also young cells are not to be found in mosquitos kept for 3 or 4 days without a second feed, which shows that the growth of the cells does not begin after feeding.

4. In mosquitos which are fed a second and third time on infected birds, *each feed is followed by a new crop of pigmented cells* - so that we may have two and even three generations proceeding in their growth side by side in the same mosquito. This proves conclusively that the origin of the cells depends upon the feed of blood.

5. No pigmented cells were found in 5 brindled mosquitos fed on infected sparrows, though they existed in 1 out of 2 greys fed on the same birds at the same time.

6. I think that the cells derived from sparrow's proteosoma differ from those from crows & larks, having a thicker capsule & more scattered pigment.

7. Staining shows (a) that the cells take methylene blue, eosin, & logwood equally. With all, when young, I find that each cell contains a number of deeper stained bodies like bullets in a bag

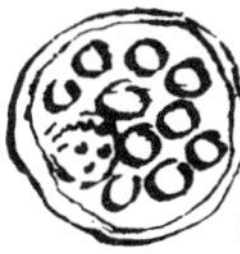

separate from a vacuole (?) containing or surrounded by the pigment; but as these bodies take eosine I hesitate to consider them as consisting of nucleinin.[1] Attempts at staining only tentative as yet, of course, & the older cells are especially difficult to deal with. A capsule is well brought out by eosine & glycerine. Meth. blue causes a deep polar staining at one pole in some cases, & occasionally this masses itself into something very like a nucleus. *Certainly* the substance of a young cell contains

(a) a capsule, (b) vacuoles, (c) pigment, (d) the bullet-like bodies.

8. I found no parasites in 3 sparrows the other day (one examination with a tired eye). Pigmented cells were found in 6 out of 18 greys fed on them. Hence I believe that one or more of the sparrows contain proteosoma. I have not had time to examine them again yet, but will do so tomorrow.

Conclusions for the week:- (a) negative results must be obtained from healthy birds; & (b) there is a check where the cells leave the stomach which must be got over. There are reasons which make me think that the cells at this point give rise to a large amoeba or something of the sort which may sporulate in external nature. It is possible that this check may cause considerable delay.

I think the cells are coccidia in the mosquito; but we must wait before deciding.

I have prepared a number of specimens for you & wished to look them over before despatching; but excitement & work fagged me so much that my eyes wouldn't hold out today & I had to go home & go to sleep all the afternoon. Feel better now, but my right eye is smarting. Anyway I will send you numbers of specimens & also mosquitos in glycerine next week.

This is a hand to hand fight with nature; she always has some nasty trick to evade me just as I am getting hold of her. But we will have it all out in a short time.

31st. The *trick* appears to be simply that I have been bursting the coccidia in making the specimen.[2] This morning I looked at a mosquito at the 11th day. The stomach was studded with huge coccidia, over 60μ without coverglass. While I looked, though formaline was added, they all burst, leaving only shrivelled capsules. Unfortunately my stock of old mosquitos is giving out.

All the above measurements have been accurately taken with ocular and stage micrometers.

I must now hurry back to work. Feel better again today after a good sleep.

Over two hundred mosquitos were fed last night. This morning I found a fourth genus of mosquito with the most singular eggs. Shall send you insects in glycerine next week.

Yours sincerely

R. Ross.

1 Chromatin.

2 *Memoirs*, 274, notes that he had not been using a strong enough salt solution. See also Letter 127.

Letter 122
02/151

Calcutta
5th April 1898

Dear Dr Manson,
I have not found sporulation only, I think, because I have not continued to look for it. On finishing my stock of twelve-day-olds I thought I had been trying to rush it too much & went back a little taking up a stock at 5 days. This showed me clearly that the coccidia reach full size of 60μ and are quite extruded from the stomach on the sixth day after feeding. In many of them at this date, a low power showed me a kind of refractive but ill defined core 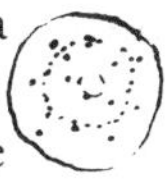; and in two of them I saw unmistakably what must be commencing sporulation, namely a division of the core into eight distinct yet ill-defined central bodies 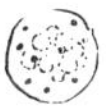. But as soon as a cover glass was applied these appearances vanished. An oil immersion, however, showed something new, namely a striated if not reticulate structure. One coccidium shows this beautifully, the radiations starting from two points (? nucleoli). The little round

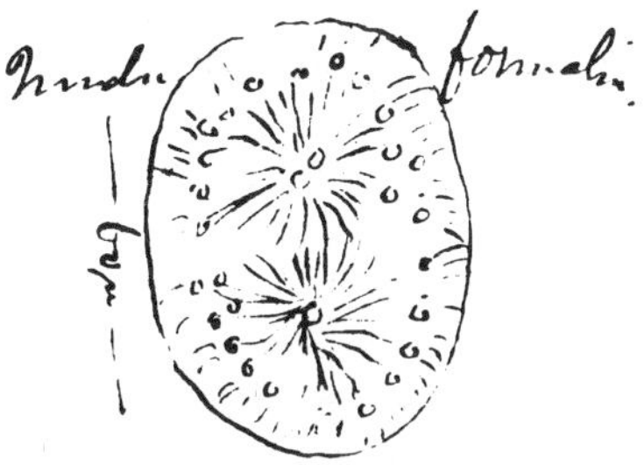

globules close to the border are found in all the coccidia of this size, but are generally scattered throughout them. But it is not time to describe structure yet, as I am only getting on with my staining. (I find that the best way to stain is by about 10 minutes exposure to weak solutions (saffranin, meth. blue, eosine, logwood, etc)).

Well having got so far I harked back, as I wanted to occupy some important posts in my rear, which I had not yet attended to. Result - formal proof of a very important question.

You remember that I had found coccidia in 5 out of 13 insects fed on three sparrows in whose blood I had found nothing after an imperfect examination. On the 2nd. I examined the sparrows again. One contained nothing in a whole specimen; the second had a *few* proteosoma; & the third had *very many* - so many that I could not possibly have overlooked them, & the bird must have been recently infected (?). This explained the coccidia & gave me a chance to make a fine experiment. I put each bird in a separate mosquito net, and released on them a number of mosquitos caught in the *same drain* & hatched out in the *same bottle*. You see the test was a perfect one as to the relation between the proteosoma and the coccidia. The insects were examined yesterday & today, and I have mounted 10 from each sparrow for you, besides putting up 8 whole insects from each bird in glycerine for you to make sections - (they will be sent by *next* mail).

Results were:-

Out of 15 mosquitos fed on the healthy sparrow I have not yet succeeded in finding *one single* coccidium.

Out of 19 fed on the sparrow with a few proteosoma & examined, *every insect* without exception contained coccidia, & some contained fairly large numbers.

Out of 20 insects fed on the sparrow with numerous proteosoma, *everyone* contained coccidia & some contained swarms of them - as many as 40, 30 & so in *one oil-immersion field*!

Thus at one stroke we get the law: -

"The number of coccidia in the mosquito is proportional to the number of parasites in the blood of the bird."

The experiment is being repeated tonight. The difficulty is of course to get a perfectly healthy bird - though perfection in this respect is unnecessary so long as the law of proportion holds. More on this in my next, when I send you the specimens.

6th April. Another law foreshadowed today. I have been obtaining uncertain results with crows. Of three which I use, I found halteridium in two & proteosoma in one. On looking through my diary I find, as I expected, that positive results were obtained only when the proteosoma crow was present (I feed on two crows at a time). On the 3rd I fed separately on the two crows with Halteridium & the one with proteosoma. Results still *negative*. Consequently I examined all the crows again today. *All* now have halteridium. Yet one (marked) certainly had proteosoma before, the typical forms, especially the rosette being present. It is a case of new infection. Evidently halteridium doesn't take in the grey mosquito (at least at this season). I must find another crow with proteosoma & then do a differential experiment which will settle the question.

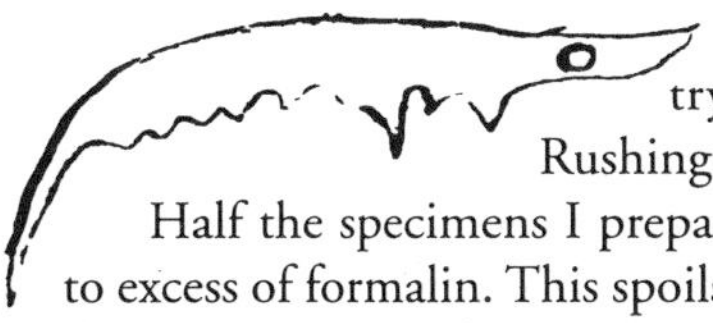

In one crow I found a huge trypanosome, nearly 40μ long! Rushing about like a lunatic.

Half the specimens I prepared for you have gone bad owing to excess of formalin. This spoils the various series; but I send you a first instalment of over thirty, illustrating the growth of the coccidia from small to full size. Better ones next week, I hope. I also send infected mosquitos of third & fourth days in glycerine (separately). Also some fed on crows with halteridium in which I don't think (I am not quite sure yet) that you will find coccidia.

From mosquitos at 30 hours I find the cells of only about 6μ *all*

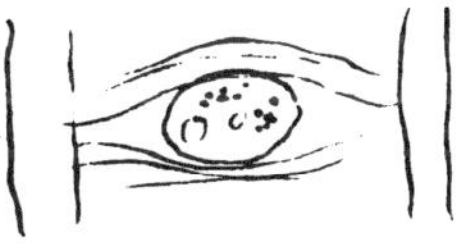

lying between the strands of muscle in the outer coat of the stomach. Nevertheless I think that they may be intracellular even in this position because I saw something burst close to one & it immediately became much more defined. These stomach cells are so delicate it is hard to say whether the coccidia are inside them or not. But one thing I know - the coccidia *all* lie in the outer muscular coat of the stomach or *just* below it.

I must give a word of warning about the specimens (it is unnecessary to you but not to others) that it is unsafe to come to conclusions at variance to mine (based on fresh specimens) until better preparations have been sent. I still use formalin, though much weaker, because, where it does not fill the specimen with crystals, it preserves the exact shape & look of the coccidia much better than glycerine & water, glyc. jelly, etc, etc. But I don't know what it may do by the time the specimens reach England. I am certain it often magnifies pigment in a most remarkable manner

turning 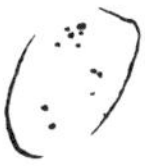 into 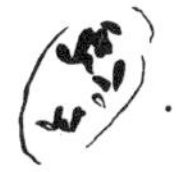 .

Also I must warn you against the nuclei of the cells of the malpighian cells which are often very like coccidia after they have lost their pigment; but the former are quite round & have a distinct nucleolus and no vacuoles.

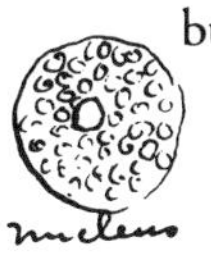

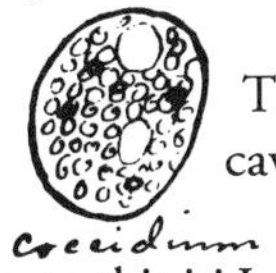

These sometimes escape into the cavity of the stomach and elsewhere.

What a beautiful discovery this is! I can venture to praise it because it belongs to you, not to me. I sometimes think it is the prettiest thing in the whole range of pathology. How simple it all is after all!

I think that something funny occurs on the seventh day; hence the complete life history may not be found all at once. Of course its discovery implies the solution of the malaria problem.

I saw what you said about Rogers' subsoil nonsense[1] & the colonial service.[2] It was amusing. What will they say about proteosoma in the mosquito?

I shall not wire to you until I find the complete life-history. I think however that you can safely announce the business (if you like) when you get this letter and the specimens. Perhaps however, better wait for my next letter; though it does not require sporulation to prove that the pigmented cells are cultures of proteosoma in the mosquito.

I wish I could get a good book on coccidia - say Labbé Sur les Coccidies des Oiseaux (Comptes Rendus de L'Academie des Sciences, Juin 1893).[3] It is no use my writing to Lewis for anything but a text-book.

I am of course forbidden to publish on this subject until I have reported to Govt. but I think some announcement should be made shortly. I will bet MacCallum will try mosquitos in a month or two.

Yours very sincerely

Ronald Ross.

1 Leonard Rogers read a paper on ground water and malarial fever to the Epidemiological Society, 18 Feb. 1898, 'The relation of variations in the level of the ground-water to the incidence and seasonal distribution of malarial fevers in India', *Transactions of the Epidemiological Society of London*, 17 (1897-98), 60-77. This was reported in *BMJ* (26 Feb. 1898), 557-558. Rogers had indicated that he doubted the 'mosquito theory'. Manson replied that the relationship between ground water level and malaria was at best coincidence or correspondence, but not 'true causation'. He went on to deny that the mosquito was simply an 'inference from analogy' with filaria. Of the five individuals reported as speaking after Rogers' paper, only Manson even mentioned mosquitoes.

2 Manson had commented on a paper read by James Cantlie on the organisation of the Colonial Medical Service, reported in *BMJ* (5 Mar. 1898), 655-656. In his remarks, Manson stressed that only a properly formulated proposal would persuade the Government to establish a Colonial Medical Service along the lines of the IMS. He objected to the education of colonial medical officers at

the Army Medical College at Netley, since colonial medical officers needed an exclusive tropical orientation, and permitted himself to suggest that a 'tropical medical school' was the solution.

3 A. Labbé, 'Sur les coccidies des oiseaux', *Comptes Rendus Hebdomadaires de Séances de L'Académie des Sciences*, 116 (1893), 1300-1303.

Letter 123
02/041

21 Queen Anne Street,
Cavendish Square. W.
22nd March, 1898.

My dear Ross,
I was delighted to gather from your last that you are at last fairly at your life's work and I wish you all success. Very likely you will find it a hard task; but remember the experience you have already had. When things seem hopeless and you are ready to throw it up the light may be just at hand. You are sure to throw a beam or two on many dark places even if the theory is not proved. But I think it will be. The rest is plain sailing and may well be left to other men.

I like the idea of your going later on a kala azar inquiry. Rogers, although he has done some good work, seems to have made a very poor fist of it at the parasite. He is reading a paper tonight at the Medico Chi. I intend going and may ask him a question or two about the marvellous biological gymnastics he has condemned the poor plasmodium to.[1] He says in his book that he has never seen crescents in Assam malaria![2] If that is a sample of the quality of his work the rest must be of very little value. We shall see.

Dont forget MacCallum's discovery of the flagellum impregnation of halteridium spheres. He has a long paper in the American Journal of Experimental Pathology[3] which is merely an amplification of what appeared in the Lancet. I think I mentioned to you what I thought was the explanation, if MacCallum is right, of the mosquito pigmented cell. Here it is again graphically.

(...)

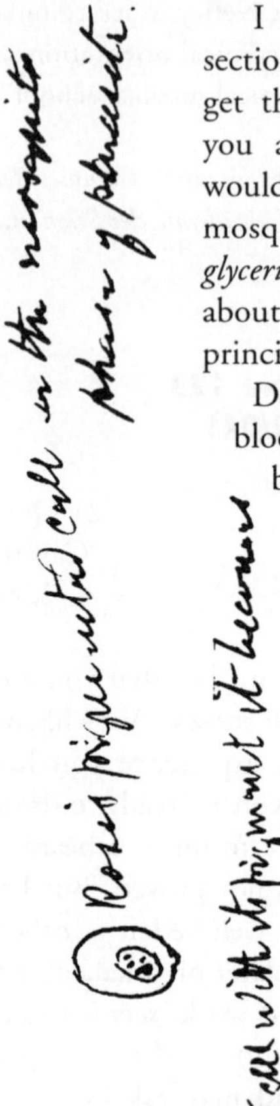

I have got some wonderful sections of filariated mosquitos. If you get the chance, and without taking you away from the plasmodium I would like to get a few filariated mosquitoes at different stages in *glycerine*; but dont put yourself out about it, for it is merely play work; the principle of the thing is established.

Dont forget to work on avian blood plasmodia. Mosquitoes bite birds regularly and they are easily experimented with and might give you material when the human article is difficult to find.

Hoping to hear of your success soon and with all good wishes in your important task I remain,

Yours sincerely

Patrick Manson

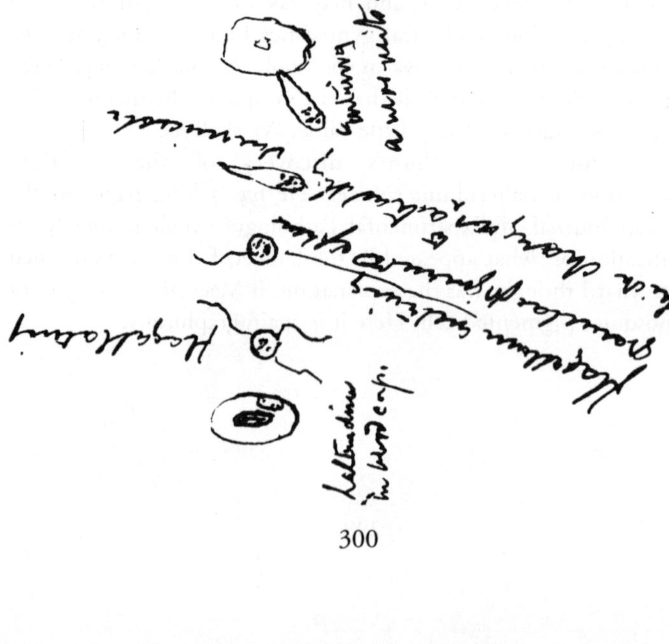

1 Reported in *BMJ* (26 Mar. 1898), 819-820. In the discussion, Manson argued that crescents were always to be found in malaria, and the fact that Rogers could not find them in kala-azar meant either that his technique was faulty, or kala-azar was not caused by the malarial parasite. Both Rogers, in reply, and George Thin denied that crescents were always found in the blood of malaria patients.

2 Rogers (1897b), 116.

3 Manson meant *Journal of Experimental Medicine*. MacCallum (1898a and 1898b).

Letter 124
02/152

Calcutta
12th April 1898

Dear Dr Manson,

My work has been rather checked this week by the mosquitos refusing to bite readily, or, what comes to the same for me, the birds learning some trick to keep them off. Hence I have neither been able to attack sporulation again or to make you many specimens, etc, though I am steadily consolidating & adding to my past work.

I send you by this mail

(a). some miscellaneous specimens of 2nd, 3rd & 4th days. Those of the 2nd day were simply beautiful when I made them, but now unfortunately the pigment has enlarged vilely in most of them (not in all). This is evidently due to some chemical reaction. I find it not only in coccidia immersed in formalin (too strong), but also in glycerine & arsenious acid. However these specimens will give you some notion of the size of the coccidia on the 2nd day (between 24 & 48 hours) after feeding; and two of them have, I think, few but *unchanged* pigmented cells. I send also some mosquitos of 4th day (I think) in glycerine.

(b). With these are the three grand series of which I wrote last week. These series alone are sufficient to establish the theory. They are:-

Series A. 10 stomachs of greys fed on sparrow with numerous proteosoma - containing numerous coccidia of the 3rd day. Associated with these is a bottle containing 8 of the mosquitos of exactly the same batch, fed & killed at the same time, but put in glycerine.

Series B. 10 stomachs of greys fed on sparrow with moderate proteosoma - moderate coccidia. Also 8 or more of the same stock of mosquitos in glycerine.

Series C. 10 stomachs fed on a healthy sparrow. No coccidia. Also 8 or more of the same insects in glycerine.

All these insects were obtained at the same time from the same drain & bred in the same bottle.

All the specimens were mounted simply in 10% formalin & sealed. Today when they leave me, they are all *simply perfect*. Each cell presents almost exactly the appearance it did when fresh, except perhaps being a little more distinct. The pigment has not become enlarged in any of them.

I have not been able to find any coccidia at all in Series C, but it is possible there may be a few because I haven't had time to look exhaustively. It is possible the sparrow had a few proteosoma, though I did not find any.

In Series B I have marked the numbers of coccidia found by a medium power in pencil on the label, thus 24 + 24, etc. They number 292 altogether in this series, giving an average of 29.2 in one insect. In Series A I have marked the numbers found in a similar manner. They amount to 1009, or an average of 101.0 for each insect.

These countings are not accurate. They were made with a Zeiss C because I have no movable stage, so that counting with an oil immersion would take me ages. Of course many more coccidia will be found by the oil-immersion. *Will you*, or *some one who has the time* count them? & will you let me know the result for my report? Don't mistake, or rather let others mistake, malpighian nuclei for coccidia. I think you will find my *proportions* fairly accurate. No. 9 of Series A has over 400 coccidia. It is the show specimen. I trust that all these will arrive safely, because they are very beautiful.

The sparrow with moderate proteosoma contained 1 infected corpuscle to 1000 healthy ones (approximately); that with many (Series A), I to 50, about. Hence the proportions in birds & mosquitos don't quite agree. Wait - I will go into it shortly. It is probably connected with the formation of flagellate bodies.

Now will you do one other thing, and that is - send these three series, A, B, & C, to Laveran 29 Rue de Montparnasse, Paris? I called his attention to the pigmented cells, and in reply he asked for specimens. I made some for him but most of them have gone bad, so that I can't send any yet awhile. I have to keep stained ones for my own information as to permanency of stain, etc, & for drawings & photography, so that it will be a charity to me if you will lend him the three series to look at and return to you. I am writing to him by this mail to announce having cultivated proteosoma[1] (as I think I should do), & I think the three series will pretty well convince him.

I know that all this time you are anxious to obtain mosquitos in glycerine shortly after feeding, so as to work out about vermicules, etc. I will send them on the first opportunity, but want all my proteosomated mosquitos for sporulation. A halteridium stock will be easy to obtain - these I hope to send next week. This has now become a merely academical question - though it is one of great interest - and I think it will easily be solved.

I want literature on coccidia badly. Perhaps I have already found sporulation without knowing it.

The three series, if they arrive in good order, will do for the meeting of the B. M. A. I hope.

13th April. Very many thanks for yours of 22nd just received. I suppose you have received mine of 22nd (wasn't it) at the same time.[2] When you wrote to the effect that light would be thrown on the matter even if the theory be not proved, you little thought that it had just been proved two days before! It was a lucky stroke, really. Brindled mosquitos appear to carry neither halteridium or proteosoma & I might have groped in the dark for months had I not happened to have come to a grey-mosquito country. Of course the theory was really proved on that memorable 20th March when I found pigmented cells in 5 out of 9 greys fed on larks with proteosoma, after a month of negative results.

As I said my week's work has not been much, but I *never* find coccidia in greys fed on crows with halteridium, & I *always* find them in greys fed on the two sparrows. Nothing is so convincing; I can say with certainty "In this mosquito there will be no pigmented cells", & almost with certainty "In this they will be present."

But another law is looming into sight - that there is an irregularity (? periodicity) in the transmissibility of proteosoma. Thus no coccidia have been obtained from a crow & a lark both containing only young forms of proteosoma 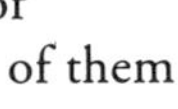 or 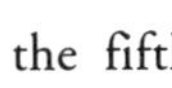 ; much to my disappointment for from one of them I had raised a stock of 70 & carried most of them to the fifth day without examining. Again my two sparrows, which seem always to contain large forms 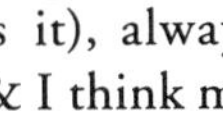 (? corresponding to crescents, though Labbé denies it), always yield coccidia (in only one insect did I not find them & I think my boy caught that one somewhere outside); but they seem to yield more of them on some nights than on others. This will be worked out easily I think. I want then to see how far *back* I can trace the coccidia. As yet I haven't found them before 30 hours, the smallest size then being about 6μ. {R.R.}[3] In fact I want to reverse your proposal & trace the coccidia back to the flagellulae or the vermicule. Then I shall be cleared for the final attack on sporulation.

Well, the theory is proved. Not a shadow of a doubt remains that we have found the alternative form of the gymnosporidia. The mosquito theory is a fact. The rest can be done by degrees, & I want to enlarge the scope of operations. By some mistake I am not allowed to travel, & they are still thinking over my request to be allowed to do so. So today I *wired* to be allowed to go to the Terai. I shall take my birds, my apparatus, and my servant, Mahomed Bux, whom I have trained to the work, with me to the low hills below Darjeeling where I have ascertained there is both accommodation & fever (in the vicinity). After looking round I shall take 10 days leave to Darjeeling where my wife is, & get some much needed rest & exercise. The next bout will find sporulation & other things, I hope.

I think you will agree it is time to knock off for a bit, especially as I must get fresh birds & can't hope to tackle sporulation for another week or more. I am dead beat with excitement & work. Shan't let myself work like this again at a temperature of 90° to 100°F.

I am living next to the laboratory with Maynard who is now acting Editor of the I.M.G.[4] He is a very good man, but was not sound on the parasite. He distrusted me & malaria work generally; but I have knocked him into shape a bit. He & everyone else here laughs at Rogers. What nonsense about subsoil water.[5] I saw your discussions at the Societies. Giles has practically annihilated Rogers.[6] If I am to tackle Kala-azar I will think it out well before hand & should like first to study purely malarial villages. *Give me advice.*

I see Thin had a knock at us at the Medical Chirurgical when he talked about Rogers' paper avoiding "speculative considerations".[7] The Johns Hopkins Hospital bulletin December 1897, page 266, also, talks about investigation guided by the "'divining rod' of preconceived idea" - with very evident application to the mosquito theory.[8]

I think you may safely disturb the security of these matter-of-fact people by announcing the cultivation of proteosoma in the mosquito. Maynard will have an editorial notice of it in the May number of the I.M.G.[9] I am to report to Govt. on the 17th May, until when I can publish nothing. The leading facts are:-

1. Pigmented cells found in greys fed on crows, larks & sparrows with proteosoma.

2. Not found in controls of greys fed on healthy men, men with crescents, healthy sparrows crows & larks, & crows & pigeons with halteridium.

3. The "pigmented cells" are found in the external muscular coat of the stomach & grow from a size of 6μ at 30 hours to 60μ at 6 days, and are probably coccidia.

4. Successive feeds of the same mosquito on the same birds are followed by fresh crops of young coccidia.

5. Similar "pigmented cells" have been found in mosquitos fed on human gymnosporidia.

This will stop the talk about preconceived ideas.

Whatever the final development of the coccidia may be, I consider the mosquito theory to be absolutely proved; and pray take this as a deliberate statement of my opinion after three years' study of the question, during which, as you know, I have kept my mind open to the opposite conclusion.

Yours very sincerely
Ronald Ross.

1 Letter from Ross to Laveran, 25 April, 1898, **RA** 02/209. Ross told Laveran of his cultivation of proteosoma Labbé from the birds' blood in mosquitoes, described his observations and said he was sending him some slides, (Gibson, 1983).

2 Actually 21st; Letter 120.

3 Ross had originally written 4μ and initialled the change.

4 See Letter 116, note 6.

5 See Letter 122, note 1.

6 A letter from G. M. Giles, 'Kala-azar', *BMJ* (26 Mar. 1898), 861, disassociated himself completely from Rogers' view that kala-azar was a purely malarious disease.

7 *BMJ* (26 Mar. 1898), 820.

8 L. F. B. 'Review of W. S. Thayer *Lectures on Malarial Fevers*' (New York: D. Appleton & Co, 1897)', *Bulletin of the Johns Hopkins Hospital*, 8 (December 1897), 265-267. The review makes no mention of mosquitoes, though Ross would undoubtedly have felt slighted by the comment, p. 265, that Italian and American investigators were the most active in the field.

9 The only editorial in May was 'Ground water and malaria', *Indian*

Medical Gazette (May 1898), 184-185. This described Rogers' theories and rhetorically asked, 'What say Drs. Manson and Ross to [them].'

Letter 125
02/042

21, Queen Anne Street,
Cavendish Square. W.
9th April, 1898.

My dear Ross,

Your letter of 21st March just to hand. I need not tell you how delighted I was to hear of your success. Dawn seems to be near. It carries the promise of a brilliant day. Depend upon it all your work will carry a rich reward to yourself and to mankind. Be very sure of your position; accumulate proofs; try for the human malaria mosquito. When the thing is certain send it to me if you like and I will take care that it is properly recognised.

It is somewhat dangerous to count chickens before the eggs are hatched but I think that after your position is sure you should hand the matter over to assistants. I think that you could demand this from the Government. I think I could work this for you through the Royal Society. Lister I know would back you up.[1] My idea is that the mosquito fauna of India and of course other malarial countries should be systematically studied by entomologists; the species described and classified. That each species should be studied in its relation to human blood parasites, especially malaria of man and animals and also at the same time to filaria. This of course is beyond the capacity of one man, of a dozen men, but the issues are so important that I dont think there will be much difficulty in finding men and funds to work it. I only hope the finishing touches will come soon so that you should have the glory and England the credit of this which will be an epoch making discovery.

I am looking forward to receiving the specimens. I hope to receive them in time for the British Medical Association meeting in July. Their exhibition will be in itself sufficient justification for the institution of the Tropical Section at their annual meetings.

The Americans will be working hard I have no doubt this summer and so too will the Italians but I think you are well ahead of them all.

I have just received reprints of MacCallum's papers[2] and also of Opie's.[3] I send them by this mail. You already know the principal facts.

By the way, this entre nous, I would not give myself away too much to Laveran. He seems to have a disposition to collar as much as he can for himself. This of course is very confidential. Send him the thing complete but not in bits as he might use your bricks to build his own house. I dont want to be ungenerous but I want you to get the full credit of work which is yours and not his.

I fancy you have work enough in front of you without adding kala azar to the burden. But were I going to do anything with the latter I would select a dozen or so well marked cases of the undoubted disease stick to them from first to last; examine their bloods every day, and their organs when they died, and work out the clinical side of the disease thoroughly along with the pathology. Then I would, if I found the disease to be malarial, study the parasite and try to find if it had any physiological or morphological peculiarities. Then I would go for its special mosquito trying to find out the geographical distribution of the species concerned and the reasons for its prevalence in the implicated districts.

Ten years hence I fancy there will be enough material for a grand book - The mosquito and disease. Get ready to write it.[4]

I have a copy of Amoebic dysentery[5] somewhere but I have a suspicion I loaned it to some unprincipled friend who has forgot to return it. If I come across it I shall send it to you. But dont worry over amoeba coli until you have done for your present problem. A. coli is a very small potato beside the plasmodium.

Wishing you every success and good health to go on with you work I remain,

Yours sincerely

Patrick Manson

By the way, if you get conclusive proofs I think you would do well to come home with them. You could then get them brought out properly, look after your own interests and, also, recruit your health, and rest.

1 Lister was President of the Royal Society, to whose Fellowship Manson was elected in 1900.

2 MacCallum, (1898a and 1898b).

3 Opie (1898).

4 Ross's *The Prevention of Malaria* (London: John Murray, 1910), appeared twelve years later.

5 Councilman and Lafleur (1890-91).

Letter 126
02/153

Punkarbari
Darjeeling Dist.
3rd May 1898

Dear Dr Manson,

I am rather afraid I have missed this mail; but will chance it.

I left Calcutta on the 17th March [sic].[1] A murrain occurred among my birds the previous night, carrying off all my proteosoma sparrows & a young crow with some kind of gymnosporidium, but I brought the rest up with me. I left my man, Mahomed Bux, at Kurseong, 5000 feet up with orders to find mosquitos & have a stock up to a week or more by the end of my leave. I then went on to Darjeeling, 8000 feet (train all the way) & took my ten days' holiday - that is I worked only about 4 or 5 hours a day. With me I took a large stock of mosquitos fed on proteosoma sparrows & another large stock fed on crows with halteridium. All the former had coccidia & none of the latter had. The former stock I carried to 9 days. Results as before - the coccidia reached 60μ on the 6th or 7th day & then no *marked* further progress (see further down). Having done this, I selected a good series for Laveran & sent them to him with a long letter & careful drawings announcing the establishment of the mosquito theory.[2] I did not tell him about the three series A, B & C which I sent you,[3] as I thought you might not like to part with them, but I suggested he might write to you on the subject. I also sent you a number of greys fed on crows with halteridium & killed early next morning for sectioning for vermicules. Lastly I made a number of drawings to scale for my report, as carefully as I could - the photos turned out failures. This was my holiday task. On the 28th I returned to Kurseong where I found my man with a stock up to 6 days - no coccidia. He had also hunted up mosquitos - a variety of grey (as also at Darjeeling). They bit well at Kurseong. I remained there two days trying to get sparrows - failed. Examined several little birds - negative. Examined 10 pigeons lately from the Terai (foot of the hills); *all* had halteridium badly - some had tabanus & lice - no coccidia in these. Couldn't do much up there, so, on 1st May, I came down here.

This place is 2000 ft. above sea & a few hundred above the Terai. Seems to be no fever here, but plenty below. Find considerable difficulty about getting birds (which I want to carry out life-history of coccidia) but hope to have some tomorrow. Shot one miner (bird not man) - full of some species - free forms. Mosquitos mostly grey here just as at Kurseong & Darjeeling. Planters are getting me fever cases. There is a small hospital of 4 beds here. Found two anchylostomiasis cases straight off & am starting cultivating dochmius according to Giles.[4] Also a horrible case of what they call cancrum oris[5] here. The pus was full of a huge fungus (? ray fungus), also swarms of flagellate organisms (cercomonas ?), also (?) *coccidia.*[6] Will examine tomorrow again.

I fancy discoveries are to be made here for the picking up - but must stick to my last.

Now to return to the proteosoma-coccidia of the 6th-7th day. My progress is greatly hampered by want of new literature on coccidia. Leuckart & Blanchard are old & I can't get Labbé's paper on coccidia of birds.[7] What are microsporidia among coccidia? I fancy the proteosoma-coccidia are going to turn out to be of this nature & that the spores will form only some days after the insect dies in water. In such a dead mosquito I found these forms (now drawn from the formalin preparation).

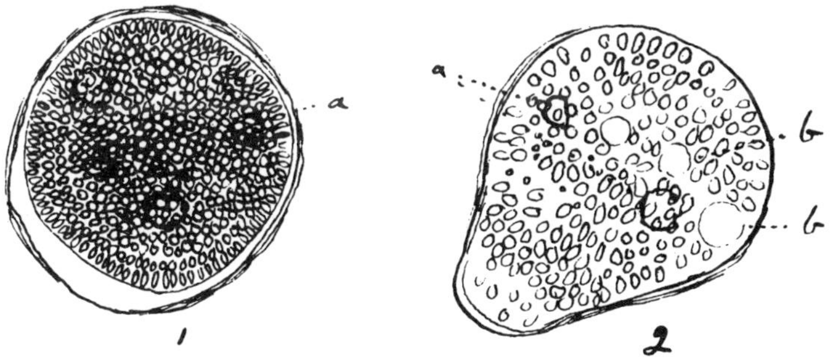

The little contained bodies are evidently elongated & are situated close under the envelope of the coccidium with their ends pointing outward especially in figure 1. This can be seen by taking the plane of the focus through the centre. By taking the plane higher or lower, the bodies are seen foreshortened. By alteration of the focus they are easily made out not to lie in the central part which contains irregular granulation & oil globules a, a, ... In figure 2 the bodies are arranged much less regularly, but still lie just under the surface. They are occasionally separated by vacuoles, b. In figure 1 the contents have separated somewhat from the capsule.

These objects may be spores. On the other hand they may be bacteria within the dead coccidia; a view which is possible because I have often seen motile bacteria in young coccidia found in mosquitos some time dead. In this mosquito the stomach tissue was full of bacteria not unlike these objects inside the coccidia.

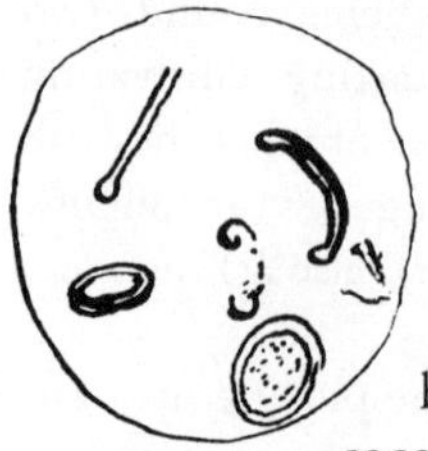

I have also found other curious things within them.

Things like hairpins, seeds, etc. It is useless to describe these. They may be involution forms & must, at all events, be worked up more before being dealt with at length. But I have drawn several diagramatically in one coccidium. Some look like free falciform bodies.

The bright refractive bodies referred to in my former descriptions are probably the same as those described by Leuckart in c.oviforme[8] because they seem to run similarly into oil globules.

I must now knock off to catch the post. No sparrows found yet. It takes a long time to settle down in a new place to work. Have written to Calcutta for sparrows & larks.

Yours sincerely
R. Ross.

1 April.
2 See Letter 124, note 1.
3 Letters 122 and 124.
4 G. M. Giles, *A Report of an Investigation into the Causes of the Diseases known in Assam as Kálá-azár and Beri-beri* (Shillong: Printed at the Assam Secretariat Press, 1890), 68.
5 Water canker or noma; gangrenous ulceration of lip or cheek.
6 *Memoirs*, 280, speculated that these might have been *Leishmania*.
7 A. Labbé (1893).
8 Leuckart (1886), 206.

Letter 127
02/043

21, Queen Anne Street,
Cavendish Square. W.
21 April, 1898.

My dear Ross,

I was delighted with your letter of 30th March and to learn of the material progress you are making. The mosquitos and preparations have not yet arrived but I suppose will turn up in due course when I shall do my best to have what is illustrative drawn, or photographed, or both. I shall have the insects sectioned and make a good search for the pigmented cells in the walls of the stomach. I daresay they will be hard to find but knowing where to look my task may not be so difficult after all. The worst of it is that the preservative media alter and shrivel so much. I hope they are in glycerine; the formaline made things so brittle that they would not section.

I write now specially to ask if you are teasing up your insects in salt solution. It struck me that as you complain of the bursting of the pigmented cells you might be using plain water merely. I had a lesson in this when mosquito-filaria hunting. The filariae in the earlier stage in the mosquito all burst and disappeared if I used water in my dissections. They kept their integrity and proportions *in salt or sulphate of soda solution, specific gravity 1040.* The mosquito juices have of course a specific gravity a long way above that of water and organisms adapted for life in mosquito cells must have a suitable organisation. Try the salt solution if you have not done so already. A curious thing about the filaria was that as the worm approached the end of its stay in the mosquito it could live & not burst in pure water. *Perhaps something of the kind may be the case with proteosoma towards the end of its stay in mosquito too.* If this should prove to be the case it is a fact that would indicate that *the next stage* of the protozoon is passed in water. Keep this in front of you.

If you send any mosquitos with proteosoma just after the feeding of the insect and when presumably the parasite is flagellating and subsequently in the vermicule form I might by luck stumble on a specimen with the vermicule entering the stomach wall. If so - Eureka.

Yours sincerely,

Patrick Manson

Letter 128
02/154

Punkarbari

9th May 1898

Dear Dr Manson,

Yours of 21st April just received. I know you are anxious for greys killed shortly after feeding on proteosoma, but, will you believe it, here I have been for 10 days, & can't get a single bird with that parasite. I am nearly wild. Sparrows all round & can't catch them. A few young ones & 2 old ones were free of it. The local idiots called Butias can't do it; I and my man have practically failed; & now I have set the police & the district magistrate on it. Fancy the whole local government trying to catch sparrows & failing! Out of 19 larks sent me from Calcutta 17 arrived dead this morning! It is simply maddening. No use shooting them of course. A planter has however made me a new trap, and the head of the police says that if he can catch dacoits[1] he can catch sparrows! We shall see.

Consequently I have done nothing in the cultivation line but the eternal negative experiments with halteridium. If I could only find the second host for this I could get on very quickly because crows and pigeons all have it & can yield more mosquitos daily than small birds can. I have examined more Tabanus flies from pigeons & lice from them & from miners - nothing found.

You say that if only you could find a vermicule entering a cell - "Eureka"; but I claim full proof already on the strength of the differential experiments plus the general structure & growth of the coccidia. I think you will admit it after seeing the specimens.

There will be no difficulty in tracing the vermicule business by ordinary dissection & washing out of the stomach; but hitherto I have kept my mosquitos to the second day for fear of spoiling my averages by missing the parasites so early as the first day. I have now done enough in the differential line & will go in for development on the first day and after the 7th day. Thanks for your tip about dissecting in salt water. I will use it. Weak formalin does fairly well in preventing bursting of the coccidia. As I told you in my last, there are signs of sporulation taking place after the insect dies in water. It all depends on getting sparrows or larks again. What an absurd difficulty!

Surgeon Gen. Harvey told me to report after three months, namely on the 17th inst. and I am wild that I shall not now be able to describe sporulation. However it may be just as well, because I ought to have some literature to go on before doing that. I want sparrows & new literature on coccidia. Leuckart & Blanchard are old, are they not?

I have now to tackle the report. Drawings are ready, but I have to make a précis of my notes - a long business. I shall claim full proof, as I said.

Not being able to cultivate I am making a careful study of Terai sickness hitherto considered to be "deadly malaria". Out of half a dozen cases only one contains a few wretched small amoeboid bodies. All have swarms of dochmius eggs besides ascaris & trichocephalus, also amoeba coli & cercomonas in many. Coin me a word like *herodiasis*[2] & you will express exactly the resulting condition. It is not one parasite but many; the wretches are being literally "devoured of worms".

Now I have no doubt that a similar condition holds in kala-azar; but it is a difficult matter to say which of all these parasites is the predominating one. So far as I can see the question can only be answered after a careful preliminary examination of chronic malaria & anchylostomiasis separately. But this will take ages.

In the meantime, if you see Surgeon General Cleghorn & he is recovered sufficiently from his accident[3] to talk about these matters, I think I would advise your discouraging my rushing off to Assam for a long time yet. The malaria problem is large enough in all conscience & is much more important than the kala-azar question. I can't do two things at once. A stock of mosquitos is quite enough work for one day; & so is a stock of patients each with half a dozen parasites, temperature to be taken (native hospital assistants are not to be trusted even to do this), diet arrangements to be made, motions to be kept separate, & so on. Both will not go into one day. Let malaria be the first thing and let me do odd jobs on the rest during odd corners of time as at present. Besides I won't be ready for kala-azar without much more careful clinical work on this terai sickness. Remember the mass of work before me in regard to finding the species of mosquitos or other suctorial second hosts for each of the gymnosporidia separately.

Perhaps however there are official reasons why I should go.

Now I must stop & get to work on my cases. I hope the specimens have arrived safely.

Yours very sincerely

R. Ross.

Have you done any more about pigment in Lymphocytes?[4]

1 Organised gangs of robbers in eastern India and Burma (now Myan ma).

2 A reference to *Acts* 12.23: 'Herod was eaten of worms and gave up the ghost.'

3 Cleghorn was then back in England, where he retired from the IMS on 25 October 1898.

4 See Letter 117, note 4.

Letter 129
02/155

Kurseong
16th May 1898

Dear Dr Manson,
I am in a vein of bad luck & haven't been able to obtain a single subject. No malaria cases. The birds which I at last was able to catch (about 20) round Punkarbari had no proteosoma & consignments of sparrows & larks from Calcutta & elsewhere arrived dead. But I have just got 15 sparrows from Calcutta & will examine tomorrow. I am consequently working all day at the report which Surg Gen Harvey told me to submit after three months.[1] It will be called "Report on the Cultivation of Proteosoma, Labbé, in Grey Mosquitos", will give full details & be copiously illustrated with drawings to scale. I claim full proof of "Manson's Mosquito Theory" & solution of problem of cultivation of the gymnosporidia & hope you & Government will be satisfied with my first three months' work. On looking through my notes (which I keep very carefully, entering every observation) I find that the result of the differential experiments is absolutely conclusive.

Out of 245 grey mosquitos fed on birds with proteosoma, 178 or 72% had pigmented cells.

Out of 41 do. fed on crescents, 154 on halteridium, 25 on a healthy sparrow & 24 on birds with immature proteosoma, or a total of 244, *not one contained a single pigmented cell.*

There is no fudge about this, & only one error - that of an insect which had been left in the net after feeding on proteosoma.

The presence of pigment & the general development of the proteosoma-coccidia, as I name them provisionally, completes an absolute proof. Hence I am justified in reporting (apart from orders) at this stage, especially as sporulation will properly belong to the second part of the enquiry.

I hope to send in the report in a day or two & will beg Harvey to let me have a copy as soon as possible, if possible with copies of the pictures, for the Tropical Section in July. I will make every effort any way to put up the subject properly for you. I fancy the detailed report to Govt. will be best. Extracts could be read, & so on; but I don't know what Harvey will say to it. I shall tell him that you want it, as I know you do.

Now for your letter of 9th April which reached me a week after 21st April. Very many thanks for it. My address should be care of Postmaster Calcutta, as the Surgeon General is at Simla.[2] The copies of

MacCallum & Opie haven't turned up, alas! - lost, I fear. It is safest to register, the Indian post-office, like other departments, being execrable.

Your letter of 9th April is full of business matters. You say that after the position is taken, the matter should be handed over to assistants, & you think you could work it through the Royal Society. Well, the position *is* taken, and I think that the sooner the affair is put on a more extended footing the better. I would suggest that, as soon as you feel satisfied of the correctness of my recent work, vigorous action be taken at once to do so. My reasons are (a) my special duty lasts only until 17th August; (b) I may be taken ill & have to go home at any moment; (c) they want me to tackle kala-azar; (d) the work is too much for one man; (e) the opportunity is a grand one (& should be seized without delay) for starting some kind of small *commission* or *deputation* with some degree of permanency, to work the general subject of *animal parasitism in India*.

I urge immediate action. These things are slow to work through; I shall have only 2 months' special duty left after you receive this letter; Surgeon General Cleghorn is now in England (address - India Office, London); strike while the iron is hot - it will never be hotter - people who know nothing of the subject will criticise; Bangalore will probably be vacant soon & the Resident has told me in writing that he will apply for me - place worth R1500 a month as against R1000 in this appointment - & once there it will be difficult for me to get out again.

Here is the programme for a Research Deputation for Indian Animal Parasitism.

Malaria. Carriers to be found for halteridium & each of the three species of human malaria - mosquitos to be classified - their habitats considered - their prevalence in different localities determined - an immense work. The sporulation of the coccidia, development in water if it exists, mode of infection of birds & men all to be determined. And a 100 other questions.

Amoeba coli, cercomonas & perhaps coccidium oviforme in men (vide Giles' report on kala-azar[3] which I trust) - immense subjects.

Worms, especially ascaris & anchylostoma, of intestine, & filaria. To differentiate between multiple infections of many parasites is alone an immense task, & I believe half the sickness usually attributed to malarial cachexia is really multiple parasitism - herodism, to coin a word.

Ulcers - an unworked field almost. Parasites of animals.

Mark this, *our present system of medicine in India is antiquated, vicious & ignorant* (as you have so often implied); it will be the duty of the Deputation to reform it, or attempt to do so. Our present diagnostic methods are those of the middle ages; what we call malaria, dysentery, hepatitis, malarial cachexia & so on may be anything. Our methods of treatment are based on the treatment of the symptoms not of the disease. We give patients tonics, diaphoretics, quinine when we should give thymol, and astringents & dieting when the intestine remains infested with parasites. Not only our hospital assistants & our assistant surgeons, but our very medical men are absolutely ignorant of the elements of tropical disease. The hospital assistant at Punkarbari had never *ever heard* of anchylostomiasis, and a young medical practitioner here, who is working in a malaria & anchylostoma country, told me himself that he had never seen the malaria parasite, did not know an anchylostoma egg by sight, & was quite ignorant of the worm and its effects.

If Chamberlain[4] takes up your ideas the Govt. of India & the Royal Society will.[5]

Don't ask for any *building* for a laboratory. We don't want laboratories, we want men. The idea of laboratories frightens government. Let us however have our headquarters together with unlimited permission to travel. We must be *together* in order to discuss matters, instruct each other, compare notes. Our headquarters should be in the hills within easy range of the terai where animal parasites most do abound. This place 5000 feet high & within two hours walk of the plain is good for a start. I can find mosquitos here; I can do double the work I can in the plains; I can recruit my health here if I get ill; I can keep my family here; I can get books & apparatus from Calcutta by rail in 18 hours; I can converse with my fellows & I can get the assistance of dozens of planters each commanding an array of diseased coolies; and I can study in numerous small hospitals. Here we are medical explorers; in Calcutta we would become mere naturalists fit for nothing but classifications, making pretty pictures & belonging to societies. Then from this place we can rush down anywhere by train. If this place does not "pan out" very well, we may work nearer the Govt. of India, Simla way. This will give us Delhi & the great cities of the Ganges valley nearer at hand. But whatever you do don't locate us in a fixed place at present. We have to travel from a moveable centre like a cycloid.

I have heard from Owen.[6] The Indian Princes Jubilee Institute is hanging fire, & the Indian Pasteur Institute seems to have fallen into the hands of C. I. G.'s.[7] These are destined for bacteriologists who I have reason to think know nothing of animal parasitism. Now, in India animal parasites are far more important than bacteria.

So this is the time to act. Put us on a firm basis & give us time for leisurely, quiet work.

It is no use piling the burdens on one back. I am now continually fidgeting at one moment because I can't get on with malaria, at another because I can't get on with anchylostoma. When I have to examine patients I think I ought to be examining mosquitos, & *vice versa.*

Thanks for your advice about sitting down over kala-azar cases. If I do so I must drop malaria cultivations; yet I agree with you that it is the only way to solve the kala-azar question. But what does it mean? Take half a dozen cases. Three blood examinations daily for haemamoebae; numerous blood countings; daily examinations of faeces; clinical notes; all to be carried out *thoroughly* & regularly (without which the cases when taken will be useless) leave neither time nor eyesight for dissecting mosquitos.

I would much rather not attempt the question at all than do imperfect work on it. Discourage the idea unless they give me at least one assistant whom I can trust to find parasites & count corpuscles & take temperatures. If I must do it, malaria will go to the wall, especially as, after Giles' reply to Rogers, there seems to be little likelihood of the disease being malaria at all.[8] The principal disease here, for a parallel, is not malaria at all; it is anchylostomiasis, or "herodism".

If however you make us a strong enough staff we will attack all the questions in due course & will do so with authority &, I hope, success.

If necessary or advisable a small laboratory or working room could be run up for R1000 from enquiries I have made.

Well, I must leave off & go on with the report, so say good bye for the present.

Yours sincerely
R. Ross.

1 Eventually published as R. Ross, 'Report on the Cultivation of Proteosoma, Labbé, in Grey Mosquitos', *Indian Medical Gazette* (Nov. 1898), 401-408; (Dec. 1898), 448-451.

2 The summer capital.

3 Giles (1890).

4 Joseph Chamberlain, (1836-1914), Secretary of State at the Colonial Office. See **Biographical Appendix**.

5 For funding malaria research.

6 Letter from Owen to Ross, 3 May 1898, **RA** 01/115. The Health Institute was delayed because the Maharana of Dholpur was injured and unable to work (Gibson, 1983).

7 The Indian Pasteur Institute was finally founded at the Hill station of Kasauli in 1900.

8 Giles (1898).

Letter 130
02/044

21, Queen Anne Street,
Cavendish Square. W.
29th April, 1898.

My dear Ross,

The slides and three bottles of mosquitos arrived three days ago. One of the slides is fatally smashed and several others are broken but can be used. The mosquitos are in good condition.

I have been very busy of late and have not had time to go through all the slides critically but I have already seen enough to be quite sure you are on the track and that the theory is safe. Some of the coccidia show up with marvellous definition the pigment, exaggerated I suppose by the formalin, being black and sharp. I will show several of the preparations to one or two friends before having them drawn and photographed. I think I will first take them to Baker's mounter to have them ringed so as to secure against evaporation, for some of the preparations have dried and as at present are useless. I fear the glycerine ones are useless.

I shall wait a mail or two to hear of further progress. Then I propose to write a short note for the B. M. J. to accompany drawings and photos. I am a little diffident about this as you say the Government has to get your report before you publish. But I don't want the Yanks or others to get before you.

I have an idea that the public would best apprehend what has been done by a diagrammatic representation of the position something in this style:- ⟶

It would also indicate the lacunae yet to be filled in the mosaic. MacCallum has supplied the fertilised stomach {? RR}[1] sphere and the travelling vermicule on its way to the stomach wall as we of course can now interpret it to be - you have done the rest but I would like you to find out the travelling vermicule stage for the crescent plasmodium, for proteosoma and quartan and tertian. I have an idea that I might find it in sectioned mosquitos plunged in glycerine about half an hour after feeding.

But don't worry yourself too much over details which other men can collect. If you wish to get these apply for some young fellow to help you and set him to this work. Meanwhile push on with the advancing parasite and try to get him the length of infectiveness. I fancy you will get him about the end of the mosquitos life as an encysted thing something like a crescent perhaps and that there will

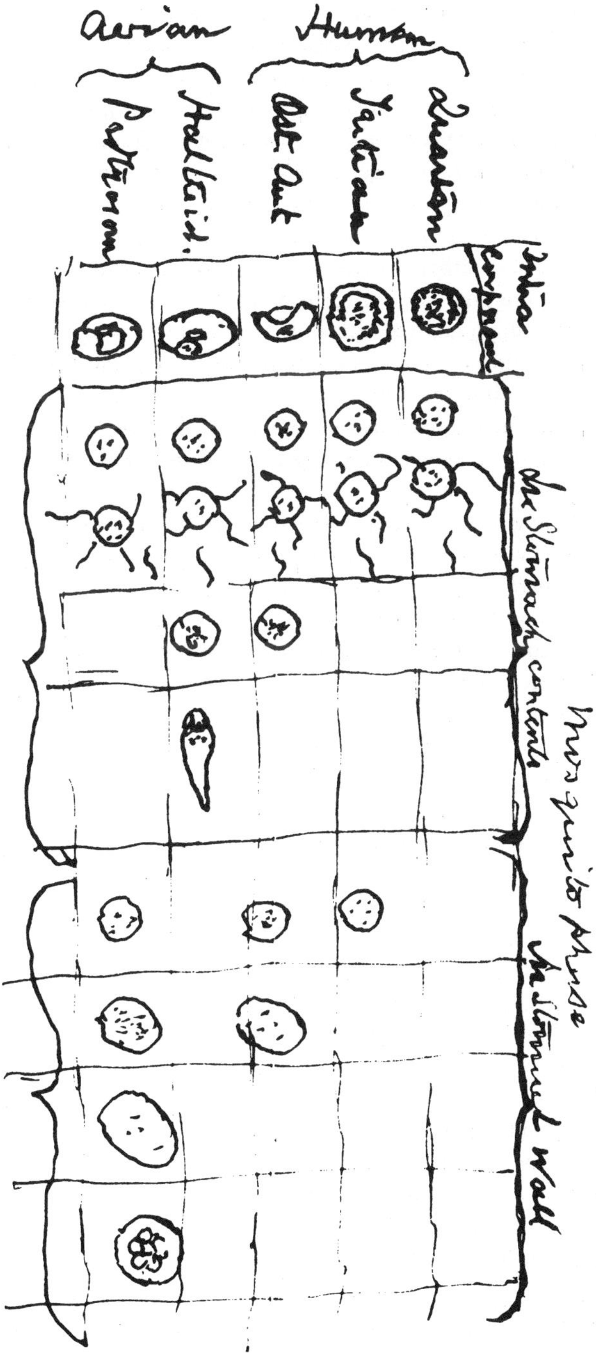
Avian
Human

be a stage of refertilisation and perhaps a travelling vermicule stage which will be the infective stage for man and other mosquitos. Possibly part of this is outside the mosquito. It is delightful to watch how the thing is panning out. What a frightful shock it would have been to us had the *Yanks done this.* {scarcely possible yet R.R.}[2] You have to thank your good angel for showing you those pigmented cells in the crescent mosquitos. And you have to thank the plasmodium that it is fool enough to carry its pigment dung along with it into the mosquitos tissues, other wise I suppose you would never have spotted him. A pity the pigment begins to disappear at the advanced stages as I gather from your letters that it does. If there is no pigment in the second generation of parasites in the mosquito you will I fear have a difficulty in finding the beasts.

Experiments on infection you could do with birds very easily. Get nestlings and keep them in an upper storey and away from telluric influences.

I shall be guided by your next letters about publishing. In case I have decided not to publish let me *know what you wish in this matter by return mail.*[3] You must have the thing out before the warm weather comes on in America and Italy. Your pigmented cells will have put them all on the scent and they are sure now to be in full cry. I would like their publications to come after yours and as confirmations.

Yours sincerely
Patrick Manson

{To Surgeon General Harvey for favour of an expression of his wishes on the subject.

25.5.98 R. Ross
Surg. Maj.}[4]

1 Query added by Ross 25.5.98.
2 Added by Ross 25.5.98.
3 Underlining added by Ross 25.5.98 leading to addition at end of letter.
4 Added by Ross 25.5.98.

Letter 131
02/156

Kurseong
30th May 1898

Dear Dr Manson,
My work has been brought to a full stop here by the *plague scare* of which you have doubtless heard.[1] The people, incited by wire pullers & encouraged by the extreme weakness of government think, or rather pretend they think, that Govt. wants to have them forcibly inoculated.[2] Every medical man becomes an object of suspicion, and you can understand that I am especially so. The coolies from two tea gardens near Punkarbari bolted in a body & the local magistrate & one of the planters have begged me not to work again just yet, and don't like my living anywhere except at Kurseong here, at the hotel. At the same time owing to the rain it is too cold here now for mosquitos to bite, so that though I have at last got some sparrows from Calcutta with proteosoma I haven't been able to feed a single insect. My man Mahomed Bux, is looked upon with worse suspicion than myself & in fact started the scare by shooting at sparrows near Punkarbari. They said there is a doctor sahib shooting coolies preparatory to inoculation! The native of India is really nearer a monkey than a man.[3] I have therefore had to wire to Simla for permission to return to Calcutta; but am going today to the house of a planter about 2500 feet to endeavour to feed mosquitos.

I don't feel quite satisfied with work. As a matter of fact I haven't examined a mosquito (infected) since 25th April. But I have done lots of odds & ends of study. The most important are that this is a bad anchylostoma country (they have been treating all these cases as malaria hitherto). It is also a halteridium country; it is *not* a proteosoma country; & so far as I have gone I have found malaria only in *two* cases, & amoeba coli in one. I have also been making post mortems on halteridium pigeons, etc etc. One very instructive case was that of a European with old malaria, of which he made little account until the last attack which presented new symptoms of vomiting & great prostration. Microscope gave at once malaria plus anchylostomiasis. The microscope is more important in tropical medicine than the stethoscope & thermometer combined, because it gives exact information about causes, whereas the others enlighten us only as to symptoms as a rule. This is my conviction now.

But my chief work has been to send in a full report on proteosoma cultivation. It took me ten days' hard work instead of three, as I had to fair copy it all myself. There are nine full plates illustrating all phases of the proteosoma-coccidia. I had the report copied (vilely) by a native writer, minus the illustrations & have sent you the copy registered. I have also begged Leslie to get the report printed off in time to send to you for the B. M. A. meeting on 26th July & have pointed out the advantage of having it published as soon as possible. There is not much time, but I hope Leslie will hurry up. If it can't be done, I have asked permission to let you make extracts from the copy I have sent for the B. M. A.

I have carefully thought out our future work & have come to the conclusion that it is *impossible* for me to attempt kala-azar yet unless I drop malaria altogether. It will only mean a similar waste of time to that which has occurred during the last six weeks. *One problem at a time.* I think then I should now make every endeavour to complete the life cycle of proteosoma, and work at haemamoeba as a secondary item. But kala-azar & anchylostomiasis should be dropped entirely. I think you will agree with me; *if so, will you write to that effect to Surg. Gen. Cleghorn?* I have already written to Surgeon General Harvey & have begged him to let me off kala-azar for the present. I don't know that he will without your backing.

As urged in my last letter I would also suggest my being put on animal parasite research on a more permanent basis as soon as possible. In my letter to Surg. Gen. Harvey[4] I asked for an extension of my present duty & I hear that *Cunningham retires on the 26th June.* At the same time I find that Bangalore won't be vacant for years, as Dobson is not to be promoted.[5] Hence I think they ought to do something for me for a permanency.

But if they intend to give me Cunningham's place *above all* don't let them do two things.

1. Don't let them *fix* me at Calcutta or anywhere else. The billet must be a travelling one with head quarters somewhere where experience shows to be best, say just above some terai (plains at foot of hills).

2. Don't let them give me other work to do such as lecturing at medical colleges. It was doing these things that hampered Cunningham so much. I could deliver courses of lectures from time to time (& would like it); but fixed employment of this kind will be ruinous to research. Also botanical, bacteriological, & other work for which I am not fit, will be as bad. Set me down specifically to solve the great problems in animal parasitism - malaria, amoeba coli, anchylostomiasis, etc. etc. Then I will do good work.

If I am hampered right & left, I won't do good work; and I think I should add that as my pension is due in three weeks I feel pretty independent. I think you will agree that back bone is necessary; my pension is my backbone; and I haven't forgotten Kherwara yet. Don't want to be undisciplined at all; but also don't want to be a jelly-fish.

Privately, it is a good opportunity to twist the tail of the Indian Government. I have just had a letter from Giles.[6] He says "I gather from your letter that they (Govt.) propose, as usual, to limit you as to time, and everybody but the densely ignorant secretariat Civilian knows that science cannot be worked in that way. The fact is that they would have no scientific work at all if they dared, and this plan of seconding a man for a few months is merely a sop to silence public opinion."

If I were you with your exceptional influence (I am only quoting your own thoughts, I know) I would do my best to force them now to take up animal parasitism properly. It has been & is grossly and disgracefully neglected, not only from a research point of view, but in actual practice - witness how they have been treating anchylostomiasis cases here as *malaria* for years. If the true enormity of this were to come to the ears of the public the doctors would be rent in pieces. It is monstrous. The education in the medical colleges is equally bad; not only medical men but also hospital assistants practically know nothing about the commonest diseases. I don't believe five per cent of the doctors out here & not .1 per cent of the assistants know what a round worm's egg is like!

What a nuisance about the specimens being so much broken! I trust succeeding samples have arrived in good order. You say you want to publish a note in the B.M.J. That is what I advised your doing in my letter of about the 14th April. There was a note in the I.M.G. for May.[7] I think *you* can make what remarks you please on the specimens & information I send you privately, though *I* cannot publish without consent of Surg. Gen. Harvey.

Yes, it was certainly the "pigment dung" in the coccidia which led me on to them; but I think I should have found them out, without it because they are such obvious bodies on the 4th & 5th days. The whole difficulty has been, not to find the mosquito phase of the parasite, but to find the mosquito. In short it is a conquest, not of observation, but of faith. Faith carried us through all the years of negative attempts with brindled & grey mosquitos. The fact that flagellation occurs *after* the blood is drawn was the finger that pointed always in one direction only; but the road was such a rough one that it required faith's boots to get along it. I doubt whether mere *observation* of vermicules, etc, would ever have done it. The vermicule found, the next thing would have been to find what became of it. Mosquitos would have been possibly tried, & ten to one the wrong species. Result negative. The road closes here, they would have cried. But we looked up & saw the finger of *theory* still pointing the same way. For the same reasons, don't expect confirmation too soon. Shouldn't wonder if every country has its own malaria-bearing species. It will be a very serious job to find them, I expect. For instance I can get no dapple wings here, and while proteosoma hasn't been seen in 50 odd local sparrows, grey mosquitos exist all over the place. This last is a very interesting fact. Then there is a deal of technique to be learned.

I think also there is much doubt about the vermicule business. Vide my report.

You also suggest my coming home. Let me first complete the life-cycle of proteosoma, if possible.

My next letter will be from Calcutta I expect. The rains are down here & I fear mosquitos won't bite even down below. If you want to send me any books, remember I have a bill at Lewis's. I have ordered your new book. *Want* Labbé on birds' coccidia badly.

Yours sincerely

R. Ross.

1 Reported in *BMJ* (7 May 1898), 1227-1228; (14 May 1898), 1290; (21 May 1898), 1353-1354, for analysis, see Arnold (1993); Harrison (1994).
2 Haffkine developed his plague vaccine in January 1897.
3 This sentence was omitted in *Memoirs*.
4 In an private letter to Harvey, 25 May 1898, Ross asked to be able to continue with malaria research rather than kala-azar, **RA** 03/125.
5 See Letter 129.
6 **RA** 06/058. Letter from G. M. Giles to Ross, 1 May 1898.
7 *Indian Medical Gazette* (May 1898), 187.

Letter 132
02/157

Calcutta
(Care of postmaster, Calcutta)
13th June [1898]

Dear Dr Manson,

As anticipated in my last I was obliged to return to this place owing to difficulties in getting birds with proteosoma & in persuading mosquitos to bite at Kurseong & Punkarbari. I arrived here on the 4th. Owing to plague scare all the bird catchers had bolted, and my sparrows from Kurseong died on returning (to their own climate!), so that I had some difficulties in getting under weigh again. At last however I have some beautiful stock of proteosoma-bearing greys & shall be hard at sporulation in three more days. The plan I shall adopt will be to examine only dead insects, as, all considered, I think the spores will form some time after death. At the same time I have a number of healthy young birds which I will try to infect by cramming malariated mosquitos down their throats. I have just ascertained beyond a doubt that birds eat mosquitos. Out of 70 which I tried to refeed last night only about 50 were found in the net (a new one) this morning.

The difficulties are minor ones - the birds are killed by too many mosquitos, the insects die in numbers at each refeed & when they lay their eggs. There is also difficulty in getting numerous sparrows here at present. But it is quite possible I may complete the life cycle of proteosoma in a few weeks.

I am also getting dapple-wings in large numbers now in *rain-water puddles*. These I am going to try on *halteridium*. Of course I am not allowed to experiment on human beings here because of the scare - at least just yet.

Your last letter received by me was dated 29th April, 6 weeks ago, so that I don't know whether all the batches of specimens have arrived safely or not. I fear your letters have been going wrong owing being addressed to c/o Surgeon General Calcutta. There is no such person; & accordingly the Post Office probably takes the opportunity to send them to Timbucktoo. MacCallum & Opie's paper has never reached me.

I am sending off to you all my old specimens used for my report. They are mostly beauties. I shall also send specimens of second day coccidia by this or next mail; and as soon as I get a sparrow with numerous parasites shall send mosquitos of the first day for sectioning.

Surgeon General Harvey has ordered 100 copies of my report, which is being run through the press as soon as possible. The plates are to be photolithographed. I hope it will arrive in ample time for the July meeting. He has however refused to *publish* the report, though he says I may send copies to experts. I don't understand the meaning of this at all & have written & asked Leslie, telling him that it is hardly possible or advisable to keep the business private.

I have seen no mention of the cultivation of proteosoma in the B. M. J. as yet, but hope it will appear soon as if not the Yanks may run in first by a fluke. I don't think *you* need hesitate about publishing a note on the subject because, as I told Leslie, the theory is yours & decidedly does not belong to the Govt. of India. In fact I would not hesitate if I were you in bringing it all out properly at the July meeting, showing my specimens, etc, & quoting from the copy of the report I sent you. Harvey evidently won't object to this as otherwise he would not have printed the report and given me permission to send it to "experts". So please do this (I will bear the consequences) unless I inform you explicitly that Surg. Gen. Harvey doesn't want it - which is not likely. Anyhow a brief notice to the effect that the work has been done will ensure priority and cannot be objected to.

14th June. Nearly 30 of my best stock died last night. It is a beautiful stock every mosquito having numerous coccidia. Also my best sparrow gave up the ghost. Owing to the heat, I expect, the coccidia in the dead mosquitos are unusually large for the period - 4th day - reaching 45µ, some of them & protruding freely. Hence I have left 20 of the dead insects to rot in water with a view to seeing what becomes of the coccidia. Sporulation *may* take place before complete growth, as in birds' proteosoma.

My servants & myself were very seedy on returning to Calcutta. Thought we had anchylostomata; but no eggs found. The heat here is awful - I shall never be able to serve in Calcutta as a permanency.

I fear I have lost time in going to the Terai but hardly expected the sparrows there to have no proteosoma, nor to be hindered by the plague scare. I might have finished proteosoma here & then come home for the Tropical Section. Anyway it is possible I may be home in September or so, if I can infect birds.

I applied for assistance. Refused of course. Things will never be done on a proper scale until a fuss has been made. Take stand on malaria, amoeba coli & anchylostoma & *pitch into them*.

15th. Just finished proofs of my report, copies of which will be sent by next mail. I enclose however proofs of my drawings, admirably done by photolithography.

No answer from Harvey yet.

Yours sincerely

R. Ross.

Specimens delayed until next mail. Will arrive in plenty of time for the meeting.

Letter 133
02/158

Calcutta
22nd June 1898

Dear Dr Manson,
I enclose letter from Leslie about the publication of my report.[1] You will see that no mention of my work must be made without the Secretary of State's assent. Copies of the reports will be sent to him by *next mail*, I trust; by which also I hope *you* will receive some; and if you care to bring the matter before the tropical section the only way to have it done will be to ask the Secretary of State's consent. However, I have never heard of this before (which seems sufficiently absurd); & my report on the sanitation of Bangalore was certainly published without S. of S's sanction.

I enclose also a registration receipt for a box containing some specimens, some of them tried old friends, others stained (wet); also a bottle of mosquitos fed on proteosoma sparrows & killed within 12 hours - in glycerine; also a bottle, on the label of which I forgot to write, containing 8 day mosquitos with mature proteosoma-coccidia. Two more mails have passed without my hearing from you, so that I don't know how past batches of specimens have sped, but I fear that they have been weak in good second-day coccidia. In this batch too the pigment of the second-day specimens has enlarged, but I shall try to send you 2nd day specimens especially, by next mail.

Leave your telegraphic address in Edinburgh when you go there for the B. A. meeting as I may be able to wire about infection of birds in time for it.

I think I am on the verge of another great advance. I have kept dead mosquitoes until they have fallen to bits - no development of the coccidia of 4th to 7th days. They resist longer than the stomach tissues but evidently degenerate - capsule shrinks, contents contract & become yellow, & ultimately bacteria enter. In the last stage of decomposition the stomach consists of a bag, the outer coat, full of bacteria, & having empty capsules of coccidia attached to it on the outside.

Hence no opening here apparently. Next the former suspicion is being confirmed that the coccidia burst in the *living insect* on about the 7th or 8th day, because in insects after that date (when fed only for the *first-time* on proteosoma-blood) only empty capsules seem to occur.

But I have found a most useful reagent - fairly strong salt solution. This brings out in a wonderful manner the *striation* of the coccidia & makes them look sometimes like caterpillars contained in an egg. Is it karyokinesis -?[2]

No, I think it likely that the striations are due to the coccidia or some of them, being packed full of *germinal threads* 10μ in length which are *scattered into the living insects' coelom.* I say this on the experience of one insect only of the 8th day examined this morning. It contained many mature proteosoma coccidia deeply striated; & also swarms of small bodies 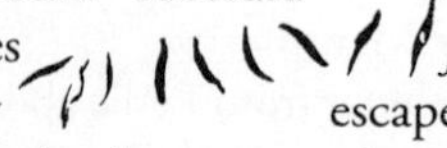 *feebly moving* in the salt solution & evidently escaped from the body cavity of the insects. I thought that by pressure I could force similar bodies out of the coccidia. The bodies are not bacteria; they taper at both ends & are broader in the centre, which appears capable of some change of shape.

23rd Have just found these "germinal rods" again in a mosquito of 8th day whose stomach was covered with empty capsules. Think I am on the track & hope to give you definite news by next mail.

I have heard from Laveran;[3] the specimens I sent him have not arrived though I registered the parcel. Yours sincerely

R. Ross.

1 **RA** 03/126, 2 June 1898. Leslie stated that the DG did not wish the report to be published until it had been confirmed by others although copies could be privately printed to establish Ross's priority. In a later telegram from Leslie (**RA** 03/141), 18 June 1898, Ross is told to order 100 copies to be printed, 50 of which to be sent to the DG (Gibson, 1983).

2 i.e. mitosis.

3 **RA** 02/183. Letter from Laveran to Ross, 28 May 1898, thanking him for describing the development of proteosoma of birds (Gibson, 1983).

Letter 134
02/045

21, Queen Anne Street,
Cavendish Square. W.
6th June, 1898.

My dear Ross,

I went to see Lord Lister yesterday[1] He promised to go over your work and give his opinion upon it; to say whether he thought it of sufficient public importance to go with to government and tell them they must go on with it. A week ago I saw Chamberlain who wants investigations made on the African fevers and who is willing to make a grant for this purpose. I told Chamberlain that important investigations were in progress in India which were about to be made public and asked him to wait for a week or two, to get Lord Lister's expression of opinion on their value before going to the Treasury for the money.

Now, therefore, send me, by return if possible, either a copy of your report to government or a precis and, if you have any very telling slides and drawings these also, to submit to Lister. When he gives me a writing to say that it is all right, as there can be no doubt he will, I shall take this to Chamberlain and say I want money. He will probably say, here you are. I shall then go to the India Office through Cleghorn or some one else and tell them what Chamberlain is doing. They will probably go one better. I will suggest a commission with you at the head of it and I will get Lister to back me up. I think this is the game but it requires to be played quickly and before the edge is off the novelty and before the Yanks and Continentals get a skimming off of the cream. You will see that Laveran will have the thing all over the place soon.

The B. M. J. has not published my notice yet. I suppose because I sent with it several drawings of your cells.

I showed the cells to Thin on Sunday. He is always full of cold water and objections.[2] He says you should sit down and work quietly for years and years until there is not a vestige of objection possible before you publish anything. I wonder how you are to live meanwhile. It has not been his policy at all events. No, we have to lever up the government and the public and then you will get the opportunities. *So send me at once if you can a statement for Lister* - drawings & more slides if you can spare them. Lister was very sympathetic and encouraging.

Yours sincerely

Patrick Manson

1 Then President of the Royal Society.

2 See, for example, Letter 23, note 2, and Letters 25 and 36.

Letter 135
02/159

Calcutta
28th June 1898

Dear Dr Manson,
I dispatched some copies of my report to you by this mail with one for Sir J. Fayrer. Will you oblige me greatly by sending it on to him. I don't know his address but will write to him as well.

I fear much I shan't be able to send you good second-day specimens as my infected birds are so much better that they don't yield good crops any longer; but will try tomorrow.

The bulk of the copies of my report are not *sewn* even yet and will never reach the Sec. of State through the Govt. of India in time for the B. M. J. Meeting.[1] The only thing to be done then is for you to send him one of the copies I have dispatched to you with Leslie's letter, & ask his permission to publish. He is sure to give it straight off.

Another advance has been made. On the 6th & 7th day the coccidia form a large number of germinal rods (?), 12μ in length. This is easily seen by using a rather strong salt solution which gives many of the coccidia *from* 5th day a striated appearance as figured in the Report, but more marked. By using pressure these coccidia are easily burst, when the rods pour out.

They are just about 12μ in length & all the same size. They taper towards each end & are therefore thicker in the middle. In salt solution after a time they show one or more vacuoles in the middle part & become bent angularly. They stain easily with Loeffler,[2] Delafield,[3] etc, and then show one or more chromatin granules toward the middle, between the vacuoles, & at the same time become broader, when they look very like small *trypanosomes*. They often possess swellings somewhere along their length; very like *flagella* do. On addition of water they tend to curl up & look like granular material. I am not sure whether they are at all motile; though I have often thought so. I think especially that they bend & straighten themselves; but these points are very difficult to ascertain because of their continual brownian movement, while it is evident that both water & salt solution kills them.

When youngish striated coccidia are burst these bodies issue attached like rays to circular cells. →

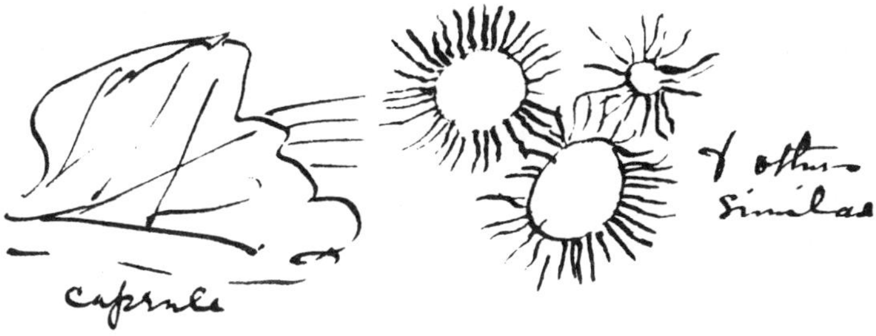

This arrangement can often be seen within the unburst coccidium. The circular cells to which the germinal rods are attached by their end stain easily like the rods, but show no sign of nucleus.

In older coccidia the rods pour out all separately & the cells are not to be found.

The rods are easily seen in large numbers in eight day mosquitos (& earlier) all round the stomach & amongst the abdominal scales. They are in the *coelom*.

The use of fairly strong salt solution has enabled me to ascertain these points, which may be taken as quite certain.

No development of the rods has yet been observed either in living or in decomposing mosquitos.

One never finds all the coccidia even when mature, to be striated, that is, to contain rods. The rest seem to contain nothing but a clear fluid with bright oil globules.

I have searched in vain in living mosquitos & dead ones for anything like psorosperms or pseudo navicellae, unless the black sausage shaped bodies (Report, Plate I, figure 20)[4] are such. These however are only rarely seen & appear there to exist only in empty capsules. I expect they are *fungi* or something - germs within germs - but am keeping my eye on them.

It appears pretty certain that on the 7th or 8th days all the coccidia burst in the *living* insect & pour their contents into the coelom.

Are the rods of the nature of *spermatozoa*, or are they *falciform* bodies. In the latter case the round cell with its radiation of rods may perhaps be the homologue of the ordinary spore of coccidia - in fact a *naked spore*.

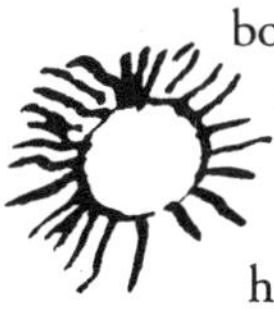

Nature probably makes some extraordinary effort here in order to complete the life cycle. What the dickens she is going to do next I cannot imagine at all. Great difficulties may however be feared owing to the absence of hard spores. But I am trying to turn the position by blind attempts to infect healthy sparrows.

Infected mosquitos have been fed on five healthy sparrows for a fortnight. On examining again the other day a few proteosoma were found in one of the sparrows - scarcely good enough. I am therefore feeding three healthy sparrows with mosquitos containing mature coccidia.

But this climate! I can perhaps stand another month of it. It is hell, simply; & the constant strain on mind & eye at this temperature is making me thoroughly ill. If I cannot infect birds or find a clear opening by the end of July I *must* clear out. Permanent work here is out of the question for me, I feel. But I shall stick on to the last gasp in order to be able to wire to you before the B. M. J.[5] meeting, if possible.

I have heard from Laveran.[6] He has received my specimens & accepts the discovery. He writes "J'ai examiné toutes vos préparations et j'ai constaté que vos descriptions étaient d'une exactitude parfaite ... il me semble pas douteuse qu'ils (the coccidia) dérivent des hématozoaires des oiseaux ... Je pense comme M: Manson que vous avez fait une découverte très importante." Perhaps however it was not very wise to put the thing in his hands at all.

29th June. I have found large numbers of germinal rods in the thorax of two mosquitos, one a *six* day & one an *eight* day one. The former contained two empty capsules & two striated (rod-bearing) coccidia; the latter contained only a large number of empty capsules. The rods lay among the scales & muscles of the thorax & showed no further development.

This scarcely looks like the spermatozoa theory. The rods appear much too numerous for this & sometimes *all* the coccidia in a mosquito are rod containing ones. They must evidently get into the insect's circulating fluid for some reason.

Now I must thank you for yours of 6th June. This reached me, being address to C/O Postmaster. But the last one before this was dated 29th April, so that I don't know how the specimens arrived. I judge that they were not very good. It must be due to the voyage as my own remain all right for months. I sent you all my best specimens last mail (except one series which I keep for demonstrations), & I hope that these, with a copy of my report will do for Lord Lister. The *best* specimens are sometimes those with the insects' scales in them, put in for the purpose of preventing the cover glass from crushing the larger coccidia.

Thin's advice to work for years & years is good. It is just what I have done. It is also good not to publish until there is not a vestige of objection possible. Here again the Report follows his advice.

My advice is that any further objections are scarcely to be recommended as they will meet with a terrible fate, I think. I don't see any line of criticism which can be taken up against the theory with any chance of success. I venture to say that there is no fact in the life history of any parasite more certain than that proteosoma in the bird becomes coccidium in the mosquito. It is quite certain. The man who criticises will die; he will knock his head against a rock.

Very many thanks for you efforts on behalf of a commission. Remember always two things - that the Govt. of India is a *mule* as regards science. It *won't* do anything unless driven. As for the I. M. S., it does not care a cent for the whole business. Remember also that if Govt. of India won't do anything I am always willing (if not anxious) to take my pension & work elsewhere & for other masters. What do you think of Egypt? Fact is we are tired of India & I feel that my health won't stand it very much longer. Besides research work will never pay me in cash out here & it will not lead to anything that will. It simply means heat & bad health - unless Govt. will put me some height up the hills, which I doubt. Monetarily my pension of £300 a year is really almost equal to my present pay of R1000 a month with the expenses of life in India with continual moves. So if there is anything going elsewhere which is open to me & is better than India, remember I will take my pension at once to get it.

Several specimens of anchylostoma eggs, trypanosomes & filariae of birds which I put up for you have, I just find, accidently been left at Kurseong.

Wishing you every luck with the Tropical Section, I remain

Yours sincerely

R. Ross.

Leave orders to forward letters & telegrams for you to Edinburgh, as the copies of the Report may come late & I may be able to wire something to you at the last moment.

1 Ross meant to write BMA.

2 Loeffler solution - 'a methylene-blue stain in weak alcohol with a little alkali'. H. W. Cattell *Lippincotts New Medical Dictionary* (Philadelphia: J. B. Lippincott Company, 1910).

3 Delafields haematoxylin, 'a nuclear stain', *ibid.*

4 Ross (1898b).

5 The Sixty Sixth Annual Meeting of the British Medical Association was held in Edinburgh, 26th-29th July, 1898.

6 **RA** 02/184, 10 June, 1898.

Letter 136
02/160

Calcutta
6th July 1898

Dear Dr Manson,

Let me in the first place felicitate you and the profession on the new Tropical Section & let me wish it every success in the future. It is started under the best possible auspices.

I hope this letter will reach you at Edinburgh. If so, it will be opportune; because I feel *almost* justified in saying that I have completed the life-cycle, or rather perhaps one life-cycle, of proteosoma, and therefore in all probability of the malaria parasite. I say almost, because though I think I have seized the final position, I have not yet occupied it with my full forces.

My last letter left me face to face with the astonishing fact that the germinal rods were to be found in the thorax as well as in the abdomen. Instead of the hard resisting spores we expected to arrive at - spores easily seen & followed - here were a multitude of delicate little threads, scarcely more visible than dead flagella and poured out amongst the million objects, which, under an oil-immersion lens, go to make up a mosquito. I dare say you imagined my consternation. I could not conceive what was to happen to the rods.

Well, I was in for a battle. It was, I think, the last stand - on the very breathless heights of science. I am nearly blind & dead with exhaustion!! - but triumphant. Expect one of the most wonderful things.

The rods were evidently in the insect's *blood.* By merely pricking the back of the thorax and letting the milky juice flow into a minute drop of salt solution thousands of proteosoma-coccidium-rods could easily be obtained. The question was what next?

I now divided my insects before dissection between the thorax & abdomen & examined each part separately. It was found that the rods were often *more numerous in the thorax than in the abdomen*; there were even cases where scarcely one could be found in the abdomen (the coccidia having evidently burst some days previously as shown by their empty capsules), while numbers (4 or 5 in a field) could be detected on teazing up the thorax & head.

Here however I was brought up standing. Sometimes the rods were more common in the head, sometimes in the thorax. I went at mosquito after mosquito spending hours over each, until I was blind & half silly with fatigue. The object was to find if possible a place or structure where the rods accumulate; or to discover some further development in them. Nothing.

On the 4th however, after pulling out the head by its roots (oesophagus etc) from the thorax, some delicate structure dropped out of the cervical aperture of the latter. This proved to be a long branching gland of some sort, looking like a coil of large intestine, and consisting of a long duct with closely packed, refractive cells attached to it. I noticed at once that the rods were swarming here & were even *pouring out* from somewhere in streams. Suddenly to my amazement it was seen that many of the cells of this gland *contained the germinal rods of proteosoma-coccidia* ***within them***. Looking further the cells of one whole lobe of the gland were simply packed with them, and on bursting the cells the rods poured out of them just as they pour out of the original coccidia.

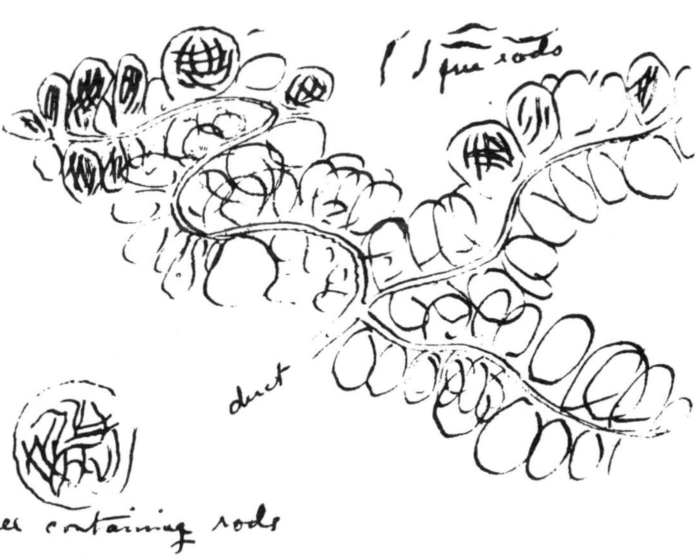

The rods were quite unmistakable, having the tapering, flattened & vacuolated structure peculiar to them. They are identified at once & no structures like them exist in the normal mosquito. Here they were in the cells of the gland. The cells were not *coccidia*. They are only 25μ in diameter, have a very thin outline & contain a perfectly clear fluid, without granulations or oil-drops such as the coccidia possess. The rods lay within them quite irregularly & motionless except for brownian movement. In one lobe almost every cell contained numbers of rods; in other lobes only one or two cells contained them. By the attachment of the cells to the central duct, it seemed quite easy for the rods to pass on occasion from the former into the latter.

Now what was this gland? Will you believe it, I examined two whole mosquitos without finding it again? What with the scales, the debris of muscles etc, I could not come upon it. A third mosquito gave the same result, until I opened up the *head* itself. There was the gland *attached by its duct which led straight into the structures somewhere between the eyes.* The cells were again packed with germinal rods.

I have found the gland now altogether in seven mosquitos. In six of them the cells were packed (especially in some lobes) more or less with germinal rods. In the seventh I could find only a small piece of gland, which was free from rods.

I still experience, however, the greatest difficulty in dissecting out the gland itself. It appears to lie in front of the thorax close to the head, but breaks so easily in the dissection that I cannot locate it properly. In the second mosquito however there was no doubt, as shown by evident attachment that the duct led straight into the head-piece, probably into the mouth.

In other words it is a thousand to one, it is a *salivary gland.*

I think that this, after further elaboration, will close at least one cycle of proteosoma, and I feel that I am *almost* entitled to lay down the law by direct observation & tracking the parasite step by step -

Malaria is conveyed from a diseased person or bird to a healthy one by the proper species of mosquito, & is inoculated by its bite.

Remember however that there is virtue in the "almost". I don't announce the law yet. Even when the microscope has done its utmost, healthy birds must be infected with all due precautions.

I say *one* cycle. I think it likely there is another. I continually observe that only a portion of the coccidia contain germinal rods. The rest, I now think, give rise to the black sausage-shaped bodies shown in plate I, fig. 20 of my report,[1] which I believe may be the true spores of the parasite meant either for free life or to infect grubs. Oddly enough, in old mosquitos these bodies also get carried away into the tissues - unless they are some disease of the insect. I will attack this next.

7th. I dissected two healthy mosquitos this morning & began by dividing the head & anterior third of the thorax from the middle third by means of a razor, and then carefully breaking up the anterior third. In both cases the glands were found & their ducts were traced straight into the head; thus:-

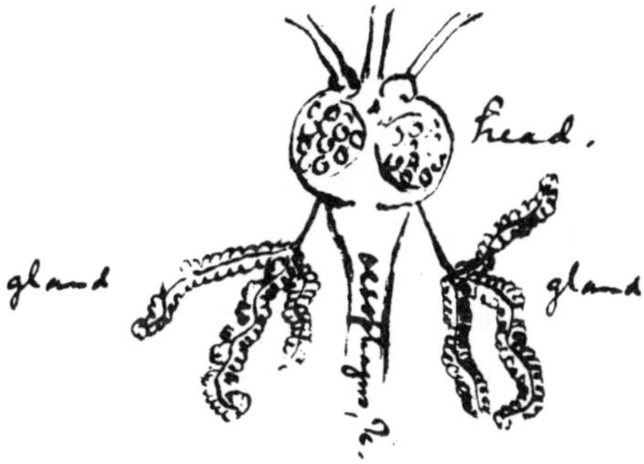

In all probability it is these glands which secrete the stinging fluid which the mosquito injects into the bite. The germinal rods, lying, as they do, in the secreting cells of the gland, pass into the duct when those cells begin to perform their function, and are thus poured out in vast numbers under the skin of the man or bird. Arrived there, numbers of them are probably instantly swept away by the circulation of the blood, in which they immediately begin to develop into malaria parasites, thus completing the cycle. No time to write more. Yours very sincerely

R. Ross.

1 Ross (1898b).

Letter 137
02/046

21 Queen Anne St.
Cavendish Sq. W.
June 24th 1898.

My dear Ross,
I have been and am still laid up with a severe attack of general gout[1] but must try and give you some idea of what has been done and what I propose to do.

In the first place be assured that your future is safe. You have done a great work and your deed will not be forgotten. You will see from the last British Medical Journal that I have secured your priority in discovery and have nipped what may have been an attempt at stealing.[2]

I must have misread one of you letters for I certainly thought you told me you had found pigmented cells in a halteridium feeding experiment. I got the copy of your report only last night - two days late for any alterations in my British Medical Journal diagram. However no great damage is done. I have only anticipated what will surely soon be found, now you have shown the way. You will note that I took care to get Laveran's, Metchnikoff's, and Nuttall's confirmation, deeming that the foreign man has more weight with our people than has the native whom we have always with us.

On Tuesday I got Lister to come to my house and had some 6 or 7 microscopes with your preparations for him to study. I was very ill at the time but struggled with clothes and told him all about the matter. He expressed himself convinced. I asked him if he would back me up in my representation to the government. He said he would and was everything you could desire in his recognition of the value of your discovery. Among other reasons I asked Lister to a special demonstration because I want him to help me in the representation I propose to make as soon as I can get to the Colonial Office and India Office.[3] I shall see, or write to, Chamberlain, who has already expressed a desire to do something in Malaria,[4] and represent to him that now is his opportunity. I shall briefly explain the nature and possibilities of your discovery and suggest that the Colonial Office approach the India Office suggesting cooperation. For a reliable and the highest possible opening on the value of this discovery I shall request him to communicate with Lord Lister P.R.S. (There is no fear about Lister's answer; I have sent him your report). I shall suggest that the Colonial Government either make a grant for the continuation of the investigation or to send over two men to be under and assist you and so qualify for working out the problem in Africa and other colonies. I shall say that time, a free hand, and adequate finances are necessary.

He will write to the India Office and the thing should be as good as done. A permanent commission appointed with yourself at the head.

Yours sincerely
Patrick Manson

I would have written more fully but am horribly weak & unfit to sit at my desk. I had to get my daughter to typewrite for me.

1 Manson suffered from gout for much of his adult life. For details see Manson-Bahr and Alcock (1927), 236ff.

2 P. Manson, 'Surgeon-Major Ronald Ross's recent investigations on the mosquito-malaria theory', *BMJ* (18 June 1898), 1575-1577.

3 See Letters 134 and 141.

4 An intimation of the Royal Society Malaria Committee.

Letter 138
02/161

Calcutta
9th July 1898

Dear Dr Manson,
One full solution of the malaria problem was obtained this morning - unfortunately just too late to catch the mail by wire to Bombay. The facts are as follows:-

Just after I wrote to you I obtained some good dissections of the gland in healthy insects. It still remains very difficult to get out nicely & almost impossible to mount for you; but by examining a number of insects I have obtained the leading facts about it. The lobes lie either in the head, neck or front of thorax (according to the fulness of the cells, I think). I think there are 18 lobes: thus

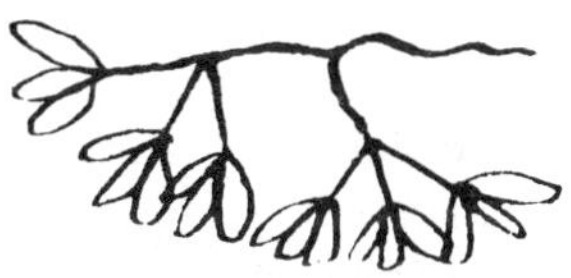

The ducts finally all join together into one large tube which runs up along the under surface of the head. In one specimen which I will send you I can trace it to its termination. When it arrives close to the origin of the mouth parts, it (the duct) passes through a kind of round shield and enters one of the long stabbing spears of the proboscis. It appears to run up *inside* this & open somewhere near its end.

There is no doubt then that the gland must pour its secretion straight into the wound made by the mosquito.

In old infected mosquitos I think that many lobes of the gland are almost destroyed by infection with the proteosoma rods. In one case the cells seem to have united into a single sack loaded with rods.

In 8 male mosquitos I have not once found any evidence of the existence of this gland.

So far then, there is a complete chain of evidence pointing to the infection during haustellation. Now for the clincher.

On the 25th June (as I think I told you) I carefully selected three healthy sparrows. Their blood had been examined three times on different occasions & always found free from parasites. On the 25th night & almost every night following I have used these birds to refeed a large stock of mosquitos which had been infected from diseased sparrows on 21st-22nd June. This was the identical stock with which I worked out the story of the germinal rods. Lately I had been finding young crops of coccidia in this stock & therefore had a presentiment of what I should observe in the birds. I wish therefore I had examined them before so as to let you know in time for the B. M. A. meeting; but I hardly expected such a knock-down result.

All three birds, perfectly healthy a fortnight ago, were now simply swarming with proteosoma, twenty parasites & more in one oil-im. field.

Again on 1st July I selected a healthy sparrow & a healthy "baia",[1] & refed another infected stock on them every night up to date. These two were examined this morning. Both had proteosoma, the sparrow a few, the baia fairly numerous.

Hence I think I may now say Q. E. D., and congratulate you on the mosquito theory indeed. The door is unlocked, and I am walking in & collecting the treasures.

For instance, proteosoma of sparrows is communicable to baias. Hence there is probably only one proteosoma, common to various birds. You see I shall give it to crows etc. Also, I have an idea indeed. What if proteosoma = spring tertian? I shall feed infected mosquitos on a man or two, & shall take it from a man to a sparrow, if it be so.

11th July. I have forgotten to say that (10) ten healthy sparrows examined on the 25th June & kept nightly in mosquito nets to keep mosquitos *out*, all remain perfectly well up to date. I told you also that on 25th June I gave infected mosquitos to three healthy sparrows by the mouth. Two of the birds died a few days afterwards (numbers of my birds have been dying) without proteosoma. The third had nothing on 1st July & was used for feeding infected sparrows; with positive results as already given. Rather a jumble, but future experiments will be more precise. It's useful to be jumbly at times to begin with.

I have now to record three more successes. Three baias (kind of bunting I think) were formerly found to contain large numbers of halteridium only - no proteosoma I am certain. They have often been used to refeed old infected stock. Yesterday they were examined again & found to contain numerous halteridium, & *swarms* of proteosoma. One bird died last night. Liver enormous & black. Heart's blood contained an enormous young brood of proteosoma. The bird's blood practically consisted of parasites. There you have it full at last.

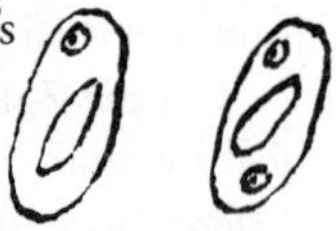

This also *proves* that sparrow's proteosoma is communicable to baias.

Having won the battle of Atbara I am now marching on Omdurman;[2] that is, I am rushing the black sausage-shaped bodies.

I wonder if the Secretary of State gave permission to publish results as soon as obtained. They ought to be published in the interest of the public. Thus the Planters' Association of Southern India have written to me asking what I have done. I am obliged to tell them that I must not say. This is very absurd. It will be worse in the future. Events will march now, and instead of keeping things dark every publicity should be given to such facts as those just found, as the communicability of malaria via the mosquito. At present my mouth is closed.

Well, I have become unbearable with conceit over tracking the germinal rods into the salivary gland. That was a grand charge! I brag openly about it!

12th July. I have just received yours of 24th & the B. M. J. of 18 June together. I am indeed sorry to hear of your illness, &, while it was very kind of you to have taken so much trouble with Lord Lister (and also in writing to me) wish that you had postponed doing so until better. I have felt inclined to telegraph & ask how you are. It was really very good of you to bother yourself, & I only hope you won't think of doing so again until quite well. We are partly selfish in wishing so, remember. However, at this distance it is scarcely possible to send wishes for even a return to health; & I can only trust that you are much better while I write. The scheme you are going to propose is admirable. No doubt the Govt. of India will jog up when Chamberlain comes along. Remember I am entirely at your disposal. The idea is grand, and I promise to throw myself into it. I have already arranged my tactics. They will be Napoleonic (!) - concentration. We shall attack one problem at a time in a body, if possible. That is the way, I am sure. See the results I am getting out of proteosoma alone. If I had remained fiddling with Anchylostomiasis or human malaria, we should not have gone quarter the distance by this time. One thing at a time, & at it full speed. - But I want to suggest my coming home for a few months - or rather you have suggested it - for the following reasons:-

1. At the rate I am now going I expect that I shall have solved the malaria problem in two months or three. I have only to fill in details of the germinal rod cycle, take photos, send you specimens, etc, & do a number of obvious infection experiments. At the same time I think I can carry out the "black body" business, grow them in water, or infect mosquito grubs with them. That will complete proteosoma. One single experiment with crescents (there are numerous dapple winged insects here now) will enable me to bring human malaria into line with proteosoma - they are sure to be just the same. This will really score all the chief points. I ought to do it in two months; it has taken me only one to work out the germinal rods cycle.

2. I should like to come home to take your advice about future work; also to read up coccidia; also if possible to go & see Labbé & Pfeiffer[3] etc; to read some papers before societies; to get some instruments I have thought of for counting eggs & gymnosporidia, etc.

3. I have had 3½ years incessant work & worry, am feeling tired & out of sorts & feel I should have a rest & get a sniff of cold before opening into such a big business as a commission.

4. If the commission is to be started my presence in England may be useful to help you to arrange details.

Now I *may* apply for furlough as you suggested; but I have just had to apply officially for six months extension of my present duty & have not yet touched kala-azar. They are sure to reply "no; you applied for six months extension; you have not yet touched kala-azar; we can't give you furlough yet; you must go to Assam."

I certainly would like & intend to run up to Assam (5 days' journey from here) for a few weeks just to have a look at kala-azar; but to deal with that disease thoroughly will take months if I mistake not. Now there appears only one way out of this difficulty (unless I go sick) & that is, if the Colonial Office & India Office come to terms, to have me sent home on duty. It will also save me money - and we are nearly ruined from having to live in hotels everywhere - family in one place, myself in another. If you think it advisable then, will you drop in a suggestion to that effect when they come to consider details with you? If however you *don't* think Govt. should be asked to send me home *on duty* & yet want me to come home, I shall certainly do so; but it will facilitate matters if you can send me a business note to the effect that the Colonial & India Offices have agreed to start a commission & that my presence in England would be useful. I could send this up to Govt. to back my application for furlough. I expect to be able to "rough hew"[4] malaria & have a look at kala-azar by October, so as to start home in November, or even earlier. In fact I may be perhaps free to go home very shortly, say September.

Your book is out here at last - reviews appearing in the lay press; very favourable, but some reviewers still hanker over the "blue mist" theories - they save so much trouble.[5] More of this anon.

Now I must thank you for the articles in the B. M. J. and all the handsome things said therein. It is useful having Laveran's, Metchnikoff's & Nuttall's assent.[6] The next thing in the B. M. J. ought to contain the full solution of the problem. I think the mistake about halteridium arose from Series 17 (vide Report p. 4, & remarks about crows p. 6). I thought I corrected myself in later letters. The remarks at the end of the leader in the B. M. J. will probably stir

Govt. to work things on a larger scale.[7] But they may wig me for authorising you to publish at all. I shall reply to the point.

Two more of my artificially infected sparrows have died from excessive proteosomiasis-swarms. I overdosed them. I hope to have a lot more birds (crows, sparrows) infected in time to wire you about the 25th. Black bodies not yet found in healthy mosquitos - probably proteosoma spores.

Remember if there is a hurry about the commission, if you want men to come out quickly & learn the mosquito business, I *will stop out here as long as you think necessary*. But personally I feel I ought to go home for six months, unless you think the reasons urgent against it. Govt. won't hesitate over sending me home on duty & will think twice as much of the commission in consequence. Bully them, squeeze them; they deserve it, and will respect the whole business much more if you do. With kind regards, wishes for return of health & all felicitations of victory.

Yours sincerely
R. Ross.

1 Later in the letter Ross refers to this as a 'kind of bunting', a small finch-like bird of the subfamily *Emberizinae.*

2 Battles of the Sudan campaign of 1898 under Kitchener. Atbara was fought on April 8 and Omdurman on September 2.

3 Richard Friedrich Johannes Pfeiffer, (1858-1945), Koch's assistant in his plague investigations in India in 1896 and malaria in Italy in 1898. He held the chair of hygiene and bacteriology at Königsberg from 1899.

4 *Hamlet*, Act V, sc. ii.

5 Anon, Review of Manson's *Tropical Diseases* (1898), *Indian Medical Gazette* (Sept. 1898), 348-350. The review mentioned that Manson cited the work of IMS officers frequently, even while castigating him for casting caution to the winds when arguing for the *Plasmodia*/mosquito theory of malaria.

6 Manson (1898b), in which he quotes Nuttall and Laveran, the latter mentioning that Metchnikoff shares his opinions.

7 A leader ('Honour to whom honour is due') in the 18 June 1898 issue of *BMJ* (pp 1607-8), castigated Robert Koch for claiming too much for himself, congratulated the Government of India for appointing Ross to his malaria research and urged the Government to retain him at his present work and 'to provide him with every assistance he may require'.

Letter 139
02/049

21, Queen Anne Street,
Cavendish Square. W.
1st July, 1898.

My dear Ross,

I have got to the end of nigh three weeks solid misery and pain. I am better at last but as weak as a kitten and tired to death. Meanwhile the world has wagged on and there has been little progress in the mosquito-malaria business. I have got the two letters, copies of which I enclose, from Lord Lister.[1] These I have sent to Surgeon General Harvey with the expression of the hope that you will get a free hand and asking him if it would be possible to get two men attached to you from the Colonial Medical Service. I mean to try for this. It will do no harm to ask; on the contrary it will show him that your work is appreciated at home. I sent him Lister's letters with the same idea. Tomorrow I hope to be strong enough to go to the Colonial Office and set them onto the India Office.

I don't know what to do about your report at the Association meeting; whether to make a precis of it or to wait for the chance of Harvey having sent out the report in full. In any case I shall have a good show of the slides and shall take care to have the matter well ventilated. The danger is to overdo the mosquito and to run the risk of boring people about it. I suppose some think I am mad on the point. Let them.

I am looking forward to your next work with very great interest. You are like Captain Cook now - sailing into unknown seas which may reveal wonders unconceived. "We were the first, that ever burst, into that silent sea" says old Coleridge;[2] original work of the kind you are on gives the feeling that the old navigators must have had when they plunged into the unknown. Wishing you good luck on your voyage and thanking you for the photo of the navigator and his wife[3] I remain

Yours sincerely
Patrick Manson

1 **RA** 02/047, 27 June 1898, Letter from Lister to Manson enclosing a written testimonial of Ross's researches and saying that he would testify directly to Chamberlain if necessary; **RA** 02/048, 29 June 1898, letter from Lister to Manson returning Ross's report saying that it is of remarkable interest and value and that Ross should be

given further opportunity of continuing his researches.

2 Samuel Taylor Coleridge, *The Ancient Mariner* (1798), pt. ii.

3 This photograph, now famous, shows Ross, his wife, Muhomed Bux and two other Indian assistants, standing on the steps of the Calcutta laboratory, behind Ross's bird cages. There are slightly different versions of it in *Memoirs*, plate VI, and Nye and Gibson (1997), plate 5.

Letter 140
02/162

Calcutta
20th July 1898

Dear Dr Manson,

I am awfully glad to hear by yours of the 1st that you are better. I was alarmed at hearing of your sickness which I know is no joke. But am sorry you have bothered yourself about my affairs while you were so ill. I trust this will reach you quite recovered.

Your letter to Harvey with Lord Lister's enclosure ought to do everything as to my being kept on at this work; but they won't give me assistance without pressure from the India Office. It is an excellent idea to send me a couple of men from the Colonial Office to learn the work. Last week I wrote asking to go home, and I should certainly like to do so; but if you think it necessary will stay out longer in order to teach your men. *Do just as you like and think fit.*

Five more birds (sparrows) have been infected. Four healthy sparrows were bitten by old mosquitos with germinal rods on the nights of the 10th-11th, and 11th-12th July. They were examined on the 15th & found all free of parasites. They were examined again on the 18th. One was free (& died of tetanus same evening); the other three now swarmed with parasites, respectively, 2, 6, & 10 in each field - proteosoma only of course.

On the 12th-13th & 13th-14th June, 5 healthy sparrows were bitten by the same old stock (3 weeks old). Two died next day & one on the 19th (no proteosoma). The remaining two had moderate proteosoma on the 18th day (sixth day of experiment).

Out of 4 control sparrows, one showed a few proteosoma on the 7th day - probably overlooked before. The rest remain quite healthy.

I have calculated by Calculus of Probabilities the chances against n birds becoming infected by accident *within a fortnight after an experiment*, on the basis of the percentage of infected wild birds I have found.[1] The chances are millions to one against 3 or 4 birds showing simultaneous accidental infection within the period. Apart from this, nine of the birds (I have infected 13) have had much more severe infections than I have ever seen before. I can therefore announce the law:-

"Healthy birds may be infected by the bites of the proper species of mosquitos which have previously fed on diseased birds."

I shall bring mathematics to bear heavily on these matters presently. Lucky I know something of the science (spent seven years over it). It will serve to knock on the head many loose ideas.

Not much work possible on the black bodies this week as I have been keeping my old stock for infecting sparrows. But I have failed to find the bodies in a large number of healthy mosquitos, so that I think they must be spores of the coccidia. They are carried by the circulation & distributed all over the tissues. The largest number of them seen by me in one insect is two or three hundred. A specimen kept for three weeks in the damp chamber shows no marked alteration or development in the bodies. They are too few to be meant to infect birds directly by the mouth or lungs. The chances would be infinity to one against one of them ever entering by those channels. What is a dead mosquito in water or dust? It is infinitesimal. Men & birds don't go about eating dead mosquitos. No, nature is too clever for such an attempt. She brings the mosquito (and the infection) straight to the man or bird & puts it nicely into his blood, so as to give it every chance. I think then that the black bodies must be meant to infect grubs. They will probably produce germinal rods & infect the salivary glands again.

I am thinking of telegraphing to you, giving the result of the infection experiments. It may help you at the B. M. A. But I think it quite right, as you say, not to bore people about the mosquito, especially as there is sure to be a great battle soon over the last results. The legions of the "blue fog" theorists are sure to be up in arms over it all. Hard hitting will be required, and demanded by the gravity of the issue at stake. You may be sure I will arm myself for the conflict with very heavy *spiked* facts. I certainly feel like a navigator according to your simile; but like one who has a fight before him before he can effect a landing.

Am trying to make you specimens of salivary glands - very difficult.

Yours very sincerely

R. Ross.

MacCallum & Opie's articles sent by you last April have just reached me.[2]

1 Nye and Gibson (1997), ch. 14, summarise Ross's mathematical excursions.

2 MacCallum (1898a and 1898b); Opie (1898).

Letter 141
02/050

21, Queen Anne Street,
Cavendish Square. W.
8th July, 1898.

My dear Ross,
I think things are going well on this side. Mr Chamberlain has written to Lord Lister to the effect that he wants something done in the malaria line and saying that the Colonial Government will bear half the expense. Lister called on me yesterday and I posted him again on the mosquito business so that he might be ready for the Committee meeting of the Royal Society yesterday afternoon which was to discuss Chamberlain's letter.[1] I suggested two medical men and an entomologist to go to India to help and learn from you who might afterwards be sent to Africa or elsewhere to take up the inquiry.[2] I think it will be all right now. At all events the Indian Government will see that whatever they think about the matter it is considered one of the first importance here.

I am having a precis of your report made and shall read it or have it read at the B.M.A. meeting at the end of the month and will have some six or eight typical slides on show. I would have had photos etc and lantern slides but I have been too ill to accomplish this and drag myself through the daily routine as well.

I am anxiously awaiting your next letters for I would like to be able to say at the B.M.A. meeting that the early stage and the sporulating stage of proteosoma in mosquito had been found.

When found, what next? I suppose following the spore into other mosquitos and into the bird. This will be delicate and difficult but to you not impossible. This worked out you will be ready to tackle human malaria.

I hope you approved of my notice in the B M J. I am sorry about the mistake in halteridium but in reading your letters I certainly had the impression conveyed to my mind that you had seen it in mosquito. Pity that McCallum and Opie have not turned up. I hope they will yet come to hand. If the Royal Society commission goes out to you I shall take care that they have a complete protozoal library.

Yours sincerely
Patrick Manson

1 At its 7 July 1898 Council Meeting, The Royal Society considered Chamberlain's letter and agreed to establish a Malaria Committee and to contribute £300 to it. (Royal Society Minutes of Council, vol. 7, (1892-98), 437-8). The Malaria Committee first met 6 days later, on 13 July. (henceforth RSMC)

2 In the event, the Royal Society Malaria Committee appointed C. W. Daniels, S. R. Christophers and J. W. W. Stephens to posts. For details, see W. F. Bynum. 'An experiment that failed: malaria control at Mian Mir', *Parassitologia*, 38 (1994), 107-120.

Letter 141a[1]
INDIAN TELEGRAPHS

8. 7. [1898]

TO	Dr Patrick Manson President Tropical Section British Medical Association Edinburgh	FROM	Ross

Post Registered Bombay

Duct of gland traced directly into mosquitos proboscis

1 Letter in the possession of Dr Gordon Manson-Bahr. The date of this telegram is a puzzle; the Edinburgh Meeting was not until the end of July and the telegram itself has been detached from the main sequence of Ross-Manson correspondence. There is evidence of 2 telegrams having been sent to the Edinburgh Meeting, see Letters 142, note 2 and 146, note 2.

Letter 142
02/163

Calcutta
27th July 1898

Dear Dr Manson,

On the 25th, some more birds having become infected, particularly a crow, I made up my mind to wire to you announcing that one complete solution of the problem has been obtained. I think it may strengthen your hand at the B. A. meeting & elsewhere, and only wish I had done it before, as I might well have done.

On the same day yours of the 8th was received. It is dated the day before my first experimental batch of birds were found to be infected. So that "following the spore into the bird" had been practically done when you wrote.[1]

I am rather sorry I opened the idea of my coming home. It may tie your hands. I had no idea that you could push things along so fast. Of course, I should like to come home, but if you have anything arranged and the men ready to come out, I must stop here. Do just as you like and think fit. Telegraph to me if necessary. "Ronald Ross care Postmaster Calcutta". (I suppose Colonial Office will pay).

The question about my coming home appears to depend on the length of the period for which your men are to be attached to me. If only for a short period, say six months, and only to learn what I know, I think it would be better to send them out statim. I could teach them, finish up odds & ends of work & get home by next March or so. But if it is to be a long business, if we are to study malaria & mosquitos over the country, work out means of prevention, investigate filariasis, anchylostomiasis, & so on, in fact do all that we are capable of, I should say let me come home first. I want to see you, & feel cold again, & to work out numerous things, such as centrifugalising for malaria germs & worms eggs (proper machines required).

Govt. of India has extended my present duty for six months (until 17th Feb. next), according to my request - I applied only for six months extension. After that I don't know what they will do.

I think it best to leave everything in your hands.

Another reason for coming home is that all the gymnosporidia must now be renamed & think it will be necessary to consult specialists on coccidia about it.

Much work has been doing. I forget how many birds have been announced to you as infected. Several fresh birds have come in, in spite of the fact that I have used very few mosquitos. The only difference caused by doing this is that some of the birds (which were not bitten) escape. Those bitten all have very severe infections, quite exceeding what is ordinarily seen. The parasites begin to appear on the 6th, 7th or 8th days & shortly reach vast numbers 5, 10, & more in a field when the bird dies. I found five young proteosoma in a single corpuscle.

I told you I would give sparrows' proteosoma to a crow. So I have. Parasites appeared first on the 9th day but have not become very numerous. They are utterly different from crows' halteridium & exactly like sparrows' proteosoma. These details however must be left for future work; and I am concentrating on the "black bodies". I find:-

1. They are not seen in healthy mosquitos

2. They are nearly always present in infected mosquitos; but not always in the coccidia. The reason is that when the coccidia burst on 8th day the black bodies escape into the coelom & are carried by the blood into all the tissues just like the germinal rods.

3. The black bodies (evidently spores) have remained quite unchanged in mosquitos dead a fortnight & in specimens kept in a damp chamber for *a month*.

4. I put one grub in a small tube with water & the remains of a mosquito containing about 100 black spores. Next day the grub was examined. Fifteen black spores (unchanged) were in its stomach.

I must now leave off as I have a terrible lot to do. I hope to rush the black spore business soon.

Today, I suppose, the Tropical Section is in full swing: I hope the telegram arrived in time.[2]

Yours sincerely

R. Ross.

1 See Letter 141.

2 Manson referred to Ross's telegram in his presidential address to the section, 'The mosquito and the malaria parasite', *BMJ* (24 Sept. 1898), 849-853. W. J. Simpson recalled to Ross in 1921 having heard it read out (*Memoirs,* 306); it was in addition to the one reproduced as Letter 141a.

Letter 143
02/051

21 Queen Anne Street,
Cavendish Square, W.
July 15th. 1898

My dear Ross,
I cannot make out what has become of my letters to you. Lately I have written almost weekly. Besides Opie and MacCallums papers I sent you a copy of my little book the day it was issued. Have you not received it? I have written regularly to keep you posted in what I have been doing to help you forward in your good work and to let you feel that you are not being overlooked

The last is that a committee of the Royal Society has your work under consideration.[1] I have lent them the copy of your report and have offered to demonstrate your specimens. The last lot arrived yesterday. I have not opened it yet. Before this I had two other lots - one a set of mosquitos fed on 3 degrees of infection - the other an earlier consignment of miscellaneous.

I have written the Under Secretary of State for India for permission to bring forward your work at the British Medical Association in Edinburgh.

I am ill again and in bed with gout.

Yours sincerely
Edith M. Manson (for Dr Manson)

Your last news of the microvermiculi is hopeful.

1 See Letter 145 note 3.

Letter 144
02/164

Calcutta
3rd August 1898

Dear Dr Manson,
Many thanks for yours - or rather your daughter's - letter of the 15th July. What an awful nuisance your being ill again must be to you. I trust you will have given up all idea of going to Edinburgh or doing any work at all: and also that this letter will find you quite recovered.

Many thanks for sending me a copy of your book; but it has never arrived. I bought a couple. The Indian post is quite untrustworthy & the clerks in my opinion, make a habit of stealing unregistered parcels. Numerous parcels addressed to me and to my wife have never reached us. It is *necessary* to register everything important for India. MacCallum & Opie's papers were left in an office for months.

I hope the Royal Society will respond to your efforts, for which many thanks.

The black spores refuse to capitulate; the result is that I am nearly dead with work again. They *don't* change in water or in dead mosquitos, though kept for periods ranging to six weeks nearly. They *don't* change in the stomach of the medium & large grubs. By feeding these on torn-up mosquitos with black spores I can get as many as I like (as many as 500) of the latter into their stomachs - but not a sign of change. I am now trying very young grubs & have also fed five healthy sparrows with the spores.

Numerous most beautiful demonstrations of the germinal rods (what *shall* we call them?) in the salivary glands; but fixed specimens almost impossible to make. Also some very good specimens of coccidia of tenth day bucking up into black spores.

Eight or so healthy birds infected. I am now working with greater exactness. For example, four birds were bitten 23rd-24th & 24th-25th July & were examined on 4th & 5th days when they were found quite healthy. On the sixth day No. 1 showed abut 3 proteosoma in a specimen. No. 2 & 3 did the same on the 7th & 8th days. The fourth escaped. Again 5 birds were bitten on the 26-27, 27-28, 28-29th July. Two showed a very few proteosoma on the 5th day (31st July), one on 6th day, & one on 8th day. The fifth has escaped to date (8th day).*

* infected today, 4th August - 9th day.

Now note. In all these birds infection began in exactly the same manner - with one or two parasites in a specimen. In all (except the last) the progress of infection has been exactly the same, namely a rapid increase until the number of germs reached is about *10* or *even more* in a thin field in four days.

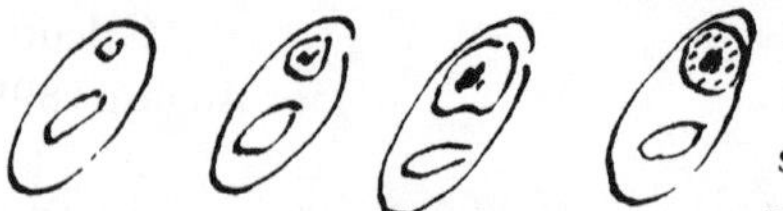

Moreover, the onset is characterised by only the small *fever* forms of proteosoma.

On the third day however the large forms, corresponding to crescents, set in.

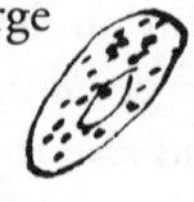

Now I have made an important discovery. These large forms are due to the *conjugation of several parasites in one*

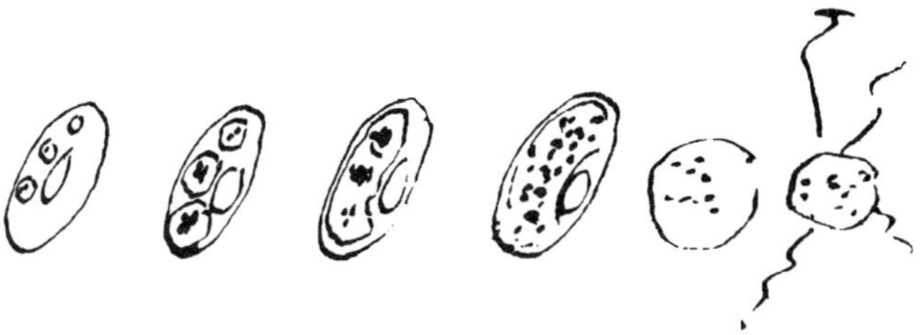

corpuscle. Good for Mannaberg![1]

The whole thing can be seen with ease. The conjugation forms only set in on about the third day of infection when the parasites become so numerous that double, treble ... infection of the corpuscles becomes common. I have frequently seen *six* parasites in one corpuscle.

Artificial infection differs from that seen in wild birds as follows:-

1. The number of parasites, which is very small at first, increases very rapidly in four days to enormous numbers.

2. The maximum number seen in artificial infection *greatly* exceeds *in almost all cases* what is ordinarily found in wild birds.

3. In art[ifcial] infection the parasites with scattered pigment (conjugation forms) are not found at first but set in on about the 3rd or 4th day. In wild birds they are generally present if the other forms are.

I very rarely find flagellation (have no time to look for it) but of course it probably occurs only in the conjugation forms.

I am dying to finish proteosoma as I am beginning to knock up more than ever. Nothing but work as hard as I can go for 2 months. Am beginning to be sleepless. Great fun all the same, as you may imagine but most trying to eyes & brain.

As you say, proteosoma should be finished & then the human germs can easily be tackled. Unfortunately that kala-azar weighs on me like a nightmare. I do hope you will be all right when this reaches you.

Yours sincerely

R. Ross.

1 Mannaberg (1894), 289-292.

Letter 145
02/165

Calcutta
10th August 1898

Dear Dr Manson,

I have not much to tell you this week. Three out of five birds fed with 7 infected mosquitos each on the 31st - many of the mosquitos containing black spores - have all remained healthy to date; while several birds *bitten* on 3rd to 4th night were attacked the day before yesterday. Apparently no outlet here. I fed many grubs of all sizes on the spores. Crowds of the spores in their stomach tube, but they are passed out & found in the droppings quite unchanged. Spores in the damp chamber remain the same. I fancy some condition of ripening is required. This obtained I fancy the spores will infect the grubs, grow into coccidia & give rise to germinal rods & spores again.

Well, I am dead beat & have asked leave to go to Kurseong for a few weeks en route for Assam. I have lost eleven pounds in weight the last two months. Work at the microscope all night; can't sleep; & feel as low as possible.

I think it a good plan when one is brought up standing to change the point of attack; so I am now going to try human malaria & some other tricks & get a little holiday at the same time. The kala-azar question has been quite changed by the discovery that proteosoma is communicable from diseased to healthy birds, & also by a recent report by Harold Brown[1] on kaladukh or kalajwar, in the Darjeeling Terai, both probably the same as kala azar. He finds malaria parasites in all the cases & reports on the varieties he finds[2] instead of giving generalities like Rogers. Hence I shall probably finish with kala-azar in a very short time. Will see kala dukh at Kurseong first.

I observed the note about the Commission in the B. M. J. of July 23rd.[3] It will be grand if the Royal Society does the business. I shall wait to hear from you before making plans; but think I should add that I expect kala-azar won't take me longer than to end of October.

I trust you are better, but fear that you were not able to go to Edinburgh.

Next week or so I hope to send you summing up of recent work, with drawings etc. I am now endeavouring to take some photos.

With kind regards

Yours sincerely

R. Ross.

About 30 odd healthy birds infected up to date.

1 E. Harold Brown, 'A Report on *Kala Dukh*, a form of fever met with in the North-East portion of the district of Purnea', *Indian Medical Gazette* (Sept. 1898), 324-330. As this was an official inquiry on behalf of the Sanitary Commission of Bengal, Ross may well have seen a version published before the *Indian Medical Gazette* article.

2 Brown's table, pp 327-30, provided microscopic analysis of blood smears from fifty patients.

3 *BMJ* (23 July 1898) 254, reported that the Royal Society had appointed a small committee to consider the causes and distribution of malaria. It was proposed that a Commission consisting of two medical men and an entomologist, funded jointly by the Royal Society and the Colonial Office, should go to India and then to West Africa to carry out the research.

Letter 146
02/052

Edinburgh,
28th July
1899 [1898][1]

My dear Ross,

Just a line to say I duly received both your telegrams[2] and letters describing the germinal rods, their incorporation by the salivary glands and the successful inoculation experiment suggested by this remarkable discovery. The news came just in time for the B. M. A. meeting & as I was requested to give a special demonstration in malaria to a combined meeting of Sections I chose your work for my theme & I hope did you justice to a very large audience. I had your slides under microscopes and your drawings as diagrams. The fat is thoroughly in the fire and you may expect soon to hear more of yourself than your modesty may care for. Lister is taking a very great interest in the progress of the investigation, the India Office in various ways has also been made conscious of the high esteem in which they - the investigations - are held, so that I think there is no need for you to be anxious about the future.

I am still ill with gout, hardly able to hobble almost but I was determined if at all feasible to come to this meeting & properly present your work, the importance of which it is difficult to overestimate. Osler was there;[3] very much interested. I gave him one of your reports.

Now you have to find how the germinal rods pass from mosquito to mosquito. In haste

Yours sincerely

Patrick Manson

1 In this and the following letter Manson wrote the wrong year (1899 & 1997 on next).

2 See Letter 141a; the other telegram is missing.

3 William Osler, (1849-1919), then Professor of Medicine at Johns Hopkins University, Baltimore. *Memoirs*, 306, also notes the presence of Raphael Blanchard and Andrew Davidson. See Mary Gibson, 'The Ross/Osler correspondence', *Journal of Medical Biography*, 1 (1993), 117-124.

Letter 147
02/053

21 Queen Anne Street,
Cavendish Square. W.
5th Aug. 1997 [1898]

My dear Ross,

Since my return from Edinburgh I have been most of the time in bed. I am much better now but frightfully weak & unable to tackle anything but necessary work. The R. S. proposals are not good - at all events to my mind. They want to send a research scholar to you & two bacteriologists I suppose to study Blackwater fever in Central Africa. This is quite inadequate and I went down expressly to the Colonial Office to say so.[1] The enclosed I have just received[2] and I shall have another try for a full commission on the original lines suggested. I hope I may succeed. Your discovery is either the most important of the "fin de siècle" or it is nothing. I shall do all I can for it on the first assumption & try to make England work it.

Look in the egg of the mosquito for germinal rods. Analogy suggests such a way of indefinite propagation in mosquito. See Koch's speech. It is the biggest piece of blatant egoism I have yet come across.[3]

Excuse a bad written letter.

Yours sincerely

Patrick Manson

I enclose a copy of resolutions at the Tropical Section of the B. M. A.[4] I was not present when they were moved & adopted. You are not forgotten. P.M.

1 The RSMC initially proposed to send a Dr R. Row to work with Ross, and Drs Todd and Christophers to Africa. (RSMC Minutes, meeting of 21 July, 1898). Manson argued in a meeting with Chamberlain and Lister (RSMC Minutes, 8 August) that the Committee needed to appoint someone with 'considerable professional experience' with blackwater fever.

2 **RA** 02/054, The letter from Chamberlain's Private Secretary, Herbert James Read, to Manson, 5 August 1898, inviting him to attend a meeting between Lister and Chamberlain (Gibson 1983).

3 Koch's speech on malaria delivered before the Colonial Society of Berlin on 9 June 1898. *BMJ* (18 June 1898), 1607-1608, reported that it could be inferred from this speech that Koch was 'the discoverer of the germ of Texas cattle fever, of the action of the cattle tick in transmitting this disease from one cow to another, of the principles by which the administration of quinine should be guided, and of many other things, including the *rôle* of the mosquito in the propagation of malaria.' Koch summarised his work to date on tropical diseases in 'Reiseberichte über Rinderpest, Bubonenpest in Indien und Afrika, Tsetse- oder Surrakrankheit, Texasfieber, tropische Malaria, Schwarzwasserfieber', published in *Gesammelte Werke von Robert Koch*, 3 vols (Leipzig: Verlag von Georg Thieme, 1912) ii, 688-742.

4 The first resolution praised Ross; the second thanked Manson. Printed in *Journal of Tropical Medicine*, 1 (1898), 24-25.

Letter 148
02/166

Kurseong
23rd August 1898

Dear Dr Manson,
I had to leave Calcutta abruptly on the 13th, much specimen making & photo taking incomplete. I had practically ceased to sleep - worked at microscope all night - & began to forget everything. Since coming here I have thought it best not to think of the germs at all. When I am in work I go too hard at it & can't shake it off my mind, with the result that I knock up in a month or two, especially in a hot climate. However the hard part of the work is over.

I fear that you also overdid it a great deal for your health at the B. M. A. meeting. Many thanks for your letters up to the 5th August & for copy of the Resolution of the Tropical Section, which is indeed flattering! I rather think however that they put the two paragraphs in the wrong order![1] The idea is of the first importance; the brain is over the hand. My function in this work has only been of the hand - that is a point I stick to. You would have polished off the whole matter in a quarter of the time I have taken. When the time comes to write the history of the whole campaign - it will have to be a separate book, not an article, I think - this will be brought into full relief, I promise you.[2]

I received Blanchard's letter which is a great honour.[3] But I fear that Harvey will insist on publishing all the work in the Transactions of Medical Officers in India. I will however answer him suitably. The subject cannot be treated in full for several months yet.

I await further news about the Commission & hope you will succeed in getting the R. S. to meet your views.

Tomorrow I am off to a place called Naksulbari[4] 9 miles from Punkarbari and in the middle of the Terai, one of the most feverish of places. It is the stronghold of Kalajwar,[5] which I take to be mosquito-borne malaria. It is said to be highly infectious. More about it next week, if I don't get touched up myself.

I must now hurry up as I want to give you the results of the last *fytte* of work. They are on next page.

I have written to Laveran, Thin and Sternberg,[6] giving them these results. To the last I have suggested mosquito nets for the troops in Cuba (cheek, but good may come of it). Dr Thin has written to me.[7] He has evidently given way to our arguments.

It was really *very good* of you to go to Edinburgh, but I fear you tired yourself too much by it. You suggest that the germinal rods enter the egg. Good idea - I will try it. But I think the black spores serve this purpose. They don't seem to infect birds by the mouth. You don't tell me whether the Secretary of State has permitted publication.

Hope the next fytte will solve the human malaria problem. With kindest regards & wishes for your health.

Yours sincerely

R. Ross.

Results of work from 4th June to 13th August.

1. The mature proteosoma-coccidia of 7th or 8th days have two methods of reproduction, by *germinal rods* & by large black *sausage-shaped spores*, found in separate coccidia. These two reproductive processes occur probably in connection respectively with the two kinds of coccidia, hyaline & vacuolated described in my report.

2. The "germinal rods" are thread-like bodies from 12μ to 16μ in length; tapering at the ends & broader in the middle, which often contains one or more "vacuoles". They stain easily with methylene blue & show one or two chromatin spots towards the centre.
3. The "black spores" vary from 12μ to 22μ or more in length, & 2μ to 5μ in breadth when mature. In shape they are crescentic, sigmoid or variously twisted. In colour they are of a deep brown throughout, but have a continuous thick black outline. Their surface often possesses several excrescences like those of round worms' eggs in the human intestine.
4. The mature proteosoma-coccidia burst in the living insect on the 7th or 8th days & discharge their contents (rods or spores) into the *circulating juices* of the insect, which carry and distribute them all over the tissues.
5. The germinal rods collect again in the salivary or poison gland of the mosquito, the duct of which runs right up one of the mandibles (or the epipharynx) of the buccal apparatus. They are evidently discharged together with the secretion of this gland into the wound made by the bite of the mosquito.
6. Thirty two birds have been infected with proteosoma by the bites of mosquitos previously fed on birds containing this parasite.
7. The function of the black spores has not yet been discovered. They have remained unchanged in water for seven weeks and in dead mosquitos for four weeks. Three sparrows to which mosquitos containing them were given by the mouth have remained healthy. They have been found in large numbers, but quite unchanged, in the stomach of mosquito-larvae fed on dead mosquitos containing them.

The details of the infection experiments are as follows:-

1. Out of 43 healthy sparrows exposed to the bites of old infected mosquitos, 15 died of diarrhoea, tetanus etc within 8 days (i.e. before the end of the incubation period) after the experiment; 22 became infected with proteosoma in 6 to 9 days after the experiment; and 6 remained not infected.
2. The only one of these 6 sparrows which was uninfected by the first experiment & which lived long enough for a second experiment, became infected on the 6th day after this second experiment.
3. One out of two crows bitten by old proteosoma-infected

mosquitos became infected with proteosoma on the 10th day after the experiment.

4 Of 4 weaver birds experimented with all became infected with proteosoma. Three of these birds originally had halteridium.

5. Out of five sparrows which originally had a very few proteosoma & which were subjected to the bites of infected mosquitos, four became infected after the usual incubation period with a fresh & numerous crop of proteosoma.

6. Two mainas[8] and four "seven sisters"[9] failed to become infected after being bitten by proteosoma-infected mosquitos.

Remarks.

In series 1, 2 & 4 of the above the invasion was characterised in *all* by the following peculiarities.

a. A very few parasites appeared on the 1st day of sickness (6, 7, 8th day after experiment).

b. The parasites increased rapidly in number every day, until -

c. On the 4th day of sickness they numbered from 10 to 30 or even more in a single thin oil immersion field, far exceeding anything seen by me in wild birds.

d. At first only the smaller forms of proteosoma, from the amoebula to the ordinary sporulating form, were seen. As, however, the parasites became more numerous, multiple infection of the corpuscles was found, as many as seven parasites being sometimes seen in one corpuscle. These appeared to fuse together (? conjugation, Mannaberg)[10] and to become the larger parasites with discrete pigment, noted by many observers.

e. The birds now either died, the liver, lungs & spleen being loaded with pigment, and almost every blood corpuscle containing one or more parasites; or slowly recovered, the number of parasites gradually diminishing.

The crow (series 3 above) & the reinfections (series 5) differed from the others in that the maximum number of parasites reached was much less than in the other cases. In series 5 there was a rush of numerous young forms on the 6th or 7th days after the experiment. Instead however of the numbers increasing to the enormous extent found in originally healthy birds infected by mosquitos, the maximum did not exceed 1 or 2 parasites in a field (of 300 corpuscles). This suggests the whole business of *immunity* for malaria.

The following are some of my results of examination of wild birds for comparison.

Out of 111 (one hundred & eleven) sparrows examined in Calcutta, only 15 contained proteosoma = 13.5%. Of these 15, only 3 had more than 1 parasite in each field; the largest number of parasites found being about 3 in a field.

Of 16 crows examined only 1 had proteosoma.

There is absolutely no doubt then that the bite of proteosoma-infected grey mosquitos can infect healthy birds.

I have not yet examined whether the germinal rods infect the *eggs* of mosquitos. I doubt it because they are evidently meant for the salivary gland; and in spite of some negative experiments, I think that the black spores serve this purpose.

This subject and the extension of these observations to human malaria & to halteridium remain to be dealt with.

R. Ross.

1 See Letter 147, note 4.

2 Ross rather changed his tune subsequently.

3 Letter from Blanchard, 28 July 1898 from Edinburgh, stating that Manson had shown him Ross's work and asking whether he could publish it in *Archives de Parasitologie*. He also mentioned that Manson had announced his results at the BMA meeting that morning. **RA** 03/160 (Gibson, 1983); *Memoirs*, 306.

4 Naxalbari is the usual spelling. Ross himself corrects it in Letter 150.

5 Kalajwar (black fever) was the same as kala-dukh, see letter 145.

6 George Miller Sternberg, (1838-1915), Chief of the Medical Staff of the United States Army. See **Biographical Appendix**. Letter from Ross to Sternberg, 24 August 1898, **RA** 86/001. There is a letter from Ross to Laveran dated 2 September 1898 (**RA** 02/211) but the letter to Thin is untraced.

7 Letter from Thin to Ross, 29 July 1898, saying that had found Ross's report very interesting and congratulating him on his work. **RA** 06/056.

8 Hindi form of 'mina'. *The Oxford English Dictionary* 2nd Ed (Oxford: Clarendon Press, 1989): 'A name applied to several different sturnoid passerine birds of India and countries further east, belonging to the genera *Acridotheres* and *Eurabes*, esp. *Eurabes* (formerly *Gracula*) *religiosa*, the common talking starling of India.'

9 *Ibid.*, 'A popular name for *Malacocercus tericolor*, an Indian bird of gregarious habits.'

10 Mannaberg (1894), 289-292.

Letter 149
02/055

21 Queen Anne Street,
Cavendish Square,
9th August, 1898

My dear Ross,

I am in an awful hurry getting ready to go on holiday for three weeks but must find time for a line to you. The Royal Society wished to send two biologists to Africa to study malaria. They said medical men knew nothing of biology. I think I have stopped this and have managed that one of the men at least shall be medical.[1] I shall nominate Daniels[2] of Demerara who has done some excellent work in many directions. I think he will be first sent to you to learn your methods and help you. The research scholar in Bombay[3] is to be sent to report on your work. Make him a convert quickly. Everything hangs on it. You have the ball at your foot if his report is favourable as it must be.

I have just had a letter from Harvey.[4] He is your strong supporter and I am sure will do all he can to help you on. He tells me that you have got 6 months extension on your present duties with the probability that you will be permanently installed to carry on science work in India. If you get a good report from the Roy-Soc I fancy you will be able to make your own terms.

I would advise you to get a skilled draughtsman to do your drawing in your next or final report on proteosoma. I suppose you can get such a man in India. These R. S. Johnnies are very much influenced by style I find. I told Lister that very few poets could illustrate their own poems. He seemed to see it. They forget that Calcutta is not London. Moreover I thought your illustrations excellent. Still we have to advance on orthodox lines it seems. You wont mind the hint.

You will note a discrepancy in my speech at Edinburgh as reported by the B. M. J. and the Journal of Tropical Medicine.[5] The fact is I was obliged to stand up to demonstrate and I was so bad with gout at the time that I dared not sit down again and had to trust to my memory for my speech not being able to see the manuscript as it lay on the table. The B.M.J.'s report is as it was spoken having been taken down by the shorthand writer; the Journal of Tropical Medicine was from the manuscript prepared the night before.

I am much better but very weak and sorely in want of the holiday of three weeks I commence this evening.

Yours sincerely
Patrick Manson

Look in ovaries & ova for germinal rods. I have had many sections made but nothing shows.

1 In fact both of them were: John William Watson Stephens, (1865-1946) and Samuel Rickard Christophers, (1873-1978). Reported in *BMJ* (17 Sept. 1898), 826.
2 For Daniels, see **Biographical Appendix.**
3 Unidentified. The visit and the report do not seem to have taken place.
4 The letter has not been found. For Harvey, (1842-1901), see **Biographical Appendix.**
5 Manson (1898c); *idem,* 'An exposition of the mosquito-malaria theory and its recent developments', *Journal of Tropical Medicine*, 1 (1898), 4-8.

Letter 150
02/167

Kurseong
6th Sept. 1898

Dear Dr Manson,
I spent a week at Naxalbari. Results poor. In about 100 persons examined malaria parasites were found only in 5 or 6, though numbers of the cases had enormous spleens with a kind of hectic fever. The cases were evidently old malarial infections. As the people always refused to stay for repeated examinations motions could not often be looked at for eggs. Not a single suitable case for mosquito feeding was obtained.

The mosquitos were dapple-wings & greys. The former breed in rain puddles exclusively I think. Hence the whole climatic variations of aestivo-autumnal. I examined numbers of both kinds caught in houses of fever cases. No coccidia or rods. As however the fever cases in question had only a few wretched young parasites in a whole specimen infection of mosquitos was unlikely. I did not see a single crescent the whole time (remember what Rogers said).[1] No rods were seen in salivary glands of many mosquitos. The dapple wings bite very fiercely. Their grubs float horizontally like sticks in the puddles, a noteworthy & very useful peculiarity.

I don't believe that fresh malaria was about at all at Naxalbari at this season. There were floods of rain which continually scoured out the puddles. People said there were very few mosquitos. Dapple wings won't live in any but the smallest puddles because the minnows which swarm in anything over a few gallons capacity devour them instantly. Malaria is probably a *very* easily preventable disease.[2] I preached mosquito-nets & an anti puddle propaganda & left. Tomorrow I am off to Assam. Please address letters to c/o Grindley & Co, Hastings Street, Calcutta. They are agents & will forward.

The real Terai disease is probably anchylostomiasis & not malaria. Many frightful cases of the former. Hospital assistant at Naxalbari had never *heard* of it! The worst cases of mere malaria with spleens touching livers looked quite cheerful & jolly.

Filaria is also present you will be *glad* to hear. I made the following most interesting observations which you may like to add to your filaria lore. While examining mosquitos I took some grey ones caught in a mosquito net within which a native catechist, his wife & one child, all with fever, slept nightly. The thorax was seen to contain something new. It was a developmental stage of f. s. h.[3] - numerous forms of all stages up to the full active stage were easily found in all of 5 mosquitos examined. Evidently our catechist was too lazy to kill his mosquito in the morning. Taking his night blood I found f. nocturna. A case of filaria diagnosed through the mosquito! - and a very easy way of diagnosing it too. I shall employ it clinically some day.

Have had a great disappointment. P. L. Simond has been here.[4] I wrote & he came down to see me. I had just gone to Naxalbari. He followed me down the line; but it was no use, he had to be in Calcutta on a fixed date & we did not meet after all. I would have given much to show him the work, and find out something about coccidia.

I have had a very nice letter from Nuttall.[5]

Have written officially to Govt. & asked for permission to publish. The present state of things is very annoying.

I thought you would not find the Royal Society rise easily to your fly. Shall be most happy to demonstrate everything to Daniels or the scholarship man; but they must *hurry up*. I must come home next February or March - that I am going to insist on. If they don't give me leave I shall take pension in order to do so; we have decided on it. Hence your men should be with me as soon as possible. I shall be in Assam in a few days . Don't expect to be able to do anything at all with kala-azar at this season. All the malaria cases will be probably stale ones - no parasites - nothing decisive. But I shall make every effort to bring at least one of the human parasites into line with proteosoma. (Am very apprehensive about not finding crescents). This done (with luck it may be done in a week or two), if kala azar turns out unfruitful,

I may come back to Calcutta by 1st Nov. where I can demonstrate to Daniels & the other man. But tell them both to wire to me of course.

I hope your holiday will have enabled you to free yourself from that horrible gout. I am all right again after about a fortnight spent up here & am ready for another fierce bout at the problem. My battle of Omdurman[6] has yet to be fought. I think it will be done this time. The black spores can of course wait until human malaria is tackled.

I see by the B. M. J. for August 20th p. 498 that Koch has gone to Italy to study malaria.[7] It is quite possible that he will at once succeed in infecting men by the mosquito if he is lucky. In the meantime I am absolutely forbidden to publish anything about my infection of birds. But Nuttall says he is going to deal with Koch. I enclose three poor photos.[8] With kind regards

Yours sincerely

R. Ross.

1 See Letter 123, note 2.

2 Although Ross subsequently modified this position, it was a future source of friction between him and many other malariologists.

3 Filaria sanguinis hominis.

4 Paul-Louis Simond, (1858-1947), of the Pasteur Institute, author of 'L'évolution des sporozoaires du genre coccidium' (1897). See **Biographical Appendix**.

5 George Henry Falkiner Nuttall, (1862-1937), see **Biographical Appendix**. His letter to Ross, 13 August 1898, (**RA** 02/214) is reproduced in part in *Memoirs*, 334.

6 See letter 136.

7 Reported in *BMJ* (20 Aug. 1898), 498.

8 Not traced.

Letter 151
02/056

21, Queen Anne Street,
Cavendish Square. W.
2nd Sept. 1898

My dear Ross,

Yours announcing your failure to get the black spores to germinate to hand.[1] Nil desperandum. Might they not be intended for deposit in water or soil, to be rained on, sunned on and nursed in this way for a time and thus to acquire germinative properties if taken up by the proper host. Try this in a test tube or otherwise.

I wd like to get some preparations of the germinal rods. It occurs to me if the veneno-salivary glands were spread out on a slip, allowed to dry, fixed with alcohol and then stained they wd. show up. I have tried sectioning your mosquitos but it is no go & I cant tell why. All the stomach wall tissues seem to shrivel up to nothing. You might try drying stomachs on slips and mounting with balsam for permanent prep[arations]s.

It is almost fixed that the Colonial Office sends Daniels of Demerara (a good man) out to you for 2 or 3 months instruction in preparation for joining 2 other commissioners the Royal Society are to send to Central Africa with a special eye to studying blackwater fever and the malaria problem there.[2] I had a great struggle to get this as the R. S. want to do things their own way, which, I am sure, is the wrong way. However Daniels will work heartily with you and at all events confirm your discoveries. I hope to know definitely about this before the mail goes out. I wish the R. S. had followed my advice more completely but every thing, every new idea, takes time to sink into even clever men's brains.

You must get ready to come home when your six months are up and be sure to come provided with a large stock of preparations. You must din the thing into the public ear over & over again before a genuine move can be started. I mean to try again however when opportunity offers.

I had three weeks in Scotland. Ten days of my holiday were spent in bed the remainder on crutches. I am much better now but walk with difficulty. Do your [illegible] up in time and don't overwork yourself.

Koch has gone to Rome to study malaria.[3] Pity he did not go there before. I sent him one of your reports which the India Office sent me.

I have hardly got into work yet since my return 2 days ago but hope by next week to be in full swing again.

Yours sincerely
Patrick Manson

8th Sept
I have now heard officially that Daniels is to be sent to you. The despatch ordering him home from Demerara has been sent.

I also learn officially that Koch & a commission are going out to India, Africa & New Guinea for 2 years to study malaria. I hope you will scoop up all the cream before they get at the milking. Doubtless your mosquito discoveries have instigated this work. In his later lucubrations Koch claims the mosquito as his own & never says a word about your work[4] - Cool - is it not?

The B. M. J. of the 17th inst. will contain a corrected part of my speech at the B. M. A. meeting on your work with one amendment.[5] I will send you reprints.

1 Letter 144.
2 Letter 149, note 1.
3 Letter 150, note 7.
4 Letter 147, note 3.
5 It actually appeared in the following issue: Manson (1898c).

Letter 152
01/168

Nowgong, Assam
9th Oct. 1898

Dear Dr Manson,
Many thanks for yours of 2nd Sept. which reached me a week ago just too late for reply by that mail. I am glad Daniels is coming out and am sure he is the man for the work. I will show him lots of things besides the mosquito business if I can. He must however hurry up as we shall certainly leave India in February, perhaps, indeed most probably, for good;[1] so that he will not have much time with me unless he comes out *statim*. My six months expire on the 17th Feb. 1899. I have asked Surg. Gen. Harvey whether it is any use applying to be kept on at scientific work but he advised me to defer my application to a later date.

I have not written for the last few mails because I have been in the agonies of the kala-azar enquiry. I arrived here on the 13th Sept. It required only a glance to see that Giles is quite wrong.[2] The definition in Tropical Diseases (derived from him) does not apply to what they call kala-azar here.[3] This is an *acute fever* beginning with a sudden onset with rigors, followed by an irregular chart, now continued, now remittent or even intermittent. After some weeks of this *both* the spleen & liver begin to enlarge & are *tender*. The fever may now leave off for some weeks during which however the enlargement of the spleen & liver increases. The fever then recurs with violence followed by great tumefaction of the organs, together with a moderate amount of anaemia, oedema of the feet, epistaxis etc. When the cases are well established, that is from 4 months after the beginning of the sickness, we have the following picture:- great enlargement & tenderness both of liver & spleen, a more or less constant symptomatic fever, a certain degree of anaemia (not very much), emaciation, oedema etc, with diarrhoea, dysentery, pneumonia as a curtain.

The motto is a "recurrent fever accompanied by enlargement & tenderness of both spleen & liver".

You will perceive that I have only to state the terms in order to get rid of the idea of anchylostomiasis.

The civil surgeon here is Dr McNaught who first drew attention to the disease in 1882.[4] If he cannot identify kala azar, who can? Besides the disease is easily identified by the family history of the patients, almost all of whom have lost relatives. Everyone, in short, knows the disease as well here, as they know cholera in other parts of India; so that there is no error of identification.

Well, unless ankylostomes can cause high fever & enlargement of the liver & spleen, they cannot cause k.a. In fact I put them out of court at once. Besides, some of my worst cases haven't got any.

Prima facie, kala azar is malaria. All the classical symptoms are there; but before I accept this view the pathology must be clearly made out. That is, parasites & black pigment must be found at the earlier stages, yellow pigment later. But here comes in the difficulty. How to distinguish k. a. from ordinary malaria during the earlier stages.

Well, I am hard at it, pricking fingers & spleens & livers, all day. There is a continuous gradation of cases here now under observation, from early fever cases with parasites from finger, & parasites & pigment from spleen but no or very slight spleens & livers; up to pronounced k. a. cases *without* parasites or black pigment, but *with* large livers & spleens.

In four post mortems on k. a. cases there was hardly any black pigment in spleens or livers in two of them, none at all in the other two. Moreover spleen blood in many living cases has *not* shown pigment.

What do you make of it?

It will be a chapter in the history of chronic malaria in malarious districts, that is in places where patients become infected over & over again.

In a mail or two I think I shall be able to give the pathology - a question of *yellow* pigment, I suspect.

Really, the cases when thoroughly established are no longer malaria. They are tumefactions of liver & spleen with continued fever - Kelsch & Kieners Hypérémies Phlegmasiques in fact.[5]

As soon as I have satisfied myself on these points I shall apply to return to Calcutta. This ought to be in a fortnight or so as I am working very rapidly with my punctures of the organs. I shall then be ready for Daniels & we will make the necessary specimens in numbers for you. But my health is very bad since returning to the heat & I don't know what may not happen.

No mosquito work done. The parasites are quartans & a species of aestivo autumnal. Crescents found in extremely small numbers in two only of the latter. Numbers of mosquitos of many species fed on both quartans & the crescent cases have shown no coccidia. I expect this is not the season.

Very glad indeed to hear you are better.

More by next letter. I must now leave off to catch post. Daniels should hurry out if he is to work with me. With kind regards

Yours sincerely

R. Ross.

1 Ross left India on 24 Feb. 1899. He returned only twice in his life.

2 Giles (1890). Giles had concluded that kala-azar was a hookworm disease.

3 Manson (1898a), 191-3.

4 Ross, *Memoirs*, 319, notes that a Mr McNaught, then Civil Medical Officer at Tura, Garo Hills, Assam, had reported on kala-azar in 1882, but that his name does not appear in D. G. Crawford's *History of the Indian Medical Service, 1600-1913* (London, W. Thacker, 1914) and that he seems not to have received any acknowledgement for his discovery. There is no mention of McNaught in H. H. Scott, *A History of Tropical Medicine*, 2 vols. (London: Edward Arnold, 1939), ch. IX.

5 A. Kelsch and P.-L. Kiener, *Traité des maladies des pays chauds: région prétropicale* (Paris: Ballière, 1889) pp 540-583.

Letter 153
02/169

Nowgong

16th Oct. 1898

Dear Dr Manson,

I have done with kala-azar & have written to ask permission to return to Calcutta to continue proteosoma. The facts are as follows.

No one can distinguish k. a. from ordinary fever during its earlier stages, but when great tumefaction of the liver & spleen are established & a fatal termination anticipated, then a diagnosis comes readily enough - it is kala-azar certainly. There are a number of such cases in hospital here & I have examined them carefully. They all have more or less continued fever, not amenable to quinine, and enormous livers & spleens. Malaria parasites are *not* to be found in their blood after repeated examinations, &, what is more definite still regarding this point, there is no black pigment in the blood abstracted from the spleen & liver during life. I have carried out methodical examinations. Out of five postmortems on such cases, one only contained black pigment to a certainty - agreeing with Gibbon's case.[1] Nevertheless kala-azar is malaria pure & simple.

I have arrived at this conclusion by a careful comparison of all cases of fever occurring here from the most recent ones to the most advanced cases of kala-azar, and by a close reference to Kelsch & Kiener.[2]

In the earliest cases just commencing, parasites are of course always found under proper conditions & the spleen always contains pigment. The ordinary species only are present. I have now found tertian as well as quartan & aestivo-autumnal - crescents occurred in only two cases. No unpigmented sporulating forms seen in the spleen. I have also observed that in some of the cases enlargement of the spleen & liver begins astonishingly early with great prostration, and this appears to be particularly the case with the *quartan* cases oddly enough.

Going a step further in the scale we have of course still greater tumefaction of the spleen & liver, especially the *latter*, together with considerable anaemia & some emaciation. Now however the acute febrile symptoms abate and at the same time parasites can be found only with difficulty in the blood from the finger. Blood from the spleen however always contains black pigment but in ever decreasing quantities.

In the next stage the enlargement of the organs continues, and a peculiar kind of regular fever, fluctuating most constantly between fixed limits, say 99° to 101°F, sets in. Finger blood now shows not a sign of a germ, but the spleen contains still a *little* black pigment, and also granules of typical *yellow* pigment. This is the stage reached on about the 4th or 5th month, a liver say of 2 inches and a spleen of 4 inches, and both very tender.

Now follows the period of great tumefaction. Neither spleen nor liver show black pigment at all. There is more or less constant fever not amenable to quinine. Ascites, oedema of feet, epistaxis, icterus, enlarged abdominal veins. On examining the liver during life yellow pigment has been found in all cases in which I was successful in taking out liver *cells*, in which only the yellow pigment lies. After however the organ is so congested that there is only a rush of pure blood up the needle - which of course yields nothing. Spleen generally shows nothing. This tale is confirmed by the postmortems, in all of which, except in one in which idiotically I forgot to look for it, there was a copious "surcharge ferruginense" of the liver, & sometimes of the spleen & kidneys.

The final stage, where recovery does not take place, appears to be destruction, fatty or amyloid, of the *liver*, with dysentery, etc.

These results simply accord with Kelsch & Kiener. See especially their remarks on the elimination of the black pigment - particularly the conclusion of the section, page 413 of the edition of 1889. They say that melanosis disappears frequently a few months after the beginning of the illness in cases which have died of *cachexia*. In other words the parasitic invasion *ceases* after a time leaving the "surcharge ferruginense" & the organs nearly ruined.

Now why does the parasitic invasion cease after a time? Certainly not in consequence of quinine, because these people don't take it. This is my theory. *Immunity* is established. Compare my results with the reinfection of sparrows. Probably these kala-azar cases become infected over & over again in the early stages by mosquitos which have bitten themselves previously - or their diseased relatives - and they would simply perish straight off unless some process of immunity were established. This is established, but the organs are left wrecked.

Hence kala-azar at the stage when it is usually diagnosed as such is in reality no longer a haemamoebiasis curable by quinine, but a kind of spleen & liver disease with the "fievre symptomatique" of Kelsch & Kiener (see page 565) & yellow pigment only. The main incidence falls on the liver.

The main point to fix the mind on is that in these severe untreated cases of malaria a species of immunity is established in a few months, which enables the system to eliminate the parasites itself, but only at the expense of profound siderosis & often ultimate distruction of the liver & in a less degree of the spleen. Compare Kelsch & Kieners cases of chronic malaria.

Among Europeans who treat themselves with quinine & are not nearly so exposed to mosquito infection & reinfection this immunity is seldom established so that they frequently have attacks of haemamoebic fever to the last, giving, of course, the usual black pigmentation.

17th Oct. Just completed another autopsy. Spleen & liver both much congested but not degenerate. Spleen, very slight traces of black pigment & some clusters of yellow pigment. Liver, profound siderosis; no black pigment. Kidneys, moderate siderosis. Intestine 200 ankylostomes, 8 ascarides, 12 flukes; also trichocephalus. Killed by diarrhoea.

The ankylostomes did not kill the man as the spleen & liver were gorged with blood, and there was no very profound anaemia.

The whole thing is a mere picture of malaria. Of course where ankylostomes are present they help toward the finale, but only as diarrhoea & dysentery do. Ankylostomes cannot cause the severe initial fevers & the immense tumefaction of the liver & spleen.

I have just examined the B. M. J. of the 24th with your speech. Very many thanks for all the handsome things said of me - much more than deserved.[3] More about it hereafter. Must leave off immediately to catch the post. Am looking forward to see Daniels. He is just the man for me. Hope you are really better.

Yours very sincerely

R. Ross.

1 J. B. Gibbon's case is reported in *Indian Medical Gazette* (Jan. 1990), 22. Gibbon's autopsy noted the destruction, pigmentation and congestion of the liver and enlargement of the spleen.

2 Kelsch and Kiener (1889).

3 Manson (1898c).

Letter 154
02/057

21, Queen Anne Street,
Cavendish Square. W.
6th October, 1898.

My dear Ross,

I was down at the Colonial Office yesterday and was told that Daniels leaves Demerara this day next week and that he will be in England by the end of the month and probably ready to leave for India by the middle of November. You may look for him about the beginning of December therefore. That will give him two good months with you, which, so far as he is concerned, should be sufficient to get thoroughly indoctrinated with your methods and views. I fear it won't be enough to get much work out of him of an original character but I have no doubt you will find him helpful. Above all it will enable him to pronounce on your work and to confirm it. I believe we will get confirmation from Italy and America before that time but it is quite on the cards that the Italians, Americans and Koch may fail to find suitable species of mosquito hosts; in which case independent testimony from Daniels will be of great use in securing a favourable hearing for you when you come home in February. Be sure to bring with you as much material as you can lay hands on. I cant get the coccidia in the sectioned mosquitos. Some other method of preparing them must be found - some method in which there is no shrinking of the tissues. I wonder if the old alcohol plan would not succeed - gradually raising the strength from 20% to 80%. Perhaps glycerine and water might succeed. You should experiment a bit in this line and also in trying to make preparations with ordinary balsam as they keep so much better. A great many of your slides have perished utterly, some are deteriorating rapidly. A good many are still in good preservation but I fear for their future. I am sending one to Rome in a day or two. I hear that Bignami and Marchiafava are going into the country to work mosquitos and I also hear that the American pack is in full cry after mosquito. We should have news soon. No letter from you last mail. I hope your health is all right.

Yours very sincerely
Patrick Manson

Letter 155
02/170

Kurseong
31st Oct. 1898

Dear Dr Manson,

Many thanks for yours of the 6th just received.[1] I am delighted to hear that Daniels will be here in December. If necessary I shall get extension of duty for a month or six weeks to work with him into March. Tell him, if he has not left before this reaches you, that he should hurry up as much as possible & that there is lots of original work awaiting him. I shall convert him in a couple of hours & then start him on unworked details all along the line. Doubtless the "events of the first day", possibly the "black spores", even the host of some of the other gymnosporidia may fall to his spear. I think I told you that an American missionary & M.D.[2] has volunteered to work with me from 15th Nov. - I will start him on specimens; and I daresay others yet may join us. I don't remember much about the mosquito I sent you for sectioning, but note that you cannot find the pigmented cells. I don't think that sectioning is very suitable for the work because for obvious reasons each section can contain only a small amount of stomach tissue. What do you think about soaking the glycerine-preserved insects in warm water & then pulling out the vitals as I do? I have got some preserved mosquitos & will try them & let you know results. Tell Daniels to bring some books on coccidia. I see two works mentioned in B. M. J. Oct. 8th page 1063.[3] He ought also to have the best kind of paraffin sectioning apparatus; but freezing will do in Calcutta in the winter months. He must wire to me from Bombay (address Grindlay & Co, Calcutta) directly he arrives, because Calcutta is so crowded in December that there will be great difficulty in getting rooms. Make him bring out various kinds of preservatives - I fear balsam won't do - I have tried it. As for the germinal rods inside the cells of the veneno-salivary glands, it will be a terrible job to preserve them. They curl up with anything else but salt solution. It is equally difficult to photograph them, as they oscillate continually; but we will make every effort to get good specimens, photos. & coloured pictures (the drawings in my report were of course only rough diagrams made in haste). This will be our first duty.

Above all ask Daniels to bring an injection syringe with the very best & *finest* platinum needles for injecting the blood of crows which have just recovered from proteosomiasis into others with a view to ascertaining whether immunity is conferred. This will be a most important branch of study for us. I observe that pyrosoma blood confers immunity in this way. The needles must be very delicate & not oxydisable. I am convinced that contrary to belief immunity can be and is established in untreated cases of malaria.

I fear you were disappointed over the results of your attack upon the Royal Society; but Daniels will do much better than most scholarship wallahs, I fancy. You must not trouble yourself in the least about obtaining confirmation of my mosquito work. Before another year has passed there will be dozens of workers all over the world. There is really no difficulty at all except *finding the right hosts* for each species of parasite. A few years more and the whole business will be established as the most beautiful of all the processes of nature in connection with disease. Malaria from beginning to end will be the "show" disease. Don't worry at all over this. I feel confident that things will now go perfectly smoothly without even the addition of another word on the subject from you or me. Your exposition in the B. M. J. for Sept. the 24th was perfection. I think that your induction of the mosquito theory was one of the grandest things in the whole range of science; the world will think so too before many months are passed. It was like Adams' & Leverrier's discovery of Neptune, only far more useful.[4]

I have had two charming letters from Laveran.[5] He makes some very caustic remarks about Koch, & evidently accepts the whole work done up to the present. Doubtless he has written to you also. He says he agrees with you that the parasites must spread from mosquito to mosquito. I fancy they do - by means of the black spores - but I beg you not to be *too* sure on the point. The more I see of malaria the graver grow my doubts as to the accepted epidemiology of the disease. It is best not to accept anything for granted. Laveran says that if I send him a résumé of my work he will communicate it to the Academy of Medicine - that is an honour which, I think you will agree with me, should not be neglected.[6]

I have one fear regarding Daniels' deputation - it is possible Calcutta may be too cold for the mosquito to bite until February! From enquiries, however, I do not think so. There is also, I hear, a winter malarial fever in Calcutta; we will investigate it.

1st November. I have just ascertained from two Calcutta men who are staying here that mosquitos are *worst* in Calcutta in the cold weather. So that is all right.

I have had a letter from Nuttall.[7] He suggests a number of possible criticisms. I have dealt with all of these in my reply. He says that a number of men he has shown the slides & report to object to my calling the pigmented cells coccidia. I said the term was provisional, but sent him the following scheme -

(...)

Scheme of Proteosoma

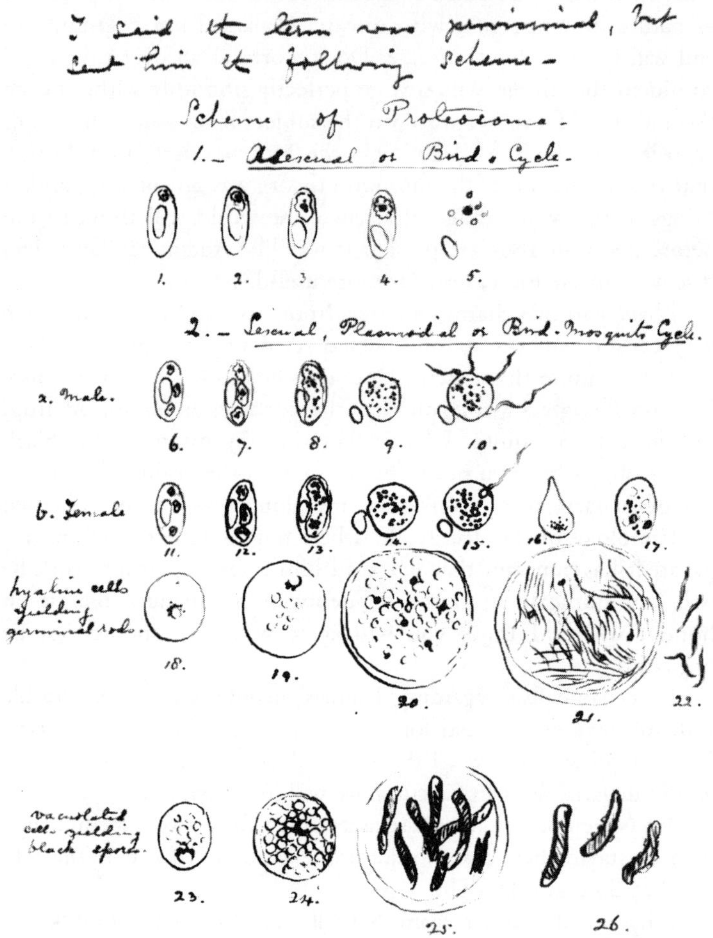

Of course all this is hypothetical at present, and the function of the black spores must be ascertained before a complete scheme can be drawn out. But on considering these drawings it seems to me that two theories are possible, depending on whether we consider that conjugation is or is not necessary to produce the MacCallum's male & female parasites figures 10 & 15.

A. If conjugation be not necessary, we may consider No. 2 cycle, the sexual or bird mosquito cycle, as representing the full life, male & female of the parasite - the youth of the parasite being passed in the bird, fecundation taking place (with the death of the male) in the mosquito's stomach, while the adult stage of the female is passed on the outer coat of the stomach wall. According to this the parasite should be a coccidium, while No. 1 cycle (in the bird only) will be simply an asexual precocious sporulation cycle.

B. If conjugation be necessary, we may look upon the discrete-pigment forms which are produced by it (the homologues of crescents) as true *plasmodia* as seen among the mycetozoa. The individual parasites in the bird coalesce to form plasmodia which are male & female & which complete their existences in the mosquito.

We should use the provisional terms proteosoma-coccidium or proteosoma-plasmodium according to the theory we adopt.

If MacCallum's work be accepted, & if the conjugation theory be proved, it may follow as a corollary that *in order to establish a sexual function, conjugation of two or more unicellular animals is necessary as a preliminary.*

All this for just so much as it is worth! The two cycles may be divided as follows.

No. I Cycle

Bird or asexual cycle	? previous sporulation cycle of a coccidium. ? solely unicellular stage of a protozoon.

No. II Cycle

Bird-mosquito or sexual cycle	? the full expression of the life history of a coccidium. ? plasmodial or conjugation stage of a protozoon.

? *Are the malaria parasites mycetozoa*?

The black spores merely contain germinal rods I think, which hatch out in the stomach of grubs and attack its cells, just as they attack the blood corpuscles of the birds, finally producing the sexual or plasmodial cycle in the imago - and so on *ad infinitum*.

Nuttall seems to think that the mosquito stage is an encysted stage;[8] but as I have pointed out the pigmented cells increase in size from 6μ to 60μ & I don't think encysted protozoa often increase in size to such an extent. On the other hand plasmodia do increase in size.

Cunningham's history of protomyxomyces coprinarius (amoeba coli etc)[9] gives a very close parallel to that of proteosoma on the plasmodial or mycetozoal hypothesis given above.

Let me know what you think of all this - it is necessary to consider the matter now. Could you show the scheme to anyone learned in protozoa - say Ray Lankester?[10]

That was a very interesting note on the mosquito in the B. M. J. of Sept 24th.[11] I see I have been robbed of the honour of discovering the veneno-salivary gland. Please observe that the pictures on pages 852 & 902 agree in one important particular - the trilobate nature of the gland.

You see I have returned here. I obtained Harvey's permission to do so. Kala-azar is evidently ordinary malaria of a severe type chiefly affecting the liver & spleen, especially the former. No more work of importance was to be done on it at this season, and the determination of the exact parasite (I think it is a quartan) would take more time than I can spare at present. The cases are not suitable for mosquito work, being, when declared, chronic. I have been told to report at once & hope to be done by the 20th when I shall attack proteosoma again in Calcutta.

How I wish *you* could come to Calcutta with Daniels for a couple of months. Could you not manage it? The journey by sea would be very comfortable & would do you good. Can you not consider it? We could return together in February. I intended to have proposed it before but foolishly forgot. It would be a change for you, and a rest. Would not the Colonial Office bear expenses?

I must now leave off to catch the post. If you could come to Calcutta you would see everything much better than in old specimens & could above all assure yourself about the infection of birds. It would be the best method of confirming my work. Do think seriously of it. I am sure Daniels will agree. You will escape the English winter.

Yours very sincerely
R. Ross.

1 Letter 154.

2 Dr S. W. Rivenburg of the American Mission in Assam.

3 F. J. Bosc, *Le Cancer* (Paris: Georges Carré et C. Naud, 1898) and Georg Schneidemühl, *Die Protozoen als Krankheitserregen des Menschen und der Hausthiere* (Leipzig: Wilhelm Engelmann, 1898). Bosc's work summarised the then fashionable theory that cancers were caused by protozoa of the sporozoa group.

4 John Couch Adams and Urbain Jean Joseph Leverrier had independently postulated the existence of another planet (Neptune)

because of perturbations in the orbit of Uranus.

5 Letters dated 12 Sept. 1898 (**RA** 02/186) and 7 Oct. 1898 (**RA** 02/187), congratulating Ross on the discovery of proteosoma in the salivary glands and resolving the question of malaria infection (Gibson, 1983).

6 A. Laveran, 'Sur un travail de M. le Dr. Ronald Ross, intitulé: Note pour l'histoire du parasite du paludisme en dehors de l'organisme humaine', *Bulletin de l'Académie de Médecine*, Ser. 3, 41(1899), 153-161.

7 Letter dated 25 Sept. 1895 (**RA** 02/215) enclosing notes with criticisms and suggestions about Ross's work (**RA** 02/216).

8 Presumably in his criticisms and suggestions above (original letter not traced).

9 See Letter 79, note 2.

10 See Letter 67, note 2.

11 'The mosquito', *BMJ* (24 Sept. 1898), 901-902. The discovery of the gland was there attributed to Professor George Macloskie, Princetown [sic] University, New Jersey, in a publication in *The American Naturalist* in October 1888.

Letter 156
02/171

Kurseong
15th Nov. 1898

Dear Dr Manson,

Just a line to tell you that I am still scribbling away at my kala azar report,[1] but that we are going down to Calcutta on the 18th. I shall put proteosoma cultivations in hand at once, so as to be ready for Daniels when he comes; but my report will keep me very busy until the end of the month. I think it will dispose of all mistakes as to the symptomatology of the disease. The fact was that when Giles investigated, the epidemic was not well defined.[2] It has become so since, and there is no doubt that the symptoms are high fever & great enlargement of spleen & liver. Even though we accept that worms may cause some toxic influence, as you suggested, they cannot produce the symptoms of kala azar. Besides the disease is quite different to anchylostomiasis elsewhere.

I cannot endorse Rogers' statement that plasmodia are always to be found in the cases, and black pigment also.[3] When Daniels comes I shall ask him to look at sections of the specimens of six cases I have brought with me. Then I propose to send the specimens on to you.

My solution is that immunity against the parasites is established after a month or two, after which the black pigment is eliminated, but the pathological condition of the organs (due possibly to the yellow pigment) remains. The disease must be malaria as every gradation from early cases with parasites & pigment in the spleen to established k. a. cases without either, existed.

I hope we shall be able to finish up the mosquito work this bout. Practically all we need do (for the present) is to find the function of the black spores and the definitive host of one of the human germs.

I see Koch has returned from Italy and that he seems to have made some wonderful discovery![4] Rogers has been made officiating Imperial bacteriologist out here and the Pioneer says he is going to find how the kala azar germ lives in the soil! I wish him luck.[5]

We are going to Darjeeling tomorrow for a day to see the great mountains which are just unfolding from their summer clouds.

I trust you have quite recovered from your illness. You must make ready for the specimens I shall send you.

I am thoroughly sick of kala azar. The time was not ripe for me to work at it and it has caused me to waste months. Remember I can stay in India until March if necessary; but I feel it will be folly for me on account of my health to attempt to stand another hot weather.

Yours very sincerely

R. Ross.

1 Ronald Ross, *Report on the nature of kala-azar* (Calcutta: Office of the Superintendent of Government Printing, 1899).

2 Giles (1890).

3 Rogers (1897b), 116.

4 'Professor Koch on malaria', *Lancet* (8 Oct. 1898), 945-946. 'One of the objects he had in view was to ascertain how far the Italian malaria coincides with the tropical form of the same malady, and he has satisfied himself that in all essentials they are identical. He has also been able to indicate properties hitherto unnoticed in the pathogenic germ of malaria as found external to man — properties possessing a distinct prophylactic value towards limiting the diffusion of the malady if not arresting it at its point of origin.' The note did not elaborate on the nature of these properties.

5 Rogers (1950), 25-36.

Letter 157
02/058

21, Queen Anne Street,
Cavendish Square. W.
30th October, 1898

My dear Ross,

I was greatly relieved by your letter of 9th inst.[1] I had not heard from you for so many mails that I began to conjure up all sorts of horrors - amongst others that you had broken down and were unable to write, or that the mosquito theory had burst up. I assure you it was a relief to be told by my wife when I came home last night that there was a letter from Dr Ross in the hall. I wish I had got it a couple of hours earlier as it would have saved me a journey to the Colonial Office where I had gone to say I thought you must be ill and to suggest telegraphing to find out. Daniels arrived two days ago and will leave for you on the 18th by P and O steamer. He is a first class man, keen as mustard, a thorough worker and with a broad mind and large experience. I am sure he will prove of great assistance to you as well as to the commission he is to join later on. After you have put him through proteosoma you should set him to work up the grey mosquito and the crescent; together you must positively settle this before you leave. I hear Koch has failed with the mosquito in Italy[2] so you have time yet to grab the discovery for England. I also hear that MacCallum is on the track and working hard.

I am very much interested in what you say about kala-azar. I conclude you regard it as malarial and I suppose the weight of evidence is to this effect. But why should the spleen and liver become so manifestly - invariably & exceptionally - involved in this particular type of malaria? I suppose that the parasite is a special one and that a peculiarity of it is that in some way it selects or damages these organs. Is it a distinct species or only a strain or variety with a peculiar type of viciousness of its own? These are points it would be of importance to settle. If it is a distinct parasite its morphological characters are worth a careful study. Did you see anything specific about them? I see you found quartan and aestivo-autumnal parasites but few crescents. It is strange that you found two kinds of parasites. It is difficult to suppose that both are causally related to the disease. It is difficult to suppose that the quartan should give rise to so much liver and spleen trouble. The facts might suggest that the receptivity of the spleen and liver to pathogenic influences was increased by malarial infection but that the specific germ which made kala-azar kala-azar was some other and additional germ. In view of Adami's recent work on micro-organisms in cirrhosis of the liver[3] I would suggest a careful bacteriological examination of the liver and spleen for micro-organisms. You might find in them some bacterium which was the real cause of the disease.

I hope you have preserved a lot of slides of the kala-azar malaria parasites for comparison with other malaria germs from other parts of India and of the world. It would be of very great service to Daniels if he could see the different varieties. The blackwater fever which he is specially commissioned to investigate seems to be like kala-azar in relation to malaria in a somewhat similar fashion.

I had a long talk with Cleghorn the other day about you.[4] He said there ought to be no difficulty in getting you permanently attached as scientific investigator and that the way to do it was through the Secretary of State. When you come home we should be able to work this easily I hope.

I have two interesting cases in hand just now which promise to turn out well. They are cases of sleeping sickness from the Congo specially imported for investigation. In both the filaria perstans is present in the blood.[5] We are looking forward to the post mortem examinations which cannot be very much longer delayed although it is quite possible that you may see the cases in life when you come home about March. I expect to find disease of the pituitary body in both and that it is caused by the operations of the filaria perstans.

Be sure not to delay unless on very urgent grounds your departure from India. You want a rest from work and in a decent climate and I am sure you would pick up a lot of new ideas and fresh information which would be of great service to you in your future work in India. I would not retire however from the service were I in your place. You are bound to be pushed forward now and as soon as the coping stone is put to the malaria pile or as soon as other men have confirmed your work which is only a matter of a few months at furthest.

I look forward with much interest to your next letter with additional information about kala-azar. Daniels will be with you about a fortnight or three weeks after you receive this. If he gets out about the first or second week of December he should have two clear months work with you.

Yours very sincerely
Patrick Manson

1 Letter 152.
2 'Professor Koch on malaria', *Lancet* (8 Oct. 1898), 945-946.
3 J. G. Adami, 'On the bactericidal functions of the liver and the etiology of progressive hepatic cirrhosis', *BMJ* (22 Oct. 1898), 1215-1218; in this paper Adami reported the cultivation of a bacillus from the livers of some patients suffering from progressive hepatic cirrhosis.
4 Cleghorn had retired from the IMS on 25 October 1898.
5 Described in P. Manson, 'A clinical lecture on the sleeping sickness', *BMJ* (3 Dec. 1898), 1672-1677.

Letter 158
02/172

C/O Grindlay & Co
Calcutta
24th Nov. 1898

Dear Dr Manson,
I am very sorry (and also flattered) that you should have been so disappointed at not getting letters from me in October. I thought however that I had missed only two or three mails, and even imagined that you might be glad of a rest from my weekly lucubrations(!) which were certainly tending to become monotonous. I was very busy over kala azar too & had nothing definite to write about, besides being very seedy as I always become on going to a hot climate.

I am delighted to hear that Daniels will be here so soon. I have just heard officially about it. It will be a pleasure & a relief to discuss the whole business with an intelligent man who takes an interest in science. Nobody here will take the trouble (as yet at all events) to look at a mosquito. Daniels will also be able to advise me in respect to his yellow pigment in anchylostomiasis - I expect it was siderosis from previous attacks of fever.

I am still scribbling away at my report. My brain is not in good working order and I am very slow over the business.

Lawrie under the name of Bugobutty Bose M. D. has crushed the mosquito theory completely in the Pioneer.[1] He practically accuses me of fabricating false evidence! The poor man has become an absurd crank. I believe the medical papers won't take his effusions.

Your book is doing wonders out here. It is a great success & everybody has a copy. Just what was wanted. I suppose a new edition will be out presently.[2] Would it be possible to give a larger number of exact references to existing literature. Such would be useful to us all. The style is as perfect as anything I know. Wish I could come near it.

Mahomed Bux comes every day to reproach me for not feeding mosquitos. I have determined to nearly finish the report first, and tell him Daniels will work him nicely. I have a nice little epidemic of malaria now going on a mile from the laboratory ready for Daniels - in the 5th Reg. Bengal Infantry - just the thing for us.

If Daniels accepts my work & it is not too late, I would strongly advise another attempt being made to send the other malaria commissioners[3] to me before proceeding to Africa.

Yours very sincerely

R. Ross.

1 Untraced, but see Letters 25, 32, 35 and 36.

2 Manson's *Tropical Diseases* (1898a). A second edition was published in 1900.

3 Christophers and Stephens went to Italy instead.

Letter 159
02/059

21, Queen Anne Street,
Cavendish Square. W.
8th November, 1898.

My dear Ross,

Charles[1] writes me he has given you the great news from the Imperial City. You are now on the mounting wave which I trust will surely lead on to fortune. Bignami should have experimented on your lines though.[2] He ought to have fed his mosquitos on crescent blood, waited a week for the germinal bodies to form and then set them to bite. I have written Charles to tell him this and I hope he will not be too late this season to try. I hope however you have anticipated him and that you can give chapter and verse, that is mosquito and experiment for tertian quartan and crescent malaria by this time.

I am not quite so sure about this kala azar business. I cannot disabuse my mind of the idea that possibly it is a double infection; a malaria infection with a something superadded. Why should it spread in the slow way it has done if there is not something specific about it. Your explanation may be the correct one but it is curious that it should be so localised, should infect particular houses and villages, and should cause so fatal a form of liver and spleen hypertrophy. If I were you I would be careful to safeguard myself in emitting the pure malarial hypothesis. I hope you will bring home livers and spleens with you properly prepared for microscopical examination. Try for a bacterium in these organs.

I sent Bignami and Charles one of your preparations each. I grudge to part with them but I think it is in your interest that the Romans should have ocular proof that you have been before them. I feel that these furrineers are inclined to filch as much as they can. This is a sentiment I only breathe to you. We will take care that your interests are looked after here.

Daniels is getting ready to leave. I have sent for him to give him his instructions from the Colonial Office. Make him thoroughly acquainted with the proper species of mosquito and see that he takes preserved specimens away with him. It wont do for him to go to mid-Africa unprovided with anything that might further the work there. Do you also furnish yourself with ample material for illustrating your work when you stand before the British public next March.

I hope you are feeling better and that you are able to place the top stone on your magnificent building.

Yours sincerely

Patrick Manson.

1 T. Edmonston Charles was a British doctor then living in Rome. He corresponded with both Ross and Manson about malarial developments in Rome, and Ross used Charles' letters as evidence in his subsequent priority disputes with Grassi and other Italian malariologists. Charles' first (published) letter to Ross was dated 4 November 1898. Ross published Charles' letters to him in 1900; he reprinted them in 1929, along with other supporting correspondence, as *Letters from Rome on Certain Discoveries connected with Malaria*, (n.p.,[1929]). The originals are still in the Ross Archives.

2 Charles' letters to Manson are apparently lost. In his first letter (above, Note 1) to Ross, he mentioned that Bignami was experimenting with human malaria, rather than confirming Ross's work on birds. Bignami's human subjects had been locked up with mosquitoes, which were allowed to bite over a period of months, 'till at last a success has just been met with'.

Letter 160
02/173

Calcutta
7th Dec. 1898

My dear Dr Manson,[1]

I have been very disappointed at the non-arrival of Daniels some days ago. I expected he would turn up by the mail of course, wrote to him to Bombay & asked him to breakfast, had mosquito ready for him & everything. No Daniels! Now I find he won't be here till the *18th*. 'Tis a pity as we have little time to spare.

Rivenburg[2] arrived ten days ago. He is a sound man though he knows little. He finds proteosoma in birds & mosquitos at once & can dissect a mosquito perfectly already.

I told you that I expected the cold weather to make a difference in the cultivation of proteosoma. It does. Luckily the vermicules take root just as before, but they *don't grow larger*. Temperature of laboratory 68°F at midday. This is a most interesting & suggestive fact. I find also that all the functions of the grey mosquitos seem to be checked. They take 5 days to digest a meal & they live half asleep without refeeding all that time. Also they bite, but bite much less readily. This is convenient in some ways as it enables us to study the second day parasites. I am having gas turned on to the laboratory in order to work the incubators. It is however quite likely that considerable difficulties will be experienced in getting the "coccidia" to sporulate & also in infecting birds. *So please look out for the necessity of having to give Daniels an extra month here* if necessary.

We are busy trying the best way to make preparations. Mere drying & the mounting in Canada balsam makes all details vanish. Only the pigment of the parasites remains visible. Staining first makes matters worse because all the tissues are stained while the parasites do not show up any better & the stain generally hides the pigment. Canada balsam will only be practicable if we find a differential stain. It is a bit of a business. After all 5% formalin seems to give the best results found hitherto; but more care must be taken in the varnishing. Some of *my* specimens have remained as good as new for six months & more.

My kala-azar report is still dragging on painfully, and has I fear, knocked the last piece of "go" out of me. It was a great mistake to put me on that difficult business at this time. I must be very cautious in everything I write & have to give notes of 75 cases. My brains seem to have solidified & advance is of the slowest, while I have taken to having constant headaches. You must expect very little more work from me until I have had a good rest; but I shall put Daniels quite through in a week, as I have Rivenburg. You will understand this, I think, when you see the kala-azar report.

I have had two letter from Charles[3] - very nice ones & will send him specimens next mail. He says your demonstration at the B. M. Association created "quite a furore".

I note your advice about kala-azar & will discuss the point carefully. Will send you specimens as early as possible. I know why no coccidia were found in the mosquitos I sent you. The "innards" of the mosquito decompose *after* they are plunged in glycerine.

With kind regards

Yours sincerely

R. Ross.

1 The first time Ross had used the familiar 'My dear' with the older Manson.
2 Dr S. W. Rivenburg from the American mission in Assam.
3 Presumably the ones dated 4 and 19 November, later reproduced by Ross (Letter 159, note 1).

Letter 161
02/060

21, Queen Anne Street,
Cavendish Square. W.
16th November, 1898.

My dear Ross,

This will be handed to you by Dr Daniels. He leaves on the 18th and proceeds direct to Calcutta to help and to learn from you. You will find him an excellent fellow socially and a first class man at his work. He is a good practical pathologist and clinicist and, in addition, he looks upon disease from the stand point of the naturalist. This, I take it, is the right way. His capacity for original work has been enhanced by the valuable circumstance that he has had to trust to himself for many years. There is no better training for a capable man. You will I have no doubt give Daniels a lot; I am sure however you will get from him a lot in return.

I am looking forward with interest and expectation to your next letters. The mosquito theory is now fairly on the ascendant; thanks entirely to you. You will be lionised when you get home.

Yours sincerely

Patrick Manson

Letter 162
02/174

Calcutta
22nd Dec. 1898

Dear Dr Manson,
Daniels has arrived at last[1] and is all you say of him. He will be of every assistance, and his advice regarding kala-azar will be of great help. I have not a moment to write as we must be off to the laboratory almost directly. Nothing new. I have only just succeeded in getting the germinal *threads* as they ought to be called into the salivary glands; but no birds have yet become infected and we are very badly off for good subjects. Sparrows have only a few proteosoma nowadays.

We shall, as soon as Daniels knows the work - which will take a couple of days, go in strong for human malaria.

My report is still going on slowly; sections of specimens still have to be cut. The thing is a positive pain to me as I get a headache if I think of work for half an hour.

Harvey spared me three minutes the other day. He is applying for me to be kept on & will recommend my leave in February. There are however many reasons against my returning to India.

Not enough specimens have yet been made for you, but I have succeeded in setting up germinal rods both dry & wet. I hope we can dispatch some *next mail.*

With kind regards
Yours sincerely
Ronald Ross.

1 On the day Ross wrote this letter: *Memoirs*, 326.

Letter 163
02/175

Calcutta
29th Dec. 1898

Dear Dr Manson,
We are so busy that I never have a moment to write to you. We have made some negative experiments with grey mosquitos on human tertian, but will shortly start others. Excuse our not sending specimens yet. Our subjects are few & poor & want all our mosquitos for

infecting purposes. Owing to Italian developments I am sending Laveran a note on the Extracorporeal Developments of the Parasites of Paludism for the Academy of Medicine,[1] and must forward all our best specimens with it. This to choke off Bignami at the outset.

I have read Bignami's stuff in the Lancet;[2] but we have profited so little by your advice to work away quietly that Daniels, Waddell[3] & I have concocted a leader for the I.M.G.[4] which will make Bignami jump a little. Try & get the B. M. J. to transcribe it (Jan. number). Next week I am sending my Preliminary Report to the B. M. J. & asking them to publish it if possible with another article by me putting the authorship of the mosquito theory straight. I shall never admit that B. has had anything to do with it & consider his attempt as most presumptuous. It is a mistake to allow this sort of thing to take hold for a moment. I shall strike back at once with full force. The theory belongs to you & Laveran absolutely. Daniels agrees with me entirely. I shall put the matter clearly in the paper, which I shall dispatch also next week, for the Academy of Medicine.

I don't accept Bignami's cases at all definitely. Even if sound they are only a confirmation of the germinal rod work. What is more I don't believe all he & the other gentry say & strongly advise you not to.

The theory was proved when the pigmented cells were obtained from proteosoma. The outline was completed with the germinal rods & black spores, excepting only the function of the latter.

The work on human malaria is only of *secondary* importance. It must be carried out separately in every malarious country and is a mere detail of the proteosoma work.

I shall be quite ready for the detractors when I come home. Haven't read Lawrie's article yet, but will make him also dance before long.[5]

We are starting photography. Birds not being infected readily at all. Mosquitos slack. But warm weather is coming on.

Kind regards & best wishes for the new year. Daniels will write next week.

Yours very sincerely
R. Ross.

1 Amico Bignami, 'The inoculation theory of malarial infection', *Lancet* (3 Dec. 1898), 1461-1463; (10 Dec. 1898), 1541-1544; A. Bignami and G. Bastianelli, 'On the structure of the semi-lunar and flagellate bodies of malarial fever', an appendix to the above article, *ibid* (17 Dec. 1898), 1620-1621. In the first article, Bignami recalled that in 1896 he had argued that 'malaria behaves itself with

regard to man as if the malarial germs were inoculated by mosquitoes'; reviewed his unsuccessful attempts, in 1894, to prove this hypothesis; and then reported his successful human inoculation experiments, from August 1898. He cited three contributions of Manson, and Ross's 'interesting observations' on birds. The article with Bastianelli dealt with the microstructure and function of the crescents and flagellae, arguing that the crescents do not have any reproductive capabilities while in the human being.

2 Laveran (1899).

3 Laurence Augustine (later Austine) Waddell, (1854-1938), Surgeon-Major I.M.S. He was then a co-editor of the *Indian Medical Gazette.*

4 'A new fashoda incident: the Italian flag hoisted on the mosquito-theory', *Indian Medical Gazette,* (Jan. 1899), 15-16. The (unsigned) leader begins 'Piracy in science is unfortunately nothing new'. The *BMJ* did not reprint it.

5 E. Lawrie, 'The mosquito and the malaria "parasite"', *Lancet* (3 Dec. 1898), 1468-1469; in it, Lawrie rejected the work of Manson, Ross, MacCallum and Laveran, in favour of his own pet theory that malaria is a disorder of degenerating white blood corpuscles.

Letter 164
02/061

21, Queen Anne Street,
Cavendish Square. W.
7th December, 1898.

My dear Ross,

I know that Charles has posted you in the progress of events in Rome.[1] You will see from the Lancet the position Bignami is taking and how there is an attempt to belittle you while exalting himself.[2] All this is very amusing and contemptible. Hold your own course and dont be influenced by it. You have plenty of friends here who know how to uphold you and your rights. Your work is the starting point of all this mosquito business; this cannot be undone. Meanwhile do your best to prove by set experiment on man that what holds good for proteosoma holds good for the human malaria parasites. Your being sent kala-azaring was a misfortune and has lost you valuable time. Now you have Daniels at your side you will have fresh incentive to push on and most valuable assistance. He is the right sort I feel sure.

Ray Lankester for the British Museum recognising the importance of the mosquito in human affairs is instituting a systematic investigation of the Culicidae. Through the Colonial Office he has sent out a circular of directions for the collection of mosquitos with a view to their scientific description by the diptera man at the Museum and I hope that soon we shall have a better knowledge of these insects. I have asked the British Medical Journal to publish this circular so that those who may not get the Colonial Office posted circular may know how to set about the business.[3]

Lawrie is again on the war-path. His latest effusion is beneath contempt. I suppose it may do a little harm with people who know nothing of the subject. The Lancet are foolish to publish such twaddle but they seem very glad to do anything to injure me.[4] The secret of this is that Curnow,[5] one of the staff of the Dreadnought, is on the contributing staff and he and others are determined to upset our School for Tropical Medicine at the Branch Hospital at Albert Docks. They are leaving no stone unturned to do this. I was sorry to see the Indian Medical Gazette had been writing with the same purpose.[6] They will not prevent the scheme going on though they may embarrass it a bit or, rather, worry those who have got a great movement at heart and have worked long for it. It is strange that there are men who wont do a thing themselves that is manifestly right and will not allow others to do it as well. You will find when you come home that you will have many warm supporters; but you will also find that you will have a lot of snarling curs who will try to snap at you and pull you down.

Peg away and keep as much of the mosquito theory for old England as you can.

Kindest regards to Daniels.

Yours sincerely

Patrick Manson

1 Letter 159, note 1, and Letter 160, note 3.

2 A. Bignami (1898).

3 An editorial in the *BMJ* (10 Dec. 1898), 1767, refers to a pamphlet issued by the Natural History Department of the British Museum, *How to collect mosquitoes (Culicidae)* (London, 1898).

4 Letter 163, note 5.

5 John Curnow, (1846-1902), Senior Visiting Physician of the Dreadnought Seamen's Hospital.

6 'The study of tropical diseases', *Indian Medical Gazette* (Sept. 1898), 343-345. The thrust of the leader was that 'the best place to study tropical diseases is in the tropics'.

Letter 165
02/176

Calcutta
5th January 1899

Dear Dr Manson,

I have sent off a copy of my Preliminary Report and also a Note on the Authorship of the mosquito theory[1] to the Editor, B. M. J. Publish them or not as you think fit. Daniels agrees with me that the Note should be published, because if we do not peg out our claim very shortly you will find that the Italians will claim all they find in it. Bignami's papers in the Lancet[2] are a bare faced attempt to steal as much as he can - I don't think much of his experiments. Remember those I tried by giving mosquito water to healthy people. Nor in fact do I feel inclined to accept everything the Italians say they are doing - such as finding the germinal threads in numbers of free mosquitos. I bet they find nothing of the kind.

I have also sent a note to Laveran, for L'Académie de Medecine in which I claim the solution of the malaria problem for you and him. He certainly proposed it first[3] - though it was only a conjection on his part - but the scientific theory depended on the function of the flagellate bodies. I have tried to make this as clear as I could in a paper to be presented by Laveran.

Most of my best specimens have been sent off to him. I think you will prefer this to getting the specimens yourself as we must capture France before the Italians can get there.

I think we shall be able to send the germinal rods next mail as we have found how to prepare them both stained & unstained. I made a beautiful specimen of the glands in which the threads occurred only in the central (? poison) lobes of the gland of each side. I think too I have got the trick of getting out the glands with certainty. Daniels has seen everything up to the infection of birds - but this is not doing brilliantly. I think only 5 birds have become infected up to date.

Daniels has cut most of the k. a. sections. No melanin, as I said. It is a nasty problem.

We shall now deliver an attack in force on human malaria. There are cases in the regimental hospital but we can't find the grubs of dappled-winged mosquitoes now, though some of these insects can be caught by hand. Mahomed Bux however, who can make a mosquito do anything, persuades them to bite in the day time simply by holding the test-tube against the skin of the patient. This will help us greatly as the people here are very frightened of this kind of thing since the plague, and don't like mosquito nets. But, after all, human malaria is only a detail of proteosoma.

Surg. Gen. Harvey has promised me my leave for six months. We start from here on the 16th February and have decided to go via Rome. Dr Charles has been most kind in writing every mail & asking me to stay with him.[4] We want to get the Indian cobwebs out of our brains by seeing things in Italy and it will cost very little more than coming home by sea.

Harvey has expressed himself very kindly about my work, and hoped I would come out again. But I fear not.[5] First my health won't stand India any longer; and next my pocket won't. We have just calculated that we shall arrive in Europe £200 out of pocket from when we left in 1895! I have had the pleasure of losing £300 or more during the last 8 years, all for the honour of serving the Govt. of India; although we have not even kept a trap & pony for the last 4 years. This is entirely due to my having to keep my family in hotels while the authorities are making up their minds as to what they are going to do and to incessant changes of station. The same thing exactly will go on if I am ever fool enough to come back here. Then the steamer companies squeeze us out of our last penny.

Don't write to me after you receive this letter, as I shall be en route at the time of the return post. I am looking forward much to seeing you - but we shall probably dally a little in Italy.

Yours very sincerely

R. Ross.

The Plague Commissioners Wright & Ruffer have seen our work. They swallow the germinal threads but stick rather at the black spores.[6]

1 They appeared in the same issue: 'Mosquitos and malaria. The infection of birds by mosquitos', *BMJ* (18 Feb. 1899), 432-433; 'Mosquitos and malaria', *BMJ* (18 Feb. 1899), 425-426.

2 A. Bignami (1898).

3 In 1884: Laveran (1884).

4 Letter of 16 December 1898, reprinted in Ross (ed) [1929] *Letters from Rome*, 25-7, (**RA** 08/030).

5 *Memoirs*, 355, for a copy of a short letter from Harvey.

6 (Sir) Almroth Edward Wright, (1861-1947), Professor of Pathology at the Army Medical School, Netley, and (Sir) Marc Armand Ruffer, (1859-1917), Head of the Egyptian Sanitary Department at Cairo.

Letter 166
02/177

Calcutta
19th Jan. 1899

Dear Dr Manson,
Daniels wrote last mail telling you how slack work is owing to the cold. He & Rivenburg have infected only 13 out of 22 birds & they all recover quickly. But we are now getting under sail with human malaria having procured (after much difficulty) two good crescent cases. We have also procured a mine of dapple-wings and are working away steadily. Unfortunately it is most exceptionally cold; so cold that proteosoma does not even take root in the mosquito on some nights. Incubation does not seem to have very much effect chiefly I think because the insects are out in the cold at nights. We are however trying every possible trick with crescents in dapple-wings & fancy we shall knock it off in the next few weeks. We have still one month to do human malaria in.

My kala-azar report is drawing to a conclusion and is partly sent to press. Daniels cut the sections and describes them. His assistance is most valuable.

He says he is writing in to confirm the proteosoma work.

I see they are trying to tackle you about the School for Tropical Medicine but don't think they will succeed.[1] I should like to write about it but don't know whether I should not do harm.

We have scarcely any mosquitoes going owing to the cold; can't make good specimens at all. But the warm weather will set in in a few days for good, I expect. Then we hope to have something of interest to write about.

Yours very sincerely
R. Ross.

1 There was a great deal of correspondence in *BMJ* and *Lancet* 1898-1899 about the proposed School for Tropical Diseases. See also G. C. Cook, 'Dr Patrick Manson's leading opposition in the establishment of the London School of Tropical Medicine: Curnow, Anderson, and Turner', *Journal of Medical Biography*, 3 (1995), 170-177, and *Idem. From the Greenwich Hulks to Old St. Pancras: A History of Tropical Disease in London* (London: Athlone Press, 1992), ch. 6.

Letter 167
02/062

21, Queen Anne Street,
Cavendish Square. W.
10th January 1899.

My dear Ross,
I am very sorry to hear you are so seedy. You must clear out at once if your health is giving way. You are much too precious to lose now and there is not much more to be gained by your remaining in India longer. You have forged the key and others must take the trouble to open the door. The Italians are hard at it as you will learn from Charles's letters[1] and we will take care here that your position in this matter is not ignored. Daniels should by this time be fairly indoctrinated with your views and methods and he is of a kind that wants only to be put in the way of work to do it and do it well. That kala-azar business was most unfortunate. Had you been left alone you would have anticipated all that the Italians are doing. Practically you had already done it and you can justly claim to have been the first to find the malaria parasite in the mosquito as well as to point out the modus operandi of that insect in diffusing malaria. All the detail will come in time, in a very short time I believe. Therefore if you are not quite well start for home at once and chuck for the time being the kala-azar report. You can finish it when you get home and a rest.

Two mails ago I wrote to Harvey telling him that I hoped he would get the Indian Government to make some recognition of the splendid work you had done.[2] I pointed out that its enormous importance was already recognised in Europe and that honours were in store for you here. I told him it would be a graceful act for the Indian Government to anticipate these. I also wrote in the same strain to Colonel Fenn,[3] whom I know, to influence the Viceroy in the same direction.[4] I dont know if any move has been already made by others. I thought I would do no harm at all events to remind them of an obvious duty.

I am glad you approve of Daniels. He ought to be of great assistance to you. I think he will do good work in Africa, for he has the knowledge and the spirit and the ability.

Yours sincerely
Patrick Manson

1 See Letter 159, note 1.
2 Letter not located.
3 Colonel Ernest Harrold Fenn, (1850-1916), RAMC, served on Lord Curzon's staff in India, 1898-1903.
4 Lord Curzon, (1859-1925), became Viceroy in January 1899.

Letter 168
02/178

Calcutta
2nd Feb 1899

Dear Dr Manson,
I think Daniels has told you of the kicks we have been getting from fortune. Three species of dapple wing fed on crescents and incubated, etc, have all absolutely failed; while the cold has cured all our proteosoma birds and it is very likely that I shall not be able to bring home specimens of infected salivary glands.

We leave here on about the 16th inst. & so have little time left for anything.[1] The last sheets of that wretched kala-azar report were sent in a few days ago. The whole thing has been as disaster for me. Of course I expected to finish it in November. But it was bad enough to put me on such work at all after the mosquito theory had been proved.

Very many thanks for your efforts toward getting me "recognition" from the Indian Government. They will I am sure be at least amused. However the only recognition which will help me will be one in hard cash, and I don't think we are likely to wring *that* from them! Without it - I say so definitely - I shall never return to this country, as I have no intention of spending any more of our slender capital on the service of humanity!

Please don't believe too much of Grassi & Cos' work. There are passages which make me think that their actual observations have been of the slenderest and that the rest is eked out by aid of my reports. Also please don't forget that crescents were cultivated by me (for an absolute certainty) in August 1897 and that all the work the Italians are now doing is only a detail and will have to be done everywhere. This will soon be done; but as Daniels says, "there will be some tall lying first."

We hope to be home on about the 20th March. I will write again before starting.

With kind regards
Yours sincerely
R. Ross.

1 Letter 171. Ross actually left on 22 February.

Letter 169
02/063

21 Queen Anne Street,
Cavendish Sq
18th January, 1899.

My dear Ross,
The romans are still active. I wrote last week to Bignami telling him we were careful of your reputation and hoping that he and his compatriots would be equally so.[1] They are all on the grab it would seem. I had a letter from Charles today saying that there are now some twenty or thereby claimants for the mosquito theory. I daresay in another month there will be fifty. It is very amusing as well as ridiculous.

I have written Daniels thanking him for his letter and suggesting he should try the artificial marsh. He will probably show you what I have written. I have also asked him to get me halteridium and proteosoma slides. I cant get them here. Dont you bother about truck of this sort but keep your energies for the weightier matters. I hope before you leave that the human malaria will be as well worked out as the avian and that the black spore business will be solved.

But dont let your wish for completeness keep you a day longer in India than your health will easily stand. Dont risk anything. Your work is practically complete and you should come home for a time.

They are getting up a tropical school in Liverpool[2] and came to me about a lecturer, etc. Amongst others I suggested your name and Boyce[3] has jumped at the idea. I dont suppose you would care for it. But I encouraged him to try for you in the hope that the Indian Government would make a better bid. I think Boyce will telegraph an offer.[4] Go with this -telegram or letter - to the I. G. and ask them if you should accept. This will bring them to make you a good offer. Pardon my Machiavellianism; but it is in your interest and in the interest of tropical medicine I have intrigued. I would like to have you at home but I would prefer to have you in India with a proper laboratory, a good position, and a free hand. There is so much work to be done there and very few who can do it.

I am glad you like Daniels. He ought to be of great assistance to you. Primed with you methods and thoughts he is sure to do some good work in Africa.

Yours sincerely
Patrick Manson

1 Letter not traced.
2 Reported in *BMJ* (28 Jan. 1899), 237-238.
3 Rubert W. Boyce, (1863-1911), Professor of Pathology at University College, Liverpool. See **Biographical Appendix**.
4 *Memoirs*, 367ff., for Ross's negotiations with the Liverpool School. Boyce telegrammed Ross once he was back in England, 25 March 1899, **RA**10/006.

Letter 170
02/179

Calcutta
15th Feb. 1899

Dear Dr Manson,
Daniels went away on the 12th for Africa.[1] Our bad luck has clung to us to the last. Anopheles pictus[2] has absolutely refused crescents, and also tertian - according to a few experiments. I cannot get a single fresh case of human malaria. These Bengalis are certainly the stupidest and most superstitious of human beings - if one can call them that. Two other dapple-wings have also refused crescents, and no other species can be got round here. I expect that the true fly is "off the water" at this season here. The Secunderabad dapple-wings were different species from A. pictus & from A. claviger,[3] though very like both.

I can't obtain a single well infected sparrow for making specimens & shall not be able to bring preparations of germinal threads in salivary glands, unless I am more lucky within the next week. If I am I shall take the mosquitoes on board ship & prepare them there; but I have little hope of it. The cold weather has almost cured all the proteosoma birds - as I think Daniels told you. This is the last stroke of ill-luck.

I am feeling better since my report has been finished & often feel inclined to stay. I am leaving hosts of beautiful experiments to the Italians & others. It is a great pity, but can't be helped.

We made an observation lately which throws doubt on the authenticity of the black spores - at least I think so - Daniels doesn't. I have reported to Govt. accordingly.[4]

I have also reported to Govt. on the practical benefits likely to arise from the mosquito theory, if they follow it up properly. Will show you a copy of the report.[5]

On board ship I shall prepare a paper giving full details of the whole work. This I may read before some society, if you like. I *may* be able to bring home live mosquitoes to illustrate it. I shall also bring some halteridium pigeons for you &, if possible, some crows - which will also do for demonstrations.

I think the paper will make all clear about the part played by the Italians - which is a very humble one. Many thanks for writing to Bignami - I await with amusement what he will answer! It was a very straight thing to write to him; but, whatever he does or says, I don't think he will run away with the credit of solving the malaria problem.

Many thanks also for remembering me in connection with the Liverpool Tropical School. Please do not forget about it, as it may be useful to me. I shall talk to you about my affairs when I see you. It would certainly be a good thing to do research in India steadily; but there are other things to be considered, and many cogent reasons why I should now leave India for good. I fear also that I may even *sell my microscopes*. My original intention was to take my pension and adopt literature - which I know will pay me better than the microscope, though I confess that it may not be so grand a thing as research on medical subjects. Now that the great problem is solved I feel I have done my duty and may sing *nunc dimittis* and look after those essential parts of clothing, the pockets.[6] I don't think a man can be called upon justly to give up too much for the chance of doing good research in the future.

But I think Daniels will now push on matters nicely.

It is evident that the study of malaria has now entered on the third and last phase - prevention. That is, we must find out how to exterminate the malaria-bearing species of mosquito. I shall have a great deal to tell you on this score. I expect we shall have to classify mosquitoes over again on the information which I have collected at odd times. I am bringing home a few species of mosquito - all I can find here, and will take them to the British Museum, with the above mentioned information.

I have just been over all my birds again - not one even decent infection. I have also been through 40 sparrows since Daniels left - all healthy. Will have up some crows in a day or two for you.

We start on the 22nd & hope to arrive on about the 20th March - all the way by sea.

With kind regards

Yours sincerely

R. Ross.

1 Where he joined up with Christophers and Stephens.
2 *A. rossi.*
3 *A. maculipennis*
4 *Memoirs*, 327-8; Ross included a comment on the last page of his Kala-azar report (Ross, 1899a).
5 Report sent to Leslie, 16 Feb. 1899, 'On the subject of the practical results as regards the prevention of the disease (malaria) which may be expected to arise from my researches' **RA** 03/243; 03/244. A version was published as 'Extermination of Malaria', *Indian Medical Gazette* (July, 1899), 231-232.
6 From the Anglican evening service, 'now lettest thou depart'. For Ross's continuing preoccupation with his pocket, see Chernin (1988).

Letter 171
02/180

City of Corinth
24th Feb.
In the Hoogly

Dear Dr Manson,
This is the last of a long series of letters to you. They began nearly four years ago.

I shall have your replies bound in a volume! The solution of the great malaria problem is history you know!

We have been two days getting out of this river, the ship being a large one; but are off at midnight. We hope to arrive on about 22nd March. My address will be Care of Mr. H. S. King & Co, 45 Pall Mall.

Bad luck lasts up to the moment of leaving. I told Daniels that he had brought a demon with him, & I fear, or rather hope, he left it behind in my laboratory. I brought a crowd of mosquitoes on board, but they are a wretched lot - about one or two parasites in every three of them - quite useless for specimens. However I am putting up the best of them on board. Not one has come to maturity as yet & scarcely any are near it. I think that the temperature must be well over 80°F for proteosoma to grow at its normal rate. Anyway I shall not be able to bring home good specimens of salivary glands (infected); but I shall write & ask Dr Laveran to let me have some which I sent him. I think Daniels has sent you one or two.

We are ever so much better after getting on board ship. Think that there was some insanitary element in our Calcutta rooms. Daniels says I am hypochondriacal! I replied that the effect on me was the same!

Anyway I hope to cease being so when we touch a cold climate.

Well, I have left many things undone which I ought to have done; but congratulate myself that the task you imposed on me is finished. You must cease *rubbing the lamp* for a little, at all events.

I am looking forward immensely to seeing you; and I have a lot more to tell you than I have conveyed by letter. I shall concoct a full history of the solution of the problem; after the publication of which things will take their right places. It was the *great induction* which did it - nothing else.

With kind regards
Yours very sincerely
Ronald Ross.

Letter 172
49/041

21, Queen Anne Street,
Cavendish Square. W.
19th March, 1899

My dear Ross,
I was very glad to get your letter of 24th this afternoon. And glad to hear you were already feeling better and trusting that your voyage will set you up for the campaign you will have to get through here. I shall of course be delighted to see you again, but so will a great many more, for you are now a famous man and an honour to your country.

Come and see me as soon as you possibly can; and before you are got at, so I may put you up to the ropes. I have just sent Boyce your address. He will probably make you an offer to boss the Tropical School in Liverpool.[1] It is a good opportunity for malaria work, and a good opportunity for consulting practice, but dont be in a hurry to close with them as your career in India is, I fancy, only beginning. But come along here as soon as you can and we will talk about all this.

I got a lot of specimens from Daniels, some of them really excellent and most convincing. None however of germinal rods or salivary glands. I have a lot of yours still in fair condition so that there will be no difficulty in getting a good set for purposes of demonstration.

Once more - Welcome home.
Yours sincerely
Patrick Manson

1 Although Ross became a lecturer, and, later, professor in the Liverpool School, his relationship with the School was never an easy one, nor did he really succeed in building up a busy consulting practice in Liverpool as Manson had done in London. For details, see *Memoirs*, ch. 19; Nye and Gibson (1897), ch. 8; and H. J. Power, *Tropical Medicine in the Twentieth Century: A History of the Liverpool School, 1898-1990*, (London: Kegan Paul, 1998), chs. 1-2.

Letter 173
02/281

44 Prince's Road
Liverpool
15th May 1899

Dear Dr Manson,
I sent you your specimens by post this morning and hope they will reach you early tomorrow. We have not had time to have any of them drawn.

I have no doubt that Fayrer's "rod in pickle" will break in his hand & wound himself.[1] I hope he will trot out Lawrie's theory by some chance.[2] The real reason for these absurdities is very apparent.

I enclose brief report of my first lecture here.[3] My wife &, I think, Boyce & others were not a little nervous regarding my oratorial powers, but somehow I was not alarmed myself; and when the time came I found myself speaking to 150 people for an hour and a quarter without a break - and also without any notes! None of them threw anything.

This was not my inaugural lecture of course. That will be a far more serious one. I shall pitch the scale high.

Two good cases of malaria in the ward.

My compliments to Mrs Manson & the young ladies.
Yours very sincerely
R. Ross.

1 Reference untraced.
2 Lawrie (1898). See Letter 163, note 5.
3 Liverpool Daily Post 16th May (**RA** 02/282).

Letter 174
02/283

44 Prince's Road
Liverpool
3rd June [1899]

Dear Dr Manson,
It is about time to write to you.

I hope you received your specimens in order, none smashed. We have been busy photographing mine, and I shall shortly be able to make you a present of a complete set of lantern slides of proteosoma. I have obtained a beautiful negative of the germinal threads.

I think you forwarded Bignami on tertian to me.[1] It is being translated. I gather he could find no black spores in the tertian parasites.

Not much doing here. I am busy reading up steadily, photographing & writing our syllabus. The difficulty with the last is to avoid plagiarising from your excellent prospectus. I have proposed including animal parasites generally in our syllabus & calling ourselves "The Liverpool School of Tropical Medicine & Animal Parasitology." The title is cumbrous & "animal parasitology" is open to question; but it seems impossible to find a better title. A school for special teaching of animal parasites as distinct from vegetable ones seems to be required. Our committee is now sitting on the syllabus.

My inaugural lecture is on the twelfth instant. You will see the subject by the card.[2] I shall discuss the possibility of extirpating malaria-bearing mosquitoes in detail, & shall send a copy of the lecture to the B. M. J., as Dr Williams asked me to do.

I have submitted proposals in writing to our Committee for a malaria expedition to Sierra Leone next August.[3] Annett,[4] our demonstrator & myself have volunteered to go, and if funds allow, to take someone with us. We propose to start immediately after the B. M. A. meeting and to return in October. Our objects will be simple:-

(a). To find at least one malaria-bearing mosquito at Freetown.

(b). To see whether its breeding pools are so isolated that there will be any hope of exterminating the insect from a small area - say that of the town.

You said that you thought you could send your £300 scholar with me.[5] Do you think that this will be possible? If so I could teach him what I know and leave him there. As I said, if funds allow, we also will take a man with us & will leave him behind until the cool weather sets in, when he can return to England to get the climate out of him. We can go out again next year and so on, until the subject is threshed out. Cost will be very small as Jones[6] will take us all out. But I have asked the Committee for a fee for myself & Annett, and also for our life insurance *if funds permit*. I think it is only right that a poor man should receive something for risking his life! As, however, the merchants here have subscribed handsomely for the school, I believe the Committee will ask the Colonial & India Offices for assistance (in respect to the expedition) - also perhaps the Belgian Government.

I am sure you will approve of the step. It is only what I contemplated when I left India. Above all things we must be quick or we shall miss the malaria season at Sierra Leone, & the Italians will be before us. The practical result is now the great thing.

In view of the expedition we have not yet taken a house here; as my wife & children will go to see friends when I am away.

I was very disappointed at not finding a *certain name* in the honours' gazette this morning. We have all been expecting it here.[7] It will come at Christmas or new year.

Did Sir J. Fayrer pick his bone with you? If so, where?[8]

Please give my kind regards to Mrs Manson & the young ladies. If you have no time to write, will you kindly order your *secretary* to tell me whether you can send your £300 scholar with me in August.

By the way, this billet can scarcely be said as yet to be permanent because they have not yet got enough funds to endow the chair. Boyce is Irish. It seems to me quite possible that the whole thing may collapse. Jones has given £350 only so long as he can afford it, he says.[9] However I shall never go back to India. I can always fall back on novel writing! Have seen no sign of private practice here, either.

I suppose the expedition should go out from the two schools conjointly - don't you think so.

I have made arrangements about getting mosquitoes but they won't turn up for some time.

Hope you are better than you were, and are not overworking yourself.

With kind regards

Yours sincerely

Ronald Ross.

We can put you up here if you care to run up for a change at all, remember.

1 G Bastianelli and A. Bignami, 'Sullo sviluppo dei parassiti della terzana nell' anopheles claviger', *Bollettino della reale Accademis Medica di Roma*, 25 (1899). A translation was carried out by the Liverpool School, *On the development of tertian parasites in the "Anopheles claviger"*, **RA** 09/005.

2 **RA** 02/286. Ross's Inaugural Lecture was published as 'The possibility of extirpating malaria from certain localities by a new method', *BMJ* (1 July 1899), 1-4. Dawson Williams became the journal's editor in 1898, on the death of Ernest Hart.

3 See Letters 185-187.

4 Dr H. E. Annett, (1871-1945), Demonstrator of Practical Pathology, Liverpool School of Tropical Medicine. See **Biographical Appendix.**

5 In fact, Ross and Annett were accompanied by E. E. Austen, (1867-1938), a Dipterologist at the British Museum. See **Biographical Appendix**.

6 Alfred Lewis Jones, head of the West African shipping firm, Elder Dempster & Co and principal benefactor of the Liverpool School in its early days. See **Biographical Appendix.**

7 Manson was created C.M.G. in 1900 and KCMG in 1903.

8 Reference untraced, but see Letter 173, note 1.

9 For details of the finances of the School, see Power (1998).

Letter 175
49/042

21, Queen Anne Street,
Cavendish Square. W.
10th June, 1899.

My dear Ross,

I ought to have answered your letter before but I have been run off my legs all this and last week - six lectures a week, three country journeys and the usual consultation office work besides the importunities of two persistent editors. I am a kind of tired of it just at present.

I think your proposal about our scholarship man a good one. On Monday we have our first school meeting and I shall bring the matter up. I thought he might be utilised to collect material for the schools and had some notion that by sending him to the West Indies he might be able to get stuff there whilst your expedition might collect West African stuff and that afterwards we might make a pool and divide the scientific swag between Liverpool and London. I cannot move however without my colleagues now and for everything of that description will have to consult the Seamen's Hospital Society.[1] A dictatorship certainly conduces to rapidity of action.

Dont be afraid about your future. Liverpool is on her honour and wont for shame, not to mention higher motives, draw back. You are right however to do all you can to strengthen your position and secure a proper endowment. Dont be afraid of private practice. It will come. But you must be prepared to wait a bit and you must be always on the spot - a definite spot and at a definite hour of each day. The medical fraternity must know where to find you and when. At first in London I had a very uphill task. I made only some [£]250 my first year or so. It came slowly at first but by degrees the stream broadens, deepens and increases in rapidity. You will advance in exactly the same way.

I was asked by Mr Hensman of the Pioneer to send you the enclosed.[2] It must be gratifying to you to find that you have sown the seed and that you are appreciated, even though it be after you have gone.

Yours sincerely

Patrick Manson

1 For the early history of the London School of Tropical Medicine, see Philip Manson-Bahr, *History of the School of Tropical Medicine in London, 1899-1949* (London: H. K. Lewis, 1956), and Wilkinson and Hardy (1998), ch. 1.

2 Missing.

Letter 176
02/287

44 Prince's Road
Liverpool
14th June 1899

Dear Dr Manson,

Many thanks for yours of the 10th. I am afraid of writing to you because you persist in answering me! You have already so much to do that you must really not answer my scribbles. Thanks for reassuring me about Liverpool - but I have no desire to leave the second city of the empire. We are very comfortable indeed here & the people are exceedingly nice and pleasant. We like everybody we have met here. Work also is flourishing. Hence I don't seriously trouble about the future. I think we have £5000 about, so that the *chair* is almost founded. Patients will come as you say.

I delivered my inaugural lecture on Monday. Lantern slides of malaria in mosquito, & microscope specimens of mosquitoes & tsetse trypanosomes, *living*, thrown on screen. People seemed to like it. We sent the lecture to Dr Dawson Williams this morning.[1]

The great thing is the expedition to Sierra Leone. It *must* start just after the B. M. A. meeting. Jones takes us free. Our objects:-

1. To find mosquitoes which carry malaria in Sierra Leone town.

2. To find if their breeding pools are so small and isolated that there is any chance of our being able to exterminate them.

This is a simple programme & we ought to do something; but we must be back in October & ought to leave a man behind until the cold weather sets in. This we can't do unless you can give us the man or unless we can get some funds from government for the expedition. Of course Liverpool has already given so much for the Tropical School that it is scarcely fair to bully her for more funds for the expedition straight off.

We *must* be in first with the practical side of the mosquito theory or else Grassi will develop it.[2] For the same reason I hope the B. M. J. can publish my lecture (if they can find space) *pretty sharp*. I think Grassi is on the practical tack now - will *bet* he is.

There were *five* cases with malaria parasites in the Tropical Ward here yesterday. The Ward has overflowed into the rest of the hospital. We have one student (caught) & several others *nibbling*.

Did I tell you that Ray Lankester is finally converted?[3] He has promised to stand sponsor for us with Govt. We want you and Lord Lister, with him, as referees as to the truth of the mosquito theory.

Have you had a card for the Royal Society for the 21st?[4] I hope so, because I have, and I want to go to it with a view to helping on the expedition.

Yours very sincerely
R. Ross.

1 Ross (1899c).

2 Grassi's work was summarised in his *Studi di Uno Zoologo sulla Malaria* (Roma: Tipografia della R. Accademia dei Lincei, 1900). See **Biographical Appendix**.

3 The Ross Archives contains no correspondence between Lankester and Ross around this date although Lankester did invite Ross to call on him in a letter of 10 April 1899, **RA** 50/006. See, also, **Biographical Appendix**.

4 The annual *conversazione* (ladies evening) reported in *BMJ* (24 June 1899), 1547. See, also, Letter 177, note 1.

Letter 177
02/288

44 Prince's Road
Liverpool
25th June 1899

Dear Dr Manson,

I was awfully sorry to leave on Thursday without saying goodbye to you. Many thanks for your kind hospitality.

I forgot to take away the specimens you said you would lend me for photography. Also the lantern slides you said you would give me. Also my razor strop! This comes of departing in a hurry.

I saw Prof. Ray Lankester. He said he would lend us Austen[1] for the expedition.

I also saw Dr Thin about my opening the discussion at the B. M. A. meeting.[2] He said that he must refer to the mosquito-malaria theory in his address, and that what he thought was my most important work in regard to it was that I had proved that not all mosquitoes can carry malaria. The rest he thought had been done by the Italians! I replied that he would have a difficulty in proving this & lent him Nuttall's paper.[3] As he asked me previously to do so, I shall give a full account of the whole business at the meeting. I daresay attempts will be made to work up the Italian claim there; in which case there will be a fight! I have got all the literature at my fingers ends - so there ought to be fun.

Lankester says that Nuttall is coming to London on the way to Cambridge on the 29th. If you see him & learn his address in town *please* let me know, as I want badly a translation of his paper.

I don't know yet whether I am coming to town on the 28th or not; but I shall certainly try to see you if I do. I believe I shall have to live with Jones & Boyce in some hotel.

Do you think you can trust your specimens, etc, to the post? If so, will Miss Manson send them to me with my strop, as I *may* not go to town yet, and don't want to waste time.

Yours sincerely
R. Ross.

1 E. E. Austen and Ray Lankester had demonstrated malaria-related mosquitoes at the Royal Society *Conversazione.*

2 Sixty-seventh Annual Meeting of the British Medical Association, Portsmouth, 1899. Ross did not attend the BMA meeting as he had set off for Sierra Leone. For Thin's address, see Letter 185, note 2.

3 Probably George H. F. Nuttall, 'Die Mosquito-Malaria Theorie', *Centralblatt für Bakteriologie, Parasitenkunde und Infektionskrankheiten*, 25 (1899), 161-170; 209-217; 245-247; 285-296; 337-346. See **Biographical Appendix**.

Letter 178
49/043

21, Queen Anne Street,
Cavendish Square. W.
27th June, 1899

My dear Ross,
I have just sent off strop, two mosquito slides and three lantern slides. The latter we may supplement by and by. When I get a little time I will select some filariated mosquito sections and send them on.

I was very much amused with your account of the interview with Thin. He will not allow that any good can come out of Nazareth. He believes any one with a long foreign name in preference to Jones of London. He is most unpatriotic and is always trying to pull us down. If he tries any game of this sort at the B. M. A. meeting I have only one question to ask him and that is Did not I show him one of your slides early last year long before any Italian or German thought of the subject and did not this slide contain the pigmented body of crescent malaria. He can only answer, yes. All the Italians have done so far as I can see is to confirm your work and to repeat in a very imperfect manner your bird malaria infection experiments, in man - experiments which were clearly indicated by yours. It is all nonsense but by keeping on writing themselves up they are hoping to get the credit of the whole business. Ask Thin if he ever read my Goulstonian lectures.[1] I dont believe he has; he thinks we know nothing about malaria in this country. We must put Nuttall on him.

I am very glad to hear that you are to have Austen with you. He will give precision to your mosquito classifications and descriptions and help you in many ways.

I dont know Nuttall's address. He said he was coming to see me and get some slides from me.

I fear you will think me slow in answering your letter and sending the stuff but I was overpowered with work yesterday and dead with fatigue at night.

Yours sincerely
Patrick Manson

1 See Letter 185, note 2, and Manson (1896a).

Letter 179
02/289

44 Prince's Road,
Liverpool
1st July 1899

Dear Dr Manson,
Many thanks for the specimens & slides. I hope to have the slides for you ready next week. We have had to put off our journey to Brussels for obvious reasons.[1]

Hope you like my lecture in the current number of the B. M. J.[2]

Yes, I am glad Austen will come with us - or rather is willing to do so. But I fear it depends on the Indian & Colonial Offices. I have proposed the matter to our committee; but it is obvious that they must keep all our funds together in order to consolidate the school. At present they guarantee my appointment only for three years, and they must put all the funds together for an endowment - so that they hesitate in giving us the luxury of a dipterist. Of course under these circumstances I must abandon my hope of getting a *fee* - & so must Annett.

I think Jones will give Austen a passage out but will kick against maintenance. Now Austen stipulated that he should be put to no expense at all, and the British Museum won't give anything. Hence if we are to take Austen we must fall back on the Indian, Colonial & Foreign Offices. About £20 from each of these will enable us to take Austen & £50 from each would make us rich! However I don't care a cent - I am going anyhow. Harvey is coming here on the 10th on Boyce's invitation.[3] Perhaps he can be roused into working India Office.

We have arranged to go out on the 5th August & return about 15th October.

Did you see the syllabus which Rees took with him?[4] I think your Committee ought to arrange with ours about the *fees* at once, or there will be a muddle.

Yes, Thin is a rare old Britisher of the usual sort. However I hinted that he better not carry his patriotism for the Italians too far. We shall be enough for him at the B. M. A. meeting.

I am busy writing out a complete account of the whole mosquito theory.[5] I have already worked up to Bignami's criticism of the

Gulstonian lectures. The thing is in full detail. I discuss every point. This shows clearly that it was your explanation of the flagellate bodies which was the *sound* & *leading* point of the theories. I then make a hash of Bignami. I am consulting original papers wherever necessary, as we have most of them.

The thing will be much too long for the B. M. A. Annett suggests publishing simultaneously in English, French & German. It requires a full paper to put everything at rest. I don't think I shall publish it however until we come back from Africa, as I then hope to add human malaria to previous work.

We shall have six weeks at Sierra Leone. I did all the latter part of the Proteosoma work including infection of birds in six weeks. Of course we shall bring back mosquitoes to England.

Yours sincerely

R. Ross.

Don't reply.

1 Presumably Ross had heard that no support for the Sierra Leone expedition would be forthcoming from the Belgium Government. See Letter 174.

2 Ross (1899c).

3 Surgeon-General Robert Harvey visited the School in Liverpool (in *Memoirs*, Ross stated that it was after his return from Sierra Leone) and suggested to Ross that he return to India to a permanent post and salary, *Memoirs*, 390.

4 D. C. Rees, Medical Tutor to the London School of Tropical Medicine.

5 Many of Ross's subsequent publications on malaria included a historical account, most fully in Ross (1910) and *Memoirs*. For his earliest one, see Letter 193, note 1.

Letter 180
49/219

21, Queen Anne Street,
Cavendish Square. W.
3rd July, 1899.

My dear Ross,

I fear you wont get much from the Foreign or Colonial Office. I dont know about the India Office although I should think they would be inclined in this way to recognise what you have done for them and to make up as it were for their scurvy acknowledgement of your work. It would be a pity if Austen cant accompany you. Stir them up through the press.

Nuttall lunched with us on Friday. He half expected to meet you in London. He told me all about Koch and his nasty ways. Nuttall's address would be care of Sims Woodhead, Cambridge.[1]

Many thanks for the very generous way you have recognised my small part in the malaria business. It is much more than I deserved. My only claim is that, in a measure, I discovered you.

Another letter from Daniels. He is doing something and I have no doubt will do more. The other commissioners dont seem to think their opportunities sufficient.[2] I wonder if they expect to find men dying of blackwater all round them.

Daniels thinks the place an excellent one for work as beyond malaria the diseases are few and therefore the problem is less complicated.

Yours sincerely
Patrick Manson

1 (Sir) German Sims Woodhead, (1855-1921), Professor of Pathology, Cambridge.

2 Christophers and Stephens wrote to the RSMC from Blantyre Hospital, pointing out that the hospital did not possess adequate facilities for their 'clinical observations.' Daniels' letter of the same date was much more positive. Their letters were considered at the RSMC meeting of 3 July, which Manson attended as a representative of the Colonial Office, (RSMC Minutes, vol 1 (meeting of 3 July 1899)). See also Bynum (1994).

Letter 181
49/044

21, Queen Anne Street,
Cavendish Square. W.
15th July, 1899.

My dear Ross,

I am sorry you are not to put in an appearance at the B. M. A. Meeting. However you have a good reason for absenting yourself. And you have a good champion in Nuttall. He is just the man and in addition to his personal weight will carry with him all the authority that attaches to the foreigner in England.[1] I hope Rho[2] will come. He has been invited. He too knows the exact history of the malaria business and, I believe, will see justice done.

Daniels sent in an excellent report to the R. S. some ten days ago. There is nothing fresh but it was evidence of much enthusiastic activity. He appears to be gradually converting his colleagues and weaning them from bacteriological methods. I suppose he has written you at length as to how things are going out there.[3]

By the way, if you have not tried the Louis Jenner stain (in Lancet of this year I think),[4] for malarial films do so. It is excellent and is the least troublesome of all the methods so far as I know. It dispenses with a separate fixing process; the stain being in alcoholic solution fixes for itself and the result is first class - a double stain - and apparently thoroughly reliable. I would advise you to use it.

One of our pigeons has plenty of halteridia, the other has none. This is just at present. A month ago it was the other way. Manifestly there is a faculty of latency about this parasite.

We too have lately had a flux of malaria cases but they have been detained at the Greenwich side[5] as we want to use them for the special education of some colonial nurses who are there at present.

Did I tell you that I had some lovely sections of mosquitos - filariated - of the same batch Annett tried. It is all in technique.

Give me the latest news before you leave. A line from Sierra Leone would be most welcome. If you strike anything good let me know at once and I will see to immediate publication. Timeo Romani, Koch. etc.[6]

Yours sincerely
Patrick Manson

1 Nuttall was an American, although from 1899 his career was based at Cambridge University.

2 Filippo Rho, from Rome, was present at the BMA Annual Meeting. Among his publications was *La malaria secondo i più recenti studi* (Torino: Rosenberg & Sellier, 1896).

3 Letter 180, note 2. Daniels had written to Ross from Blantyre on 24 April 1899 (**RA** 50/015) saying that he had found 2 species of anopheles different from those in India but complained that no mosquitoes had been prepared for him prior to his arrival and now it was the cold season. He wrote again from Fort Johnston on 5 June 1899 (**RA** 50/027) saying that it was too cold in Blantyre for mosquitoes to bite but now he had no suitable cases of malaria. (Gibson, 1983).

4 Louis Jenner, 'A new stain for rapidly fixing and staining blood', *Lancet* (11 Feb. 1899), 370.
5 The main *Dreadnought* Hospital at Greenwich as opposed to the Branch Hospital at the Albert Dock.
6 I fear the Italians, Koch, etc.

Letter 182
02/290

44 Prince's Road
Liverpool
23rd July 1899

Dear Dr Manson,
Thanks for yours of the 15th. Delighted to hear of Daniels' report.[1] Wish he had not written that letter to me, or that I had not shown it to Sherrington.[2] He evidently did not like the place on arrival. I am afraid some confusion has been caused in your counsels. Sherrington says that Michael Foster[3] speaks about Christophers' fever[4] being a great confirmation of the mosquito-theory - how? Did you read my "outbreak of fever" in the current B. M. J.?[5] What do you think of it? I wrote to the "captain" of the boys' brigade, but have had no reply. Mr & Mrs Parker were most reliable people who knew almost everyone concerned.[6]

We have long been trying Jenner's stain. It is very good. I stained flagella with it - faintly blue. But we must have Romanowsky[7] for the nuclei of the zygotes.

Our pigeon never lost the halteridium quite. The parasites only decrease & increase in numbers - chiefly according to external temperature, I think. I noticed exactly the same thing when I took my birds to the hills last year (forgot to mention it in my report on kala-azar) - though not so marked.

We start on 29th Saturday - am afraid I can't come & see you before going. The B.M.A. has given us £100 which will do us nicely.[8] Expect to get weekly letters from a pupil again. We ought to spot the mosquito in a week - if we don't I shall be in a rage. Jones wanted to give us a big dinner for farewell - I wouldn't have it - "Let him not that on his harness boast himself *girdeth on his armour*, etc".[9]

Your man Bennett[10] comes here tomorrow - Plenty of crescents for him. You must not be hard on Annett about your filaria sections. Can't expect him to do it on first trial.

Hope you got your lantern slides - also your two specimens (returned) - all right. The slides show what is required. I have sent a set to Laveran, Nuttall, Thin, & Crombie. To you they are a present from the *School.*

I have been very busy with Professors Herdman F.R.S. (zoology)[11] & Harvey Gibson (botany)[12] getting out the absolutely correct nomenclature for the malaria parasites. Have sent a brief paper to Nature - but don't know whether they will take it.[13]

The life history is as follows:-

1. *Amoebulae* or *myxopods* in corpuscles become (a) *sporocytes,* (b) *gametocytes*
2. Sporocytes produce asexual *spores*
3. Gametocytes, male & female. Male produces several *microgametes*; female consists of one *macrogamete.* One microgamete fertilises the macrogamete in stomach of mosquito. Result a *zygote*

3.[sic] Zygote pierces wall of stomach & grows attached to outer coat. Nucleus divides into several *zygotomeres* (compare figures in my report). Each zygotomere produces a *blastophore* covered with *zygotoblasts*.

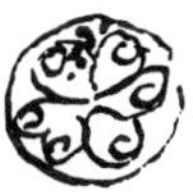

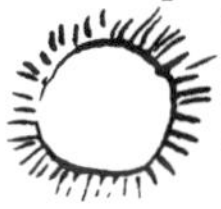

The blastophores disappear leaving the capsule of the mature zygote packed full of zygotoblasts.

4. The zygoblasts escape & are seen to be *flagellulae* or *mastigopods.*

5. They enter salivary gland & become amoebulae.

This terminology is sound and is partly used by Mesnil[14], & Grassi & Dionisi. I am not certain about the "black spores", consequently do not touch them. Herdman says that the word spore should apply only to asexual reproduction. I therefore invented zygotoblast (which he accepts) for the sexually produced offspring of the zygotes.

How do you like this?

The little buds one finds by the side of the crescent spheres are homologues of the *polar bodies.*

We have also tackled the classification of the parasites of men & birds. We *must* stick to Grassi's confounded specific names; but I suggest two genera as below.

Family: Haemamoebidae, Wasielewski.

Genus 1: *Haemamoeba*, Grassi & Feletti. The gametocytes are shaped like the sporocytes before the spores are produced.

Species 1: *Haemamoeba Danilewskii*, Ross. Syn. *Laverania Danilewskii*, Grassi, Feletti; Halteridium Danilewskii Labbé

Species 2: *H. relicta*, Grassi & Feletti - Syn. *Proteosoma Grassi*, Labbé.

Species 3: *H. malariae*, Grassi & Feletti. Quartan.

Species 4: *H. vivax*, Grassi & Feletti. Tertian

Genus II: *Haemomenas* (blood-moon), Ross, gen. nov.
The gametecytes have a special (crescentic) shape.
Species: *Haemomenas Praecox*, Ross. Syn. *Haemamoeba Praecox* Grassi & Feletti - etc. -The aestivo-autumnal parasites.

There is no reason why the birds' parasites should be put into separate genera, as Labbé does; and zoological rules demand that the *specific* names *first* given should be adhered to. Labbé's terms must therefore be abandoned. So must Grassi's genus Laverania which is wrongly conceived - applied only to H. Danilewskii & to crescents. Haemomenas is a good descriptive term. (μενας - moon)

It would be very useful for educational purposes to have uniform nomenclature. I think we can venture now to adopt one. Tell me if you will adopt the above. It has been carefully prepared and is zoologically correct.

Grassi calls the gametocytes, gametogenes - which is bad. Sporocytes & gametocytes go so well together. He employs zygote, which is correct. The term "sporozoites" & "sporoblasts" (Grassi) are not correct as they contain the word *spore*. Zygotoblasts is best.

Now for the question of *priority*. The rule is that the man who discovers the life-history of a single member of a group claims priority for that of all the members of the group, unless these other members have a markedly different life-history - in which case they won't continue to belong to the group. The malaria problem was a purely zoological problem & is amenable to zoological laws of priority. In finding the development of the zygotes of H. relicta (Proteosoma) we claim priority in finding the history of the zygotes of the *whole group* - unless the other members of the group differ. But they do not differ. Hence Grassi & Co can make no claim whatever to priority in this respect. All they can claim is to have extended our results partially to *Haemomenas praecox* (of which I found the first stages in 1897), & wholly to *Haemamoeba vivax*. This is an altogether secondary achievement - being merely confirmative. Medical men who are not zoologists don't understand this, unless it be crammed into them. If there is any nonsense talked at the Association meeting, I think this statement will put it right. I have just written to Dr Thin & put it to him in the same words.

Unless this rule be adhered to it is evident that all priority in discovery would go to the winds. For instance quartan has not yet been traced in the mosquito. Unless this rule holds, the man who will discover it, will have an equal priority with ourselves, Grassi, Bignami & Bastianelli, & Koch - a *reductio ad absurdam*! The whole difficulty lay in *first* finding the development of *any one* of the parasites. From the zoological point of view it does not matter a cent whether this parasite is one of birds or men. And the problem was a zoological problem.

Dr Thin tells me that Nuttall will open the discussion immediately after the Presidential address. I don't think there will be much discussion about priority. But there may be. Anyway it does not matter much. Nuttall will fix the main facts.

We have the most beautiful case of aestivo-autumnal tertian (?) here. Swarms of parasites - Am staining them with Romanowsky.

Must leave off. Will send you material from Africa, of course.

Yours sincerely

Ronald Ross.

None of the slides has been "retouched" *at all*.

1 See Letter 181, note 3.

2 C. S. Sherrington, (1857-1952), then Professor of Physiology at Liverpool and President of the Biological Society of Liverpool. See Letter 181, note 3.

3 (Sir) Michael Foster (1836-1907), Professor of Physiology at Cambridge and a member of the Royal Society Malaria Committee.

4 Although this presumably refers to correspondence from Christophers to the RSMC, there is no reference to it in the Minutes. The first report which the Committee received from Christophers and Stephens was received in December, and was published as J. W. W. Stephens and S. R. Christophers. 'The malarial and blackwater fevers of British Central Africa,' *Reports to the Malaria Committee of the Royal Society*, Report No 2, (London: Harrison and Sons, 1900) 12-42.

5 R. Ross, 'An outbreak of fever attributed to mosquitos', *BMJ* (22 July, 1899), 208.

6 In his letter to *BMJ*, (above, note 5), Ross had recounted a story told him by Mr and Mrs Parker on his voyage home from Calcutta. It concerned a Boys' Brigade which went to camp in October 1898, in Barrackpore Park, near Calcutta. The boys declined to use mosquito nets whereas the officers employed them. All of the boys came down with malaria, but the officers, who were sleeping in the same bungalow, remained free of the disease. The 'captain' was not named in Ross's letter.

7 Dimitri Romanowsky, (1861-1921), the Russian parasitologist, published the account of his stain in 1891. It is translated from the original German, as 'On the question of parasitology and therapy of malaria', in B. H. Kean, Kenneth E. Mott and Adair J. Russell, eds., *Tropical Medicine and Parasitology: Classic Investigations* (Ithaca, Cornell University Press, 1978), 2 vols., I: 35-44.

8 The Council of the of the British Medical Association voted the sum of £100 towards the expenses of the expedition, at its meeting on 12 July 1899; reported in *BMJ* (15 July 1899), 167.

9 Misquoted from 1 Kings, 20:11.

10 Unidentified.

11 (Sir) William Abbott Herdman, (1858-1924), Professor of Natural History at Liverpool.

12 Robert John Harvey-Gibson, (1860-1929), Professor of Botany at Liverpool.

13 R. Ross, 'Life-history of the parasites of malaria', *Nature* (3 Aug. 1899), 322-4.

14 Félix Mesnil, (1868-1938), a French parasitologist who worked with Laveran on trypanosomiasis. A Laveran and F. Mesnil, *Trypanosomes et Trypanosomiases* (Paris: Masson, 1904).

Letter 183
49/045

21, Queen Anne Street,
Cavendish Street. W.
25th July, 1899.

My dear Ross,

I had deceived myself into the idea that I wrote thanking you for the lantern slides which you so kindly sent me last week. I evidently had mixed up my last letter with my intended letter. Senile decay coming on apace. The lantern slides are excellent and will be of great use to me in teaching. My Daniels' slides came all right. The germinal rods on the lantern slides show up very distinctly. There must be a method for fixing and staining these with certainty and precision.

I dont think you are altogether right about the influence of temperature in determining the amount of halteridium in peripheral pigeon's blood, for one of our pigeons, which formerly showed great profusion of parasites, is useless now; whereas the other, which when you were here had very few, has at present an abundant infection. Both live in the same cage. There must be another factor.

I did not mean to be hard on Annett about the mosquito sections. I only wanted to pull the pathological leg. The cause of Annett's failure was principally in using paraffin and not celloidin.1 The heat in the paraffin process seems to spoil the filariae in the tissues.

I like your terminology and classification and will adopt it I think. The only objection that occurs to me is that it is perhaps a little premature for there are several gaps in our knowledge still that have to be filled in before we can be quite sure as to where we are and what is what. For example:- Your gametocyte may be the result of conjugation of two sporocytes or of bodies indistinguishable from sporocytes; in which case they are not sporocytes as they do not culminate in the formation of spores but of gametocytes. Then when the amoebulae enter the human body is there no stage passed through before they enter the corpuscle? Then what about the life of the parasite - the reproductive life which facts imply - outside the human body and probably in successive generations of mosquitos? I do not despise your black spores. Nature does not labour systematically for that which is nought. In framing your nomenclature provide for future expansion in the directions I indicate. Meanwhile I shall adopt it provisionally as I consider it the best. These big words are fearfully confusing. I think I will have a diagram made with schematic representation of life history of the parasite and names attached to each stage, and have it hung up in permanence on the wall of the laboratory so that it may sink into the mind of the student.

I suppose zoological laws make it necessary to stick to Grassi's names though I consider them ugly and ill chosen. The beast is no amoeba any more than it is a plasmodium. Then to apply the name H. malariae to quartan is utterly wrong and misleading. Why not call it H. quartana. I like your name for genus 2 "Haemomenas", but Grassi's praecox is weak. Dont you think you should include the pyrosoma bigeminum? It is evidently of the same order of beasts.

By the time you return I will have elaborated probably a diagram planned to teach your names and the order of events in the life history of the parasite.

Our building is getting along fairly well as far as the school is concerned, but the hospital is not likely to be ready for occupation until the spring of 1900. A pity this but it cant be got ready sooner.

Take care of yourself in that God forsaken country to which you go. Be specially careful on your way home. I am gradually learning that one of the most dangerous times is when the ship on the way home passes the Canaries and begins to enter cool weather. Then blackwater is apt to develop. Remember this and have your warm clothes ready in anticipation of sudden change of climate. Lots of men die at that time. Only last night I had official intimation of such an occurrence. So take care and dont waken up in the next world complaining that you had no warning. The plasmodium has a special grudge against you and doubtless is looking out for a chance to wreak its revenge..

Wishing you all good fortune and hoping to hear of fresh triumphs I remain,

Yours sincerely

Patrick Manson

Pray remember our pathological requirements in the shape of any morbid material, blood films, etc. etc.

1 A preparation of pure pyroxylin used to imbed material before cutting and staining.

Letter 184
02/291

44 Prince's Road
Liverpool
28th July [1899]

Dear Dr Manson,

Just a farewell line to you. My kind regards to Mrs Manson & the young ladies. I enclose you a rough copy of my paper in Nature, which will appear on August 3rd - *private* until then.[1] Dr Charles writes to tell me that the Italians have incriminated all the Italian Anopheles but have absolved the Culex.[2] This ought to make our task easier in Freetown. Austen has arrived & is very keen. We have got one Romanowski to work at last & so ought to have good cytological results as soon as we get on the zygotes again. Sorry I could not run up to town to say good bye. Expect to hear from us in three weeks.

Yours very sincerely

Ronald Ross.

Off early tomorrow.

1 Ross (1899e).

2 Letter from T. E. Charles dated 22 July 1899, **RA** 08/044.

Letter 185
02/292

Sierra Leone
20th August [1899]

Dear Dr Manson,
Just a line to tell you that we have struck oil nicely, and have cultivated the quartan bug in a small black Anopheles. You will see details in an account in the B. M. J.[1] The quartan zygote is just like the others. We have not yet found a single crescent, doubtless owing to quinine & partial immunity. Nor have we found a single Anopheles larva except what we have hatched ourselves. I have urged Jones to try and get a man sent out to continue our work. But he must arrive before the 20th. Sept. to learn our tricks etc, if he is to do any good.

I read Thin's opening speech.[2] It was all right about the mosquito theory, but dreadful stuff about the Tropical Schools. His attempt was too obvious.

I hope to bring a lot of Anopheles home & will give you some. I think the betting is that these Anopheles carry all kinds of fever.

I have not a moment to write more - so please excuse me. We are all quite fit. Hope you are the same.

Yours sincerely
R. Ross.

Just found mature zygotes in 2 more large Anopheles from Wilberforce hospital.[3] Makes 4 infected insects out of 13. Hence the large Anopheles must also be malaria bearing.

1 A Correspondent [i.e. Ross], 'The malaria expedition to Sierra Leone' *BMJ* (9 Sept. 1899), 675-676.

2 G. Thin, 'The etiology of malarial fever', *BMJ* (5 Aug. 1899), 349-354. Although Thin devoted more space in his Presidential Address to the BMA Section of Tropical Diseases to the Italian contributions to malaria than to those of Ross and Manson, he stated that Ross's own work 'at once and forever removed' doubt about the role of mosquitoes in transmitting malaria. He also argued that the Army Medical School at Netley should have been converted to a civilian school of tropical medicine, and that this would have rendered redundant the two new ones at London and Liverpool. For other opposition to the Tropical Schools, see Cook (1995 and 1992, ch 6).

3 Wilberforce was a suburb of Freetown.

Letter 186
02/293

Sierra Leone
8th Sept. 1899

Dear Dr Manson,
The steamer has come in unexpectedly and I have time to scribble only a short note. We have practically done our work now, having discovered the haunts of Anopheles. It is just as I said in my lecture.[1] They are puddle-breeding mosquitoes & require permanent, stagnant puddles containing algae - that is, as a rule. Such puddles are comparatively rare, because most puddles either dry up quickly or are scoured out by rain. As a matter of fact Anopheles breed here mostly in two small flat places which can be easily drained. I won't bother you with details as yet (though I don't know what I won't do when I see you!) because we are sending full information to the B. M. J. & Lancet.[2] Next mail I hope to send photos of puddles.

In one respect our work has been poor - in express feeding experiments with Anopheles. At first the R. A. M. C. men refused to let us feed any but mosquitoes hatched from Larvae on their cases; and now we can't get a good case for love or money. The reason is that all the soldiers (& we can't get civilians to work with) are filled up with quinine as soon as they are taken sick. We have found crescents in only two cases! & then too scanty to give results with mosquitoes. I can detect the tertian & quartan zygotes in the Wilberforce mosquitoes to a certainty but am not sure about the aestivo-autumnal. Rather annoying, isn't it. But it is morally certain that this Anopheles carried aest. aut. as well.

Jones wired me that Ould is coming out & will be here on about the 15th.[3] He can try to work these details if we haven't time.

Major Nathan,[4] the Governor, is keen about it all. I have advised him to keep a native on purpose to hunt up Anopheles pools & kill mosquitoes. I hope the ch. med. officer here, Prout, will follow up.[5] He seems inclined to do so. The R. A. M. C. men won't do a thing to help us & take no interest. Ignorance & conceit! We have just killed a puddle full of Anopheles larvae with *3i* of oil. Of course drainage would be better. I hope you are quite well & not doing too much work. All of us have escaped fever - nets.

Yours sincerely
R. Ross.

1 Ross's Inaugural lecture: see Letter 176, note 1.
2 Ross wrote anonymously as 'A Correspondent' to *BMJ* (9 Sept. 1899) 675-676; (16 Sept. 1899) 746; (30 Sept. 1899) 869-871; (14 Oct. 1899) 1033-1035. Similar reports were also published anonymously in *Lancet*: (Sept. 9. 1899) 743; (16 Sept. 1899) 806; (30 Sept. 1899) 912; (14 Oct. 1899) 1041-2, though Ross wrote that these were written by Annett in consultation with him, *Memoirs*, 378.
3 Dr Robert Fielding-Ould, (1872-1951), see **Biographical Appendix**.
4 Matthew Nathan, acting Governor of Freetown.
5 William Thomas Prout. For details of Prout's subsequent career at Liverpool, see Nye and Gibson (1997), ch. 8.

Letter 187
02/294

Sierra Leone
15th Sept. [1899]

Dear Dr Manson,
We have now nearly completed a map of the Anopheles puddles in & round the town. They are comparatively very few - just as I said would be the case. One man could oil them all twice a week without difficulty. We all think that if such oiling were to be continued steadily for a month or so, a blow would be dealt to the whole genus Anopheles here from which they could not easily or quickly recover. They evidently have many enemies, & with man against them won't do well.

The great difficulty is the apathy & inertia of the medical profession. None of the R.A.M.C. men here, for instance, have taken any interest in our work, while, on the contrary, the Senior medical officer nearly wrecked us from the first. Prout & Berkeley[1] *say* they will help, but what will they do when we have gone? I fear I cannot answer for them. It was our hope, do you remember, to make Sierra Leone a test place by killing the Anopheles and watching results. I fear however I cannot answer for the faculty here.

Strachan[2] at Lagos is much more keen. He has found Anopheles there at once & sent us some. They are *just like those* here - probably the same species causes the fever all down the coast. He has also found the larvae - in the roadside puddles.

Ould has arrived here full of ardour. As soon as he picks up the work, he will go on down the coast, to Accra and Lagos. I think Strachan will undertake the practical work, with his assistance.

We start back by next mail, and I shall run down to town to tell you all about things. I think we now know exactly how to spot malarious foci & to prevent malaria - thanks to the original grand induction.

Rains are breaking & Anopheles may shortly disappear. We have just had certain proof that the larvae perish on the drying up of a puddle, but when the next shower comes a fresh crop appears.

With kind regards

Yours sincerely

Ronald Ross.

Ould may not be able to do any work of importance if the Anopheles vanish at the end of the rains.

1 Dr Berkeley, one of the two medical officers in Freetown.

2 Henry W. W. Strachan, Principal Medical Officer of Lagos.

Letter 188
49/046

21 Queen Anne Street,
Cavendish Square. W.
12th October, 1899

My dear Ross,

Are you back?[1] If so I hope you are all right and not yourself the victim of the merry mosquito. You have held up the torch once more and I heartily congratulate you. You have once more gone one better than the Italians who together with Koch are busy apparently snarling over your work each claiming it as his own. It is a ludicrous spectacle.

When are you coming up to town? Your bed is waiting for you here.

Our school is fairly on its legs with some ten or twelve students. The residential system is much appreciated all the rooms being occupied. I only wish we had built more of them when we were at it. I think the school is to be a great success.

I suppose you have brought back tons of material. Any scraps you can spare throw at us.

I would have written you several times in acknowledgement of your letters but did not know my replies would catch you. Two men are coming back from British Central Africa.[2] Daniels like the good man he is means to stick to his guns finding plenty of material where the others say they were starved. The other two will be sent out to the West Coast so soon as they get back.[3] I don't think they have accomplished much. I hope I am wrong but accounts have not been encouraging.

Come up to town or let me hear from you soon.

Yours sincerely

Patrick Manson

1 *Memoirs*, 382, says that Ross arrived back in Liverpool 'about 3 October'.

2 S. R. Christophers and J. W. W. Stephens.

3 In fact, they next went to India.

Letter 189
02/295

42 Prince's Road
Liverpool
13th October [1899]

Dear Dr Manson,

I was delighted to get yours of yesterday, and purpose to run up to town as soon as possible & occupy "my bed" for a night or two. Since returning I have been seized by the inevitable cold in the head & throat - a cold of the worst virulence - and am nearly dead. Should prefer malaria!

I have much more to tell you about than I can communicate by letter under two hours writing - so wont attempt the latter feat. Not much material. A few live Anopheles which however probably won't live.

Have had a charming letter from Thayer. He says he has found Anopheles in the most malarious part of Baltimore, & some of these from the room of a malaria case contained *zygotes*. This is great, isn't it? His letter is dated August 24th, so I suppose they have done more by this time. He adds, "It has seemed to me that the Italians have not emphasized sufficiently the fact that their work has been nothing but an adaptation & repetition of your experiments."[1] I shall show his letter to Thin! Sorry to hear about the malaria commission. They had bad luck, poor men. Fortune favoured us - that is all. Very glad about the London School. We have three pupils up to date, I believe. Your opening lecture was grand.[2] More when we meet.

Yours very sincerely
R. Ross.

1 William Sydney Thayer, (1864-1932), physician at Johns Hopkins Hospital, Baltimore. See **Biographical Appendix**. Letter to Ross, 24 Aug. 1899, **RA** 49/224.

2 P. Manson. 'The need for special training in tropical disease', *BMJ* (7 Oct. 1899), 922-926.

Letter 190
49/048

21, Queen Anne Street,
Cavendish Square. W.
16th Dec. 1899.

My dear Ross,

The enclosed from the Colonial Office will interest you.[1] It came last night.

I am going to Palermo on the 27th & will visit Rome en route and try to stay there for a few days to find out the position. Is there anything you wd like me to attend to in particular. Let me know in time.[2]

Have Elliott & Fry sent you proofs of photos?[3] They sent 3 to me on approval. I don't know if you have seen these yet. Say.

Nice mess in S. Africa!!![4] Are we rotten?

Yours sincerely
Patrick Manson

1 **RA** 49/049, notice of a telegram from Daniels to the Colonial Office which read "Crescents develop in anopheles described".

2 Manson's visit to Italy proved to be the initial source of the breakdown of his relationship with Ross. Manson was one of a party of doctors, and reports of the visit in *The Times* called Ross an engineer and minimised his role in the malaria story, in favour of the Italian contribution. After Manson failed to protest to the newspaper, Ross did himself. (*Memoirs*, 392-3).

3 Untraced.

4 The Boer War broke out in October.

Letter 191
49/050

21, Queen Anne Street,
Cavendish Square. W.
14th February, 1900.

My dear Ross,
All right about the microscope. I dont fancy the name Plantation Parasitoscope; why not "Planter's microscope"? He can use it for any purpose. If you give it too special a name wags will make fun of it - call it shitoscope and the like - as is the way with the facetious griffin.

I have been over your "Instruction etc" very carefully again.[1] They are admirable but I think you should revise them. Evidently they were written currente calamo, and as things so written often are, are very graphic and to the point. They are so good that I would like you to give them a final polish. I have taken the liberty of sending you my copy with some pencil notes for your consideration and, if you see fit, adoption.[2] The Colonial Office have asked me if I thought they should be sent out to the colonies and be placed in the hands of all men going out to Africa and other malarious parts. Of course I shall say Yes. But I am anxious before doing so to have you give it the final polish I suggest and to make one or two slight additions. It will do a lot of good and may lead to some useful additions to knowledge.

I had a letter from Daniels the other day.[3] He had traced the crescent through an Anopheles but I have not yet seen his detailed report.

I told Baker to make an alteration in the way of fitting in the slides and covers.[4] I hope he has done this, as the first model I saw was very imperfect in this respect.

I hope Mrs Ross will come up with you and I hope she will bring a change of weather. I have a beastly cold and feel a rag.

Have you seen Dantec's book.[5] It is terribly long winded and uninteresting.

Yours sincerely
Patrick Manson

By the way I had a long interview with Leslie the other day. He is home on a two years' holiday. I reproached him with allowing you to leave India without due reward and without an effort being made to retain your services. I think they are conscious of their shortcomings in these respects and I think they are penitent. In fact Leslie said they would have you back again tomorrow and give you anything you liked to ask for in the way of work and a good salary.[6] I fancy something in the way of recognition is in the air - at all events I urged it - and I fancy you have only to lift your little finger to get the directorship of one of the new laboratories. I have no authority for saying this; I only write of my impressions gathered from conversation.

1 Anonymous [R. Ross], *Instructions for the Prevention of Malarial Fever, for the Use of Residents in Malarious Places* (Liverpool: The University Press of Liverpool, 1899). Published as Memoir 1 of the Liverpool School of Tropical Medicine.
2 Apparently not in **RA**. However the work reached a sixth edition by 1901.
3 The Letter has not been traced. Daniels' various reports were published by the RS in their *Reports to the Malaria Committee of the Royal Society*. C. W. Daniels, 'Development of "crescents" in the "small dark" Anopheles prevalent in British Central Africa', *Reports to the Malaria Committee of the Royal Society*, 5th series (1901), 41-44.
4 Baker manufactured Ross's microscope; See Letter 7, note 9.
5 A. le Dantec, *Précis de Pathologie Exotique: Maladies des Pays Chauds et des Pays Froids* (Paris: Octave Doin, 1900).
6 Leslie was Harvey's secretary: Ross's comment, *Memoirs* , 391, was 'of course, I could only refuse again.'

Letter 192
49/051

21, Queen Anne Street,
Cavendish Square. W.
8th. Mar. 1900

My dear Ross

Many thanks for your report & especially for the inscription.[1] It will be placed among the family heirlooms. I have not had time yet to read it - but it looks thorough & workmanlike.

I wish you wd send me, if you have not destroyed it, the copy of No. I memoir with my suggestions in the margin.[2] Is there any chance of the latter being incorporated. I want to know for Colonial Office purposes.[3]

Yours sincerely
Patrick Manson

When will your speech appear & where?[4]

1 R. Ross, H. E. Annett, E. E. Austen, *Report of the Malaria Expedition of the Liverpool School of Tropical Medicine and Medical Parasitology* (Liverpool: The University Press of Liverpool, 1900). Published as Memoir 2 of the Liverpool School of Tropical Medicine.

2 See Letter 191.

3 Ross, *Memoirs*, 391, states that Boyce and Milne thought the amendments could not be made on account of expense and that as far as he was aware the Colonial Office did not take up the work. However the Liverpool School had received an order on 18 June 1900 from the Colonial Office for 400 copies of the Memoir, *Liverpool School of Tropical Medicine Historical Record* (Liverpool: The University Press of Liverpool, 1920), 19.

4 Ross, on the invitation of Sir James Crichton-Browne, presented a lecture 'Malaria and mosquitoes' to the Royal Institution on 2nd March 1900. It was published in *Nature* (29th March 1900) 522-527, also by the Institution and the Liverpool School and was translated into French for the *Revue Scientifique*.

Letter 193
49/220

21, Queen Anne Street,
Cavendish Square. W.
16th March, 1900.

My dear Ross,

Many thanks for your reprint from the Medical Annual.[1] It is a first class piece of work and I am very grateful to you for the full justice and more than justice you have done me as regards my very small share in the mosquito-malaria theory. You have assessed the Italian and Koch share in the matter very correctly and I hope settled the historical part of the discovery for good and all.

You may have seen from the papers that I had a lecture at the Colonial Institute on Tuesday.[2] The debate after the paper was amusing in the extreme. There are still doubters and still believers in blue mists.

I have not been able to get to the Colonial Office this week but next week mean to have an afternoon there when I shall find out about the number of your pamphlets they are likely to require. I think you should make the alterations, or something like them, I suggested as, if the Colonial Office take it up it would be well to have it as nearly perfect and practical as you can get it. Daniels has recently sent me some slides of his Anopheles with zygotes. They are quite convincing. I am circulating them among the members of the malaria commission.[3] Lister saw them today and is convinced.

I am beastly busy with my second edition[4] and distracted with proofs and cuts and the rest of it. How I do hate book making.

Yours sincerely
Patrick Manson

1 R. Ross, 'Malarial Fever', *The Medical Annual and Practitioners Index* (Bristol: John Wright & Co, 1900), 342-357. Ross's historical account was more temperate than his later ones.

2 Manson's address dealt with the necessity of studying tropical diseases and the possibility of their extinction; reported in *BMJ* (17 March 1900), 655.

3 By then consisting of Lord Lister, (Sir) Clifford Allbutt, Sir Michael Foster, Sir John Kirk, E. R. Lankester, Manson and Mr Lucas (representing the Colonial Office). There is no reference in the minutes to Daniels' slides.

4 P. Manson, *Tropical Diseases: A Manual of the Diseases of Warm Climates*, 2nd Edition (London: Cassell, 1900). It appeared in June 1900.

Letter 194
49/052

21, Queen Anne Street,
Cavendish Square. W.
27th March, 1900.

My dear Ross,
Dont be foolish. Stick to your present guns. Leave fiction to the kail-yarders and the like.[1] Your malaria work will live; novels are very ephemeral, even the best of them, and I fancy a man soon gets written out in that line. Go on with your present work. It will pay better in the long run. Are you looking after private practice?

It is not quite right or fair for the Liverpudlians to blame the Colonial Office. I have no doubt the Liverpool course will be recognised soon.[2] I have given my vote for this from the beginning and I feel pretty sure that Mr Chamberlain is in favour of it.

I have had such a wrestle with my new edition. I begin to see the end but the worry of placing illustrations, changing references and other piffling work sometimes drives me nearly distracted.

I looked for your paper in Nature today but did not find it.[3] I suppose next number will give it.

By the way; have you a set or two of your illustrations in your report to spare. I want to have them framed for the use of the school and dont want to break up my own copy. I like to teach by pictures and I like to have them hung on the wall for the student to study at spare moments.

I have a fine guinea worm case just now and have secured a lot of embryos and infected cyclops. Would it be of any use to you to send you any of the latter.

Are there any of my filaria infected mosquitoes about the laboratory. I find I sent Annett nearly all the first four or five days old infections. If you come across them you might send me a few.

Yours sincerely
Patrick Manson

1 Presumably a response to a Letter from Ross which is lost.
2 In two letters sent in February 1899, Chamberlain stated that the Government could not give financial aid to the Liverpool School and that doctors appointed to the Colonial Office must be attached the Hospital at the Albert Docks for at least two months, *Liverpool School of Tropical Medicine Historical Record* (1920), 12; Power (1998).
3 See Letter 192, note 4.

Letter 195
49/053

21, Queen Anne Street,
Cavendish Square. W.
4th Ap. 1900

My dear Ross,
I read your paper in Nature last night: It is first rate. You paid me more than my due I fear.

I am writing Rees[1] to lend you Cyclops. He has a lot. We are very hard up for malaria and beriberi cases just now. We are still the victims of underground conspiracy and malevolence, but are prepared to be patient & wait for the inevitable.

You have placed the Italians & Koch in their proper position about malaria. Pity you don't have the paper done into German and

Italian. It would do a lot of good for it is unanswerable and gives dates and facts as they really transpired. I suppose you wd have no difficulty in getting a first class German or Italian paper to publish it.

Yours sincerely

Patrick Manson

1 See Letter 179, note 4.

Letter 196
02/054

21, Queen Anne Street,
Cavendish Square. W.
8th June, 1900.

My dear Ross,

This from Thin.[1] I shall do what I can to get the signatures from staff & perhaps students.

My impression is that the R. S. will suggest delay until their commissioners at present in Africa report finally. The R. S. might feel its hands being more or less forced and that they are not given the opportunity to play the game off their own bat. However that is for the Council I suppose to say.

Meanwhile I shall get the signatures. My own of course I cannot for official reasons append.

Have you seen Marchiafava & Bignamis reprint from XX Century Pr of Medicine.[2] Lord - they magnify themselves and belittle everybody else as much as possible. I could hardly believe my eyes when I read. The latest thing in robbery is attributable to Grassi. You recollect the filaria in mosquito's proboscis. Grassi claims that as his!!!!! What next?

When are you coming up to town again? I am frightfully driven at present with practice, work, school etc etc.

Yours sincerely

Patrick Manson

1 A letter from Thin to Manson (**RA** 50/128) regarding the petition to Lord Lister organised by Ross asking the Royal Society to call upon government departments to support the destruction of mosquito larvae as part of the duties of sanitary personnel (**RA** 12/042). Thin, however, agreeing with the principle of the destruction of

mosquitoes, thought that this petition might upset the heads of the government medical departments (Gibson, 1983).

2 E. Marchiafava and A. Bignami, 'Malaria' in Thomas L. Stedman (ed.) *Twentieth Century Practice: An International Encyclopedia of Modern Medical Science*, vol 19 (London: Sampson, Low, Marston, 1895-1900), 1-522.

Letter 197
49/055

21, Queen Anne Street,
Cavendish Square. W.
12th June, 1900

My dear Ross,
I forget when the Malaria Commission is supposed to terminate their labours. There is a meeting next Tuesday when I hope to hear of some decent results.[1] Daniels is still in Brit. Cent. Africa & has now gone off after tick fever.

I think with you the mosquito business should be hurried up - but how? People, including R.S., Governors & the rest want educating up to the acting mark. It can do no harm to try over & over again. Unfortunately there is so much war on that a hearing for anything else is difficult to get. I think the Mal. Com. is finished this year, or next spring. I shall let you know positively soon. I hear from Sambon[2] that Grassi's new work[3] is in great part occupied with a polemic against you & Koch. Why you I dont know - unless it be that you wiped his eye.

Yours sincerely
Patrick Manson

Have they asked you to do Malaria for the new edition of Quain?[4] I told the editor to do so. They pay fairly well.

[The following added by Ross]
Yet Manson accepted the dedication of this very book of Grassi's and afterwards pretended he did not know that it attacked me infamously. R. Ross

1 The Committee meeting of 19 June 1900 received reports and letters from Daniels, Christophers and Stephens. See also Letter 198, note 1.
2 Louis Westenra Sambon, (1865-1931), was investigating malaria in the Roman Campagna. See **Biographical Appendix**.
3 Grassi (1900a).
4 R. Ross, 'Malarial disease', in H. Montague Murray (ed.) *Quain's Dictionary of Medicine*, 3rd edition (London: Longmans, Green & Co, 1902), 947-958.

Letter 198
49/056

21, Queen Anne Street,
Cavendish Square. W.
15th June, 1900.

My dear Ross,
I was at the Colonial Office this afternoon and ascertained that the Malaria Commission's commission concludes in October unless the importance of their results justifies prolongation.[1] I do not know that it does, not having seen any recent report. I may hear more at the R. S.'s malaria commission meeting on Tuesday next; if so I shall let you know.

Bad news from Daniels. He has had a dose of Blackwater fever and is on his way home.[2]

You must read Marchiafava and Bignami's article in the Twentieth Century's Practice of Medicine.[3] It is very good except that it is prolix in parts and is all for themselves.

Yours sincerely
Patrick Manson

1 Although it extended its brief and title to sleeping sickness and, later, other tropical diseases, the Commission continued to function.
2 Curiously, there is no reference to this at the 19 June 1900 meeting of the RSMC, and Daniels stayed in Africa until the end of the year.
3 See Letter 196, note 2.

Letter 199
49/057

21, Queen Anne Street,
Cavendish Square. W.
20th June, 1900.

My dear Ross,

The R. S. Committee which met yesterday will, I presume, reply to the petitions.[1] I fancy that the Colonial Office and the Indian Government will be asked to name a town where systematic mosquito destruction can be tried, and that medical officers and others will be informed of the benefits expected to accrue from such measures, the Royal Society endorsing the importance of the measure. I presume a letter to the two government departments concerned will be sent in presently.

Your appointment to Elder Dempster[2] will do you a lot of good. It will presently lead to other substantial additions to your income. These things once started gather volume.

Grassi has not so far as I know claimed in print Low's discovery.[3] Sambon told me that he said that he had told me all about it in Rome which is neither more nor less than a d—-d lie.

If I hear more in detail of the action of the R. S. about the petition I shall let you know; particularly if they make a recommendation to the Foreign and Colonial Offices.

Yours sincerely
Patrick Manson

Did Dr Murray, who is editing the new edition of Quain's Dictionary ask you to do malaria? I think I told him to.[4]

1 See Letter 196, note 1.
2 The shipping line of Sir Alfred Jones.
3 G. C. Low. 'A recent observation on filaria nocturna in culex: probable mode of infection', *BMJ* (16 June 1900), 1456-1457. George Carmichael Low, (1872-1952), then Craggs Scholar at the London School of Tropical Medicine. See **Biographical Appendix**.
4 Letter 197, note 4.

Letter 200
02/296

Llandulas, North Wales
9th August
[1900]

Dear Dr Manson,
Many thanks for sending me the letter which you found in your pocket book (!). I enclose a very interesting telegram received from Annett's expedition through our secretary Milne.[1] You will see that they have evidently found active *Filaria nocturna* in proboscis of Anopheles. The expedition is at Bonny, up country, where it takes, I believe, months for letters to reach; and from this fact as well as from Annett going to expense of wiring I suppose that he was not aware of Low's discovery when he made the observation. If so he will be third in the field. I have told Dawson Williams.[2]

No, the fishing is bad. River flooded & fish gorged with worms. I sit on the bank waiting for flood to subside.

I forgot to ask you several things. 1, what are lathyrism & manioc poisoning - where is the literature?[3] 2nd. Have you seen Blanchard "Instructions a l'usage des médecins, des naturalistes, etc"?[4] - & ought not this important work to be noticed by the B. M. J.?

I had an awful journey on the 3rd. Did not reach home until 11 p.m. Couldn't find the house & thought I would have to sleep in a ditch, in the middle of the storm.

10th August -

Have just been sent a paper containing your lecture at Aberdeen.[5] Certainly one of the best things you have ever done. Exactly what was required. Governments *must* be pressed on or else they will do nothing for a long time yet. Even after your lecture Lord Aberdeen remarked that there are lots of mosquitoes in Canada without malaria. Our next difficulty will be papers like the enclosed in the Englishman.[6] Please read it, and when you get a sight of Rogers' report, go for it. I have always said that R. is no good - he has not got the brains nor the reliability.[7] Fancy using the spleen test to prove that malaria is carried by drinking water! Why my regiment in Secunderabad, though it was socked with malaria had no spleen at all.

I have had a telegram from Blanchard saying "Section de bacteriologie vous adresse challeureuses felicitations pour descouvertes sur paludism." I wish I knew what section of bacteriology. I believe there are several congresses in Paris.[8]

Hoping you are having good sport.

Yours sincerely

R. Ross.

Grassi's polemics force me to write a full account of my malaria work from the beginning up to present. I think this is the best thing to do. I shall take the opportunity of saying what I think not only about Grassi but about other matters.

If you don't take care Govt. of India will push Rogers views against yours.

1 Alan Hay Milne, Secretary of the Liverpool School.

2 Editor of the BMJ. For the controversy surrounding the discovery of the etiology of sleeping sickness, see Maryinez Lyons, *The Colonial Disease: A Social History of Sleeping Sickness in Northern Zaire, 1900-1940,* (Cambridge: Cambridge University Press, 1992).

3 See Letter 201.

4 R. Blanchard, 'Instructions à l'usage des médecins, des naturalistes et des voyageurs, rédigées au nom de la Commission du Paludisme', *Bull. Acad. de Méd.* Paris, 3rd ser 44 (1900), 6-58. It does not appear to have been noticed by the BMJ.

5 Manson had delivered a lecture, 'Malaria: a sanitary problem' at the Public Health Congress, held at Aberdeen, 2-7 August 1900; reported in *Lancet* (11 Aug. 1900), 458 and *BMJ* (18 Aug. 1900), 451.

6 Reference untraced.

7 Leonard Rogers, 'Abstract of a paper on the relationship of drinking-water; - water-logging and the distribution of anopheles mosquitoes, respectively to the prevalence of malaria north of Calcutta', *Indian Medical Gazette* (Sept. 1900), 345-349. Although Rogers recognised that Ross's work had proved that malaria 'may be communicated to man through the bites of mosquitoes which have some days previously bitten another case of malaria', he argued in this paper that proper, filtered water supply had a stronger (negative) correlation with spleen rate than the mere presence of *Anopheles.*

8 International Medical Congress in Paris, 2-9 August, 1900.

Letter 201
49/058

Littlewood Park, Alford
N.B.
20th Aug. 1900.

My dear Ross,
Your letter of 9th inst. was forwarded but I have been so busy slaying things I have had not time to answer. Lathyrism is a form of spastic paraplegia brought on by eating the vetch *Lathyrus sativus* - there is some a/c of it in Aitkens Practice of Medicine[1] & in recent French books the names of which I cannot recall. The disease runs in parts of India & in Algeria. *Manioc poisoning* is really prussic acid poisoning caused by eating the bitter manioc before it has been thoroughly steeped in water. There is very little literature but you will see some a/c of it in one of the British Guiana Medical Annuals[2] & in other papers I cannot refer to at present.

Rogers is decidedly off the line. When his paper comes to hand we will see what we can do.[3]

I had a similar telegram from Blanchard & supposed it referred to my Aberdeen paper, but believe now there has been some mistake. I suppose the Govt. of India will lean towards the wind which entails least expense. The Colonial Office will, I fancy, follow truth & let the Govt. of India go its own road, to the devil or elsewhere. If somehow Sambon, Low and Company come through all right there is no fear our side will prevail.[4]

Yours sincerely
Patrick Manson

I leave this on Tuesday & get home on 1st Sep.

1 William Aitken, *The Science and Practice of Medicine* 2 vols, 5th ed. (London: Charles Griffin and Company, 1868), i, 860-862.
2 J. H. Conyers, 'Cassava poisoning', *British Guiana Medical Annual and Hospital Reports*, 7 (1895), 91-94.
3 R. Ross. 'Captain Rogers' recent investigation on malaria', *Indian Medical Gazette* (Dec. 1900), 461-462. L. Rogers, 'A reply to Major Ross's criticism', *ibid.*, 463. Ross criticized Rogers' assumption that spleen rates were an accurate measure of active malaria. Rogers replied to Ross's 'fatherly' comments that he had been ordered to survey a large area for practical purposes, not to investigate the mode of malaria transmission.
4 In a famous experiment, Carmichael Low, L. W. Sambon and an

artist Terzi camped out in the highly malarious locality of Castel Fusano, in the Roman Campagna, and by mosquito avoidance through screens and sleeping nets, were able to remain well. L. J. Bruce-Chwatt, 'History of malaria from prehistory to eradication', in Walther H. Wernsdorfer and Ian McGregor, eds., *Malaria: Principles and Practice of Malariology*, (Edinburgh, Churchill Livingstone, 1988), 2 vols., 1, 1-59.

Letter 202
49/059

21, Queen Anne Street,
Cavendish Square. W.
14th Sept. 1900

My dear Ross

Many thanks for Annett's letter - which I return.[1] Ask him from me to try feed a *day* feeding mosquito or other insect on *diurna* blood, and then try the same species of insect on *nocturna*. If my idea of specific difference be correct then the intermediary hosts will be different & the insect suitable for one will be inefficient for the other.

The men in the Campagna are well.[2]

Yours sincerely
Patrick Manson

Thanks for the papers. Lankester's is very scientific.[3]

1 Letter untraced.

2 Letter 201, note 4.

3 Probably R. Ross and R. Fielding-Ould, 'Diagrams illustrating the life-history of the parasites of malaria', *Quarterly Journal of Microscopical Science*, 43 (1900), 571-579, and E. Ray Lankester, 'Note on the morphological significance of the various phases of haemamoebidae', *ibid.*, 581-588. Lankester compared the reproduction of the malaria parasite with that of other coccidia and other single-celled organisms. See, also, Joe Lester, *E. Ray Lankester and the Making of Modern British Biology* (Faringdon: British Society for the History of Science, 1995) 147-149.

Letter 203
50/172
Telegram

Langham Place 12.11pm   Received at 1.14pm   Pembroke Place

17 September 1900

Ross Thompson Yates Laboratory University College Lpl
Son?[1] developed tertian keeping him without quinine 48 hours can you come verify

Manson

[added by Ross] infection of Manson's son with mosquitoes brought from Italy on 17 Sept 1900. I could not go. R. Ross

1 Telegram torn - loss of text. Manson's son Patrick Thurburn Manson had been bitten by malaria-infected mosquitos on 29th and 31 August, as part of an experiment by Manson to prove the malaria-mosquito theory, whereby volunteers were bitten by infected mosquitoes brought from Italy. See P. Manson, 'Experimental proof of the mosquito-malaria theory', *BMJ* (29 Sept. 1900), 949-951.

Letter 204
49/060

21, Queen Anne Street,
Cavendish Square. W.
18th Sept. 1900

My dear Ross,
I have just received your letter. I fear it is too late for you to come on as Bernie[1] has had 20 grains of quinine and although the infection was a very definite one it was not severe and parasites (benign tertian) were few. As I had got the testimony of 5 witnesses already I did not like to tell you to come up. Bernie was bitten by 3 lots of anopheles - in July (end of) - Aug. (end of) and last week. The end of Aug. lot did the trick. Last Thursday he felt ill temp. going to 102° - continued high temp - that day & Friday but never over 102°.

Saturday morning apyrexia. Hitherto as after many & long examinations of the blood I found no parasites I concluded he was probably suffering from a mild influenzal attack such as I am suffering from myself at present. So his temperature being normal at 2p.m. I went to the country. Soon after I left he had chills followed by high fever - 104° - delirium & later profuse sweats. Sunday morning apyrexia - fever Sunday afternoon followed by drenching sweats. On Monday morning on my return apyrexia. I examined his blood & found half grown tertians and one tertian gametus. Repeated examinations during the day by myself & others confirm this. Fever to 103° yesterday afternoon - splenic pain & splenic enlargement. Patient limp and as he is going up next month for his London M.B. I thought it time to squash the infection - so when his temperature fell to 100 he had his quinine.

This now is proof which is incontrovertible and will appeal to the meanest and most combative intellect.

Yours sincerely
Patrick Manson

1 Manson's son; see Letter 203, note 1.

Letter 205
49/061

21, Queen Anne Street,
Cavendish Square. W.
4th Jan. 1901

My dear Ross,
Many happy returns of the New Year - better of the century.

I have been expecting the copy of your Policlinico letter re Grassi[1] - I have not seen his assistant's indictment of him yet. I had hoped he wd send me a copy.[2]

I think you may safely drop him now. Lister put the points correctly and fairly & his verdict is final & is sure to be accepted by the public.[3]

The Colonial Office is having a small Commission to consider how to set about the practical application of mosquito malaria work. I shall let you know the result. It sits on 23rd inst. Are there any points you wd like insisted on? Let me know.

Yours sincerely
Patrick Manson

1 In an attempt to defend his work, Ross initiated an exchange of Letters between himself and Grassi in *Il Policlinico.* R. Ross, 'Le scoperte del prof. Grassi sulla malaria', *Policlinico*, 7 (1 Nov. 1900) 550-552; G. B. Grassi 'Per la storia delle recenti scoperte sulla malaria' *Policlinico*, 7 (1900) 593-600. R. Ross, 'Le scoperte del prof. Grassi', *Policlinico*, 8 (1901) 274-284. G. B. Grassi 'Replica del prof. Grassi', *Policlinico* 8 (1901), 284-288, (Gibson 1983). See *Memoirs*, 411-412, and **Introduction**.

2 Letter 209, note 1.

3 Lister had studied the claims of the Italians and Ross and gave an account of Ross's discovery of 1897 in his annual presidential address to the Royal Society. He concluded "Thus was in truth established the mosquito theory of malaria" (*Memoirs*, 412-3).

Letter 206
49/062

21, Queen Anne Street,
Cavendish Square. W.
7th Jan. 1901

My dear Ross,

Many thanks for your note. Could you send me one or two *points* bearing on the work of the proposed Committee on

Destruction of Ms
Prevention of bites
Situation and character of houses
Especially on what you think of the style of living in W. Africa as contrasted with E. Indian life.

I don't know yet what the proceeding will be. Fancy it is only a preliminary to find out how the Governors & lay public will jump.

Yours sincerely
Patrick Manson

Have got Policlinico.[1] Good.
P.M.

1 Letter 205, note 1.

Letter 206a[1]

School of Tropical Medicine
Thomas-Yates Laboratory
University College
Liverpool
13th January 1901

Dear Dr Manson,
I make the following brief notes regarding my opinions as to the prevention of malaria.

I. ***Public Measures***; that is measures to be taken by local governments, and municipal and sanitary authorities.

(a). *In Towns*

1. *Measures against mosquitoes.* Such seem to me to be the measures which are likely to do the greatest good to the greatest number of persons *in towns* for the least expense. They can certainly be carried out *to a large degree* in every town; they will benefit all classes equally; they can be effected without reference to the prejudices of private persons; they will add largely to the public comfort, and they will minimise the necessity for all kinds of private measures. Action should be taken against all varieties of gnats. The following are the particular steps required.

(1). Gradual obliteration of breeding pools, etc, as funds allow, and where practicable. Management of drains, streams, etc, so as to prevent accumulation of water favourable to gnats.

(2). Appointment of native agents to empty out tubs etc; to oil pools, wells etc; & to persuade inhabitants to take action.

(3). General clearance of undergrowth in towns, as funds permit.

(4). Municipal byelaws to prevent owners & tenants of premises from keeping stagnant water or rank vegetation about their houses.

(b). *In Rural Areas*

Little can be done in rural areas except the proper management of public rest houses where such exist. These to be built some hundreds of yards away from villages; to be well screened by wire window screens. Vicinity to be kept cleared of undergrowth & pools. Site to be carefully selected.

(c). General Public Measures

1. All public buildings - hospitals, gaols, asylums, barracks, etc. - to be treated as noted above for rest houses.

2. Gradual formation of separate cantonments for Europeans &

troops, on the Indian plan, with large, airy, well built houses, whitewashed walls, and screened windows if the climate permits; each house to be surrounded by a large, well-cleared compound, the servants quarters to be placed at a distance. Merchants, etc, to be encouraged to live within the cantonments. Drainage, site & clearance of undergrowth to be of course carefully attended to.

II. ***Measures for Isolated Communities.***

Especially for gangs of coolies, for soldiers & prisoners. In addition to as many of the above as are practicable, the free use of quinine is to be insisted on.

III. ***Measures for Medical men.***

1. All malaria cases to be isolated in nets - the isolation and treatment to be continued sufficiently long after the fever has ceased.

2. Window screens for hospital wards; destruction of mosquitoes, both larvae & adults; etc.

3. Instruction of educated persons on the subject.

IV. ***Measures for Travellers.***

1. To avoid sleeping in native houses or where natives have recently slept.

2. To prefer good tents to native accommodation.

3. To take the greatest care regarding the rise of the mosquito net.

4. To select camping sites at some distance from villages.

V. ***General Private Measures.***

1. Always to sleep in good mosquito nets.

2. To employ *punkahs*,[2] whenever possible; both during the day, and, in addition to the net, during the night.

3. To whitewash the walls.

4. To screen the windows.

5. To clear the garden.

6. To destroy all larvae which can be found in or round the house.

7. When it is impossible to avoid being frequently bitten by mosquitoes, or when the locality is very malarious, to take a good dose of quinine once or twice a week.

Remarks

It is doubtful whether there is much more malarial disease among the natives in Africa than there is among the natives in India. On the other hand, there is no doubt that the Europeans suffer far more in Africa than in India. I ascribe this to the fact that in Africa the Europeans have not learnt how to live in the tropics so well as the brothers in India have; and especially because

1. They often neglect the mosquito net.

2. They generally neglect the punkah.
3. Their houses are often wretched shanties.
4. Their houses have no compounds.
5. They live amongst the natives.
6. They do not select good sites even when these are available.
7. They are totally ignorant of the real nature of disease.

Yours very sincerely
Ronald Ross.

1 Letter in the possession of Dr Gordon Manson-Bahr.
2 A fan.

Letter 207
49/063

21, Queen Anne Street,
Cavendish Square. W.
15th Jan. 1901

My dear Ross,
Thanks very much for memo re prevention of malaria.[1] The C. O. sent me the official printed one this morning. They will be very helpful. I find we have to go slow and if we are to do good wait for the laggards, convince them & carry them with us and make them think *they* are driving the coach. Otherwise passive opposition which means failure. All the C. O. are with us, but the fellows out there I fear are sceptics, indifferent or jealous.

I shall send you Roy. Soc. papers soon. I have been overpowered with accumulations of work. I as yet have not had time to get the necessary [illegible] & learn method of procedure & traditions.[2] I was afraid, being so young a member I might not be the right man to propose you - but others think otherwise. You are I should think sure of election, although, I am told perhaps not the first time of being put up. You see the turn of the Society.

Be sure to send me the translation of Grassi's reply.[3] You might ask him if he knew all about proteosoma years ago why his sense of humanity did not force him to divulge things so pregnant with good for mankind.

Yours sincerely
Patrick Manson.

1 Letter 206a
2 Manson had proposed Ross for Fellowship of the Royal Society. He was elected on 6 June 1901, at the first time of asking. Other signatures on his ballot paper included James Crichton-Browne, Lauder Brunton, David Ferrier and H. Charlton Bastian (Election Papers, RS).
3 Letter 205, note 1. The manuscript translation of Grassi's reply 'For the history of the recent discoveries on malaria' survives in the Ross Archives, RA 09/038.

Letter 208
49/064

21, Queen Anne Street,
Cavendish Square. W.
24th Jan. 1901

My dear Ross,
I was very grieved to see the intimation of poor Myers' death.[1] If there are any particulars to hand I suppose they will appear in the medical papers tomorrow.

Thanks for your papers.[2] I dont know if they will be required. I shall keep them ready & take advice.

Your running comments on Charles' letters are good reading.[3] The facts as set forth (innocently enough) by Charles are absolutely conclusive against Grassi's pretensions. I wonder what his next wriggle will be. I am having his Policlinico letter translated for the fun of the thing: shall send you the translation if you care to read his slurs of yourself in English. I think I know his game but have forestalled him I think. Anon I shall tell you about it.

Yours sincerely
Patrick Manson

1 Walter Myers (c1872-1901) died of yellow fever at Pará, Brazil, whilst investigating the causes of the disease for the Liverpool School. The School named a lectureship in his memory, which Ross subsequently held. See Letter 227, note 3.
2 In connection with Manson's proposal of Ross's election to the Royal Society.
3 See Letter 159, note 1.

Letter 209
49/065

21, Queen Anne Street,
Cavendish Square. W.
30th Jan. 1901.

My dear Ross,
Many thanks for the papers which I return herewith. I have just read a translation of Grassi's reply to your letter in Il Policlinico. When a man takes to abuse & says he is enjoying himself he is in a bad way. Calandruccio's French pamphlet is crushing.[1] Pity a man with Grassi's talent and power of work shd behave as he does. Instead of fame he will get the reputation of and go down to posterity as a scientific barahhab.[2]

I dont know what will be the outcome of the Col. Off.'s meeting last week. The old Governors are not enthusiasts and are too prone to find difficulties and objections. Good news of activity from Hong Kong.[3]

Yours sincerely
Patrick Manson

1 Sauveur [Salvatore] Calandruccio, *Unicuique suum, Prof. J.* [sic] *B. Grassi* Written in French and translated in *Journal of Tropical Medicine* 4 (1901), 214-221. In this letter, Calandruccio, who had studied and worked with Grassi in the 1880s, accused him of appropriating for himself research which he (Calandruccio) had carried out on *ascaris*, termites and other organisms. His comments were not taken seriously by the Italian research community. (Personal communication, Prof. Bernardino Fantini.) See, also, *Memoirs*, 398-99, and Letter 232, note 2.

2 Perhaps means barathrum (OED: an insatiable extortioner.)

3 See J. C. Thomson 'The prevalence of mosquitoes and malaria in the colony of Hong-Kong', *Lancet* (12 Jan. 1901), 126-127.

Letter 210
08/090

21, Queen Anne Street,
Cavendish Square. W.
4th Feby, 1901.

My dear Ross,
Grassi's Studii goes forward to your address tomorrow. Return it when done with it.

I cannot fix the date on which I sent the specimens to Rome - probably just before Nov. 8th 1898.

Yours sincerely
Patrick Manson

Letter 211
49/066

21, Queen Anne Street,
Cavendish Square. W.
February 11th, 1901.

My dear Ross,
I am very sorry I cannot attend the meeting at Liverpool tomorrow. Needless to say my sympathy is with every effort to ameliorate the deplorable health conditions in West Africa.[1]

If anyone seriously thinks about it the secret and source of the relative backwardness of that country is malaria. In virtue of recent advances in knowledge we have it in our power to mitigate or, even, altogether to suppress the scourge. Why has this not been vigorously attempted? My answer, based on recent experience, is "*unbelief; unbelief founded on ignorance*". There will be no general action on the malaria mosquito theory until we get the cooperation of the public and this we wont get till the public believe. Our first point of attack therefore is ignorance. Every layman, and for that matter, doctor thinks he has as good a right to an opinion on the mosquito business as you or I. He is as capable of reasoning, he thinks, as you or I. Granted. But he altogether ignores the all-important circumstance that he has not been to the trouble to inform himself of the facts on which our reasoning is based. Did he possess these facts he would have arrived at exactly the same conclusion that you and I have. Therefore, your first effort must be to force the facts on him. When he grasps them he will be ready enough to act on them.

Urge on the meeting the importance of attempting a relative immunity from malaria. In my many encounters with scoffers I am constantly being told that it is impossible to escape altogether mosquito bites. I admit this. But if we reduce the number of mosquito bites by one half, *pro tanto* we diminish the chances of infection. If one mosquito in 1000 is infected and a man, through carelessness, is bitten 10 times a night he is infected 3 times a year; but if by care he manages to escape being bitten all but once a week, it will be 10 years perhaps before he is bitten by an infected mosquito and become a malarial. This you should impress on the meeting. It puts malaria protection on the same footing as vaccination against smallpox, or a pure water supply in regard to typhoid.

Had I my way, and were I an employer of labour on the Coast, I would make all my employees pass an examination in the mosquito malaria theory, believing that if they understood it they would act upon it. This sounds fanatical. Perhaps. But remind your audience that what seemed madness yesterday may pass for wisdom tomorrow. Ignorance is very often the mother of death.

From the backwardness of our people in taking this matter up I fear that the Germans, Italians and especially the Americans will once more show us how to apply our own discoveries. My patriotism squirms over such a possibility. I hope much from the practical business like energetic and self reliant methods of treating questions relating to their interests which have made Liverpool people what they are.

I shall be very much interested to learn what of practical [word missing] is to come from the Liverpool meeting.

Yours very sincerely
Patrick Manson

1 For the resulting deputation to Joseph Chamberlain, See Letter 212, note 1.

Letter 212
49/067

21, Queen Anne Street,
Cavendish Square. W.
20th March, 1901.

My dear Ross,
I went to the Colonial Office at 11 o'clock and was told the deputation[1] was put off till 12. As I had made 3 appointments

between that hour & 1, having put the patients off once before I was obliged to leave before your arrival. However I heard all about it & about Michelli's[2] speech at the tiffin[3] afterwards. Although the immediate result is not very great the ultimate effect of strong stirrings up cannot fail to do good. If the Governors feel they are under criticism they will bestir themselves - of course pretending all the time they are above being influenced by such means. Nothing new here. Sending out six men for plague duty at the Cape - do you know any *experienced* man - £760 a year & passage, send him along.

Yours sincerely
Patrick Manson

1 Joseph Chamberlain received a deputation at the Colonial Office from the Chambers of Commerce of London, Liverpool and Manchester and the Liverpool School of Tropical Medicine, represented by Ross, on the subject of health and sanitation in West Africa. (Nye and Gibson (1997), 98 and *Memoirs*, 433ff.).

2 (Sir) Pietro James Michelli, (1853-1935), Secretary to the Seaman's Hospital Society and to the London School of Tropical Medicine.

3 Lunch (anglo-indian).

Letter 213
49/068

21, Queen Anne Street,
Cavendish Square. W.
4th May, 1901

My dear Ross,

Just got your note telling me of your nomination to the R. S. I am very glad.[1] India will follow now with long delayed acknowledgement.

I hope you will come to me on Wednesday.

Yours sincerely
Patrick Manson

1 Ross was elected FRS on 7 June 1901.

Letter 214
49/069

21, Queen Anne Street,
Cavendish Square. W.
5th May, 1901

My dear Ross,
I wish you would send us a few millionaires. I hope your experiment will turn out well.[1] Dont begin till you are very sure of success - otherwise things would get a bad set back by a seeming failure. We cant spare Daniels.[2] Rees has gone to the Cape[3] & there is no one who could take Daniels place available.

Come & stay with us next time you are in town. I am on the war path again I think.

Yours sincerely
Patrick Manson[4]

1 In June, Ross returned to Sierra Leone, having secured a donation of £1000 from James Coats, jr., to fund the expedition.
2 Charles Wilberforce Daniels had been appointed Superintendent and Medical Tutor at the London School of Tropical Medicine on the resignation of D. C. Rees. He was seconded for service on the Royal Society Malaria Commission.
3 D.C. Rees resigned the above position in March 1901 and left on 6 April for plague duty at the Cape.
4 RA 49/070. In an attached note Manson regretted being unable to accept Alfred Jones' invitation. Jones had suggested a banquet to be given for Ross following his election as FRS.

Letter 215
49/071

21, Queen Anne Street,
Cavendish Square. W.
10th Sept. 1901.

My dear Ross,
Herewith a translation of Golgi [sic[1] Grassi] by Sambon. Sambon has seen the preparations (one) and says it is true. Thus

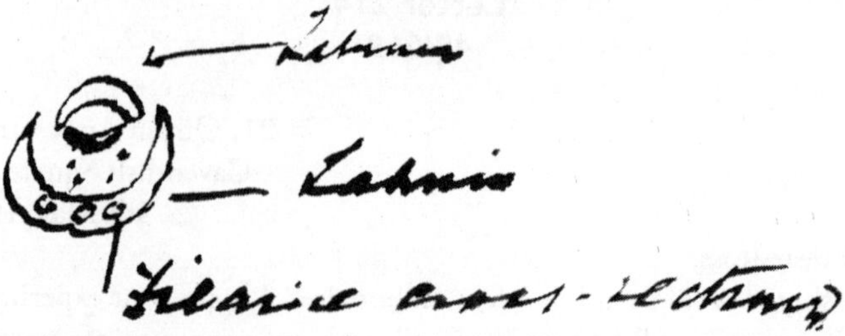

I am not convinced yet - nor shall I be till I see the actual preparation.

Yours sincerely
Patrick Manson

Please return the paper (translation) as soon as possible

1 See Letter 216: on the probability that the references to the translation are the same, Manson slipped when he wrote Golgi.

Letter 216
49/072

21, Queen Anne Street,
Cavendish Square. W.
11th Sept. 1901.

My dear Ross,
I have just received a letter from Sambon & Low saying that Grassi has modified his paper on the filaria proboscis business and now, while claiming a good deal for himself, fully admits Lows priority in demonstration.[1] So tone down what you may say about it. Sambon says Grassi has come round again.

Yours sincerely
Patrick Manson

Please send me the M.S. translation as soon as you can. The modified translation will be published.

P. M.

1 An earlier paper by B. Grassi and G. Noè, 'The propagation of the filariae of the blood exclusively by means of the puncture of peculiar mosquitoes', *BMJ* (3 Nov. 1900), 1306-1307 had appeared in

English. We have been unable to trace any publication of the translation mentioned here. See also Letter 222, note 2.

Letter 217
49/144

21, Queen Anne Street,
Cavendish Square. W.
11th Sep. 1901

My dear Ross,
I hope you have got back none the worse for the West Coast[1] & that we shall see you up here soon & get the news.

I saw Antrobus[2] of the Colonial Office today & speaking about the Commission[3] we agreed that it might be well to postpone the visitation until you had some idea as to how the present experiments in sanitation at S. Leone & Lagos are to issue. What do you think?

I hear nothing of Grassi. Do you?

Yours sincerely
Patrick Manson

Hope family events are all right.[4]

1 Ross returned from Sierra Leone and Lagos in early September.
2 (Sir) Reginald Laurence Antrobus, (1853-1942), Assistant Under-Secretary of State for the Colonies, 1898-1909.
3 Letter 212, note 1 and *Memoirs*, 436-7.
4 Rosa Ross was pregnant with their fourth and final child, Charles Claye Ross, born on 13 October 1901. See Letter 219, note 1.

Letter 218
49/073

21, Queen Anne Street,
Cavendish Square. W.
14th Oct. 1901

My dear Ross,
I dont know anything about the enclosed.[1] I suppose it is intended for some German man. I have been so busy I have not got through my paper reading for the last three months & have not yet tackled Smith & Taylor on B.W.[2] I hope to do so some day. Durham is off to Christmas Is. after beriberi & my son follows on Wed.[3]

When are you coming up to town again. Be sure to come here. Daniels believes in your mosquito campaign but is *very very very* strong on not risking failure & in *concentration* on one place. This conquered the British public will do the rest; this a failure & goodbye for years to mosquito sanitation. Verb. sap.

Yours sincerely
Patrick Manson

[Added, Ross's hand] Koch, Deutsche Medizinische Wochenschrift 1899, 1900

1 Possibly Koch's reports of the activities of the malaria expedition to Italy, the East Indies and New Guinea, published in *Deutsche Medizinische Wochenschrift* (see Ross's annotation). These are reproduced in *Gesammelte Werke von Robert Koch*, 2 vols in 3 parts, (Leipzig: Verlag von Georg Thieme, 1912) 2, ii, 389-434.

2 Frederick Smith and M Logan Taylor, 'Two cases of Blackwater fever', *Lancet* (21 Sept. 1901), 776-777.

3 Herbert Edward Durham (1866-1945) led the London School of Tropical Medicine expedition to Christmas Island to investigate beriberi, on which expedition Manson's son Patrick Thurburn unfortunately died in an accident. See also Letters 203 and 204.

Letter 219
49/074

21, Queen Anne Street,
Cavendish Square. W.
18th Oct. 1901.

My dear Ross,

My wife & family join me in congratulations on the arrival of the son[1] & hope all is well. You must look after private practice now. Got him to educate.

Annett sent me your Part II.[2] It is excellent & most valuable although some bits I dont quite agree with.

You see we are opening our mouths very wide. I hope we may get the £100,000.[3] We could turn it to good purpose I am very sure. Our class is too large & we have had to turn away a good many. Isn't this a pity.

When come you to town. Your bed is ready.

Yours sincerely
Patrick Manson

1 Charles Claye born 13 October 1901.

2 Presumably Part II of the Liverpool School of Tropical Medicine Memoir V by M. Logan Taylor *Second Progress Report of the Campaign against Mosquitoes in Sierra Leone* (Liverpool: University Press, 1902). Ross had published the first part of this report (*First Progress Report of the Campaign against Mosquitoes in Sierra Leone*) in 1901.

3 A meeting was held by the Seamen's Hospital Society for the purpose of obtaining further funds (£100,000) to enlarge the London School of Tropical Medicine and place it on a sound financial basis. Reported *Lancet* (26 Oct. 1901), 1144-1145.

Letter 220
02/305

21, Queen Anne Street,
Cavendish Square. W.
8th Nov. 1901.

My dear Ross,

Many thanks for the letter from Bathurst.[1] You should get Dutton to represent the matter to the Governor or to address the Colonial Office officially. Are you coming up to the Roy. Soc. dinner? When is the book to be by me & when will you require letters.[2] The latter I will hand to you when next in London but, remember, they are mine - heirlooms.

Yours sincerely

Patrick Manson.

1 **RA** 13/066, 13 Oct. 1901. J. E. Dutton wrote to Ross describing the sanitation and breeding places of mosquitoes in Bathurst, The Gambia.

2 Ross had asked for the letters which he had sent to Manson from India.

Letter 221
02/306

21, Queen Anne Street,
Cavendish Square. W.
24th Nov 1901

My dear Ross,
I shall get Edie[1] to send off your letters tomorrow morning. Mine I fear will require a good deal of editing before they are fit for the press & some of yours where they refer to certain men in India will also be better for the pruning knife.

Yours sincerely
Patrick Manson

1 Edith M. Manson, his daughter.

Letter 222
49/075

21, Queen Anne Street,
Cavendish Square. W.
21st Jan. 1902

My dear Ross,
Many thanks for your Mosquito Campaigning.[1] It is good reading. When I came to the bit about Grassi & the Italians it quite took away my breath. I fear some of them deserve it. Have you seen Noè's paper (Grassi's assistant) on the filaria mosquito business. This beats the malaria peculations. He claims that owing to *Italian* labours the scientific method for filarial prophylaxis has been discovered!!![2] Cockfighting is not in it. If you have not seen the paper I will send it to you. He pats Low on the back but insinuated Grassi had done it before & knew all about it.

Yours sincerely
Patrick Manson

1 The reference is unclear. Ross published *Malarial Fever, its Causes, Prevention and Treatment* in February 1902, but it made no strong claims against the Italians. See, also, Letter 225, note 3.

2 Giovanni Noè, 'Sul ciclo evolutivo della Filaria bancrofti (Cobbold)

e della Filaria immitis (Leidy)' Recherche fatte nel Laboratorio di Anatomia normale della R. Università di Roma ed in altri Laboratorî Biologici', viii (1900-1901), 275-353, cited in L. W. Sambon, 'Remarks on the life-history of filaria bancrofti and filaria immitis', *Lancet* (16 Aug. 1902), 422-426. In this paper, Sambon reviews the history of filarial disease research and the role of mosquitoes in its transmission, arguing that Grassi and Noè claimed far more priority for themselves than was warranted by the facts. Ross published a Letter in *Lancet* (13 Sept. 1902), 775, supporting Sambon's interpretations.

Letter 223
49/076

21, Queen Anne Street,
Cavendish Square. W.
23rd Jan. 1902

My dear Ross,
I have sent the paper to Sambon but will forward it to you tomorrow evg.[1] The translation I have is merely a precis of the new facts detailed & omits the lies & cheek - so it is not worth sending. I shall ask Sambon to translate the lies & insinuations.

Yours sincerely
Patrick Manson

Observe Grassi is now using Noè as his stalking horse.

1 Letter 222, note 2 for the outcome of Sambon's activity.

Letter 224
08/100

21, Queen Anne Street,
Cavendish Square. W.
13th Feby 1902

My dear Ross,
Yours of 12th to hand this a.m. I wrote you in the evg. of 11th addressing to your house telling you that I did not know what Grassi was to say in his book & accepted the dedication in good faith.[1]

Sambon I have not seen lately. I had hoped he wd lend some notes on the points in Grassi's book. Sambon is not very reliable as regards such things. Means to do it but don't do it.

You might mention that when I visited Rome the investigation of the mosquito in filaria infection was in progress[2] - that the specimens I showed Grassi were some I had made shortly before I saw him, that Annett had tried his hand in it not very long before and that Low was then at work or about to begin work on the material I had given him. It is still open to question if Grassi's explanation of the mechanism of infection is correct - the detail, however, is a matter of small importance - the principle - infection through the bite of the mosquito is ***the*** discovery & Grassi had nothing to do with this further than to confirm Low's work. The rest is all detail requiring only a little perseverance to elaborate. A laboratory boy could do this.

Yours sincerely
Patrick Manson

1 Grassi had dedicated his *Studi* to Manson.

2 These details are recounted in Sambon's article cited in Letter 222, note 2.

Letter 225
49/077

21, Queen Anne Street,
Cavendish Square. W.
12th April 1902

My dear Ross,
I was sorry to miss you when you called. Edie apparently made a mess of her letter.[1]

I am glad to hear of your approaching advent & hope the new move will lead to great things.[2] I believe it will.

What about poor Liverpool?

I have just heard that the Committee of Management of the Seamens Hospital Society have agreed to double the size of the London S. of T. M. and that the work is to be taken in hand at once. We must get you in there in some capacity. How would it suit you to be a sort of free lance - to give two or three lectures or more each session on new subjects or new ideas. This wd spare you routine drudgery of lecturing on a set group of diseases, yet wd force you to formulate floating notions and wd give the School the eclat of your name.

Yours sincerely
Patrick Manson

Thanks for malaria,[3] shall read it tomorrow.

1 This letter is untraced.
2 Ross, dissatisfied with his employment conditions, had resigned his post at Liverpool and accepted an appointment to head a new department of animal parasitology at the Jenner Institute (eventually the Lister Institute).
3 Presumably R. Ross, *Malarial fever, its cause, prevention and treatment* (Liverpool: University Press, 1902).

Letter 226
49/078

21, Queen Anne Street,
Cavendish Square. W.
20th June 1902

My dear Ross,
So you are back again. Very sorry you cd not manage the Jenner Institute.[1]

I have told the Colonial Office to refer a colonial patient to you for survey. I thought you might not object to earn a guinea but if this sort of work does not suit you let me know and tell me a good Liverpudlian who could be trusted in any similar case. Are you coming up to Coronate?[2]

Yours sincerely
Patrick Manson

1 Ross resigned his position at the Jenner Institute on 1 June 1902, having found the conditions of his appointment unsatisfactory. For details, see *Memoirs*, 460 ff. and Nye and Gibson (1997), 103-7.
2 The Coronation of Edward VII, scheduled for 26 June but ultimately postponed until 9 August because of the King's emergency abdominal surgery on 24 June.

Letter 227
49/079

21, Queen Anne Street,
Cavendish Square. W.
26th June 1902.

My dear Ross,
I am very glad to see your name in the list of Coronation Honours but resent the grade they have put you in.[1] Surely you have done more for country and humanity than Lipton[2] et hoc genus omne.

I am as before and shall stick there, I doubt not, till the end of the chapter. My chief regret is that wife & friends are disappointed.

I am very glad they have done well by you in L'pool.[3] You should have a brilliant time before you now. Without anxiety & plenty of opportunity & time to look about. My worry now is uncertainty of health and care about providing for the rainy day which may come at any time. I have been at it for 38 years now & have hardly a right to look for a longer innings.

Yours sincerely
Patrick Manson

1 Ross was awarded the Companion of the British Empire in Edward VII's Coronation Honours List.
2 Sir Thomas Lipton, the millionaire grocer, was created a baronet in the same list.
3 Ross was reappointed at Liverpool to the post of Walter Myers Lecturer with a salary of £600.

Letter 228
49/080

21, Queen Anne Street,
Cavendish Square. W.
8th July 1902

My dear Ross,
Many thanks for your kind invitation but as I have relatives in Manchester I must stay with them or in a hotel otherwise I shall give offence. They are funny.

Just heard from Low. He had got as far as Aden & was nearly frizzled up by the heat.[1]

No special news. Very busy. Yours sincerely
Patrick Manson

The Lancet, so far, have done nothing with Sambon's paper on Grassi.[2] I suppose they are afraid to whack the skunk.

1 George Carmichael Low was leading the Royal Society's first sleeping sickness expedition to Uganda. He travelled via Aden from where he wrote to Manson on 24 June 1902, G. C. Cook, 'Correspondence from Dr George Carmichael Low to Dr Patrick Manson during the first Ugandan sleeping sickness expedition', *Journal of Medical Biography*, 1 (1993), 215-229.

2 Sambon (1902).

Letter 229
13/157

21, Queen Anne Street,
Cavendish Square, W.
24th Nov. 1902.

My dear Ross,

I see from this morning's paper that you have been awarded a Nobel Prize & I heartily congratulate you on this substantial recognition of your work.[1] I very much wish you had not been a cosignatory of that letter in the B. M. J. & Lancet of Saturday.[2] It is absolutely wrong & unjust. I have not written a word about the trypanosome business. I have spoken of it in public 3 times - once at L'pool, once at a laboratory meeting of the Path. Socy reported in last Lancet very briefly,[3] once at the School. Each time I fully acknowledged Dutton's work & never once claimed any discovery for myself. I hoped confirmation, such as I have given, would add to rather than detract from Dutton's find.

Yours sincerely
Patrick Manson

1 Ross was awarded the Nobel Prize for Medicine on 10 December 1902; Ross had received the news on 3 Nov. 1902. Nye and Gibson (1997), ch. 7.

2 R. Boyce, R. Ross, and C. S. Sherrington, Letter to the Editor. 'Note on the discovery of the human trypanosome', *Lancet* (22 Nov. 1902), 1426; in this letter the authors support the claims of Everett

Dutton. Manson had never himself stated that his and C.W. Daniels' case was the first.

3 Reported in *Lancet* (22 Nov. 1902), 1391.

Letter 230
08/103

The Liverpool School of
Tropical Medicine
B 10, Exchange Buildings,
Liverpool
17th Feb 1903

Dear Dr Manson,
I see that Grassi is again on the warpath.[1] I shall probably not discuss his twaddle again, but may have to point out publicly that in claiming to give the full literature he has made a number of important omissions. For instance his quotation, No I, is not from me but from an abstract of a paper by me.[2] In his quotation II (my paper of Dec. 18th 1897) he has entirely omitted your drawings of the pigmented cells & the remarks of yourself, Thin & Bland Sutton. He has also failed to give your important paper of June 18th 1898 which preceded all his own work, and also the opening remarks of my Report on the Cultivation of Proteosoma.[3] The effect of this is of course to give a wrong impression of the whole business. I see also that he has again dedicated his paper to you obviously in the hope that he will induce many of his readers to suppose that you (who know the facts) endorse his views. Did he ask your permission to be allowed to dedicate this work to you? If he dedicated it to you without your permission will you allow me to say so publicly if necessary?

Believe me
Yours sincerely
R. Ross.

1 B. Grassi, *Documenti riguardanti la storia della scoperta del modo di trasmissione della malaria umana* (Milan: A. Racanti, 1903). Grassi's pamphlet reproduced eighteen articles or parts of articles, including eleven from Grassi and his colleagues, and four from Ross, along with a running commentary by Grassi. The offending dedication (see Letters 232 and 233) read: *A PATRICK MANSON scopritore del*

ciclo evolutivo della filaria e geniale iniziatore delle recenti scoperte sui parassiti malarici, [un] *rispettoso omaggio di* B. GRASSI. (To Patrick Manson discoverer of the evolutionary cycle of filaria and genial initiator of the recent discovery of the malaria parasite, respectful homage of B. Grassi)

2 Abstract of Ross (1896d) reported *BMJ* (8 May 1897), 1179.

3 Ross (1898b).

Letter 231
08/104

21, Queen Anne Street,
Cavendish Square. W.
18th Feby 1903

My dear Ross,
I have not read Grassi yet. Leave him alone. You waste powder & shot & time if you return to the charge. Your position is addressed and emphatically & publicly acknowledged.

Yours sincerely
Patrick Manson

Letter 232[1]
08/109

University College,
Liverpool
February 20th. 1903

My dear Dr. Manson,
I too have not read Grassi's book, and, as you suggest, will probably take no notice of it. But I wrote to you in your own interests and not in mine, because your name on the title page of this book, as well as its predecessor, will naturally lead those who do not know you to infer that you believe in, or at least sympathise with his views. If you think over the matter, you will I fancy see that the person to whom a book is dedicated cannot always disclaim all approval of the contents of that book. Of course this might be done with reference to a purely scientific work; but where the work is of a polemical nature, and especially where it is entirely devoted to attacking a single person, the position may be very different. For example, as an illustration,

suppose that a person A. issues a libellous book upon another person B. and dedicates this book to a third person C. whose authority and position is such that his name on the title page will support the libels of A., and suppose that C. has accepted the dedication of this work either with a previous knowledge of its contents, or at least with some notion of the purpose of the work—— then do you not think that B. could lay an action for damages against C. for knowingly assisting to propagate the libel of A? I think you will find that lawyers will hold this view. Of course as I have said, I have not read Grassi's book carefully, and do not know whether it is libellous, and mention this supposition only as an illustration. But whatever the legal aspect may be, there is morally no doubt that when a person accepts the dedication of a polemical attack on another person, he practically approves of that attack. And this view will be much strengthened if as in the present case, the book is the second work of a similar nature which A. has dedicated to C. in the hope of pushing home his attack on B. You will remember that at the Committee of the Royal Society which considered Calandruccio's affair,[2] it was specifically mentioned that your name on the title page of Grassi's work supported his views; and you will also remember the letter which you wrote to me on the point.[3] Your name on the title page of a second book will greatly strengthen this opinion, in spite of your letter. Of course those who know you will simply suppose that you still disclaim approval of the book; but I am sure that the vast bulk of readers who do not know you personally will undoubtedly consider that Grassi has your entire approval; and as the book has evidently been poured through Europe and America in shoals, the effect may be a damaging one to me. In fact it appears to me quite obvious that Grassi has dedicated both his books to you for this very purpose.

I do not know whether the book was dedicated to you with or without permission. Whatever the fact may be, people will certainly suppose that permission was granted; and, I am writing to you not in my own interests, but only for the purpose of warning you of the inferences which I think will be drawn. I shall take no action myself unless you ask me to do so, and shall leave the matter entirely to you. Please make any use of this letter which you may think necessary.

Believe me

Yours very sincerely

[R. Ross]

1 First typed letter from Ross to Manson; **RA** 08/110 is a draft of letter with a few minor alterations.

2 Calandruccio wrote to the Royal Society in November 1901, arguing that the Darwin Medal, which the Society had awarded Grassi in 1896, should have been shared between them, since Calandruccio had done much of the work for which the medal was awarded. Both Physiology and Zoology Committees of the RS investigated Calandruccio's charges, but concluded that there were no grounds on which the Royal Society could adjudicate between the two men and declined to support Calandruccio's claims. The matter was officially closed by the RS Council on 19 June 1902. (Royal Society, Minutes of Council, Vol. 8 (1898-1903), 255, 264-5, 304-7.) See also Letter 209, note 1.

3 Letter 209.

Letter 233
08/105

21, Queen Anne Street,
Cavendish Square. W.
21st Feby 1903

My dear Ross,

Although Grassi had my permission to dedicate his first paper to me, he neither asked nor obtained my permission to dedicate to me this last polemic. I dont agree with your A. B. C. argument. Did it hold good a man might be dragged into all sorts of controversies against his will and be forced to have Italian and other books translated at great expense and be obliged to read them when he had plenty of other and more important work to do.

I am in no way responsible for Grassi's statements. I don't know what he says in this new book, but in a paper published by him some time ago on filarial disease his "facts" (historical) in many instances were all wrong as were also many of his interpretations.

Yours sincerely

Patrick Manson

Drop him. You can say he used my name without my permission I mean in this second work, but I dont like to be mixed up in any paper and useless squabble.

Letter 234
08/106

21, Queen Anne Street,
Cavendish Square. W.
5th Mar. 1903

My dear Ross,

Many thanks for the specimen which I shall return tomorrow morning. It is a revelation of malignity. Some years ago (vide 1st ed of my manual[1]) I recommended a somewhat similar way of exploring for crescents - wash haemoglobin out with water, fix with alcohol, stain with blue methylene. It is all right with an experienced hand but as the novice did not know dirt from deformed crescent or amoebule I discarded it. The modified Romanowski you advocate is an improvement but as with my method is not for the novice. In extreme degrees of infection it is not necessary & in feeble infections perhaps not absolutely to be trusted. However it is a method & I shall try it in practice.

Re that infernal nuisance ~~Golgi~~ Grassi. I mean to write a letter of repudiation to B.M.J. & Lancet but I hate war and publicity of this sort.[2] More especially as he is generally discredited & it seems an act of supererogation. However I suppose it must be done.

I have had a very low down time with gout lately but am better now.

Yours sincerely
Patrick Manson

1 Manson (1898a), 30-31.

2 Letter from P. Manson to the Editor, 'Professor Grassi's recent pamphlet', *Lancet* (28 Mar. 1903), 923.

Letter 235
49/081

21, Queen Anne Street,
Cavendish Square. W.
19th Mar. 1903.

My dear Ross,

Prodeegious. Many thanks for the slide. You must come to the B. M. A. Swansea meeting. It is quite close to L'pool

Yours sincerely
Patrick Manson

Letter 236
49/082

21, Queen Anne Street,
Cavendish Square. W.
15th Apr. 1903.

My dear Ross,
Captn Gill, n.i.a. army medical service[1], who has had large experience of Cuban and Manila malaria will hand you this. He is anxious to make your acquaintance and to see something of the Liverpool School.

Yours sincerely
Patrick Manson.

1 Unidentified.

Letter 237
49/083

21, Queen Anne Street,
Cavendish Square. W.
3rd July 1903

My dear Ross,
Many thanks for your telegram of congratulation.[1] Your turn next. Pardon delay in acknowledging but I have had so many letters to write last few days I have had no time to overtake them - threatening writers cramps.

Yours sincerely
Patrick Manson

1 Manson was appointed KCMG in 1903.

Letter 238
49/084

21, Queen Anne Street,
Cavendish Square. W.
16th June 1904.

My dear Ross,
Many thanks for you Nobel Prize essay.[1] It reads like a novel. I am very much obliged for the generous treatment you mete out to me. I hardly deserve the kind things you say about me.

For the last 3 months I have been practically bed ridden - gout. I am about again but very lame and living in perpetual dread of a relapse. I fear I am done for now. I had hoped for another 5 or 6 years lease of health but at present the prospects are poor. However, I shall keep the flag flying as long as I can.

Yours sincerely
Patrick Manson

1 R. Ross, *Researches on Malaria being the Nobel Medical Prize Lecture for 1902* (Stockholm: P. A. Norstedt & Soner, 1904).

Letter 239
02/307

21, Queen Anne Street,
Cavendish Square. W.
20th Dec 1906.

My dear Ross,
Before sending the letters to the R. Col. I wd like to see the copy.[1] I have an indistinct recollection of some rather sharp criticism on Govt or other individuals - and one or two other things it might be undesirable to expose to the public eye. Please therefore send me either the letters or the copy before processing further.

Yours sincerely
Patrick Manson

1 See Letter 241, for evidence that Ross had proposed to place their correspondence in the library of the Royal College of Surgeons, of which he was a Fellow.

Letter 240
02/308

21. Queen Anne Street,
Cavendish Square. W.
21st Oct. 1908

My dear Ross,
Your letters though long delayed are none the less welcome. When the balance arrives & if you are kind enough to give me a copy of mine I would like to deposit them in the library of the School of Tropical Medicine along side Lewis' note books[1] which I presented to the school some time ago. They will have an interest and value in years to come to some medical Dryasdust writing the history of malaria when we are dead and gone - the bugs hunting us & not we the bugs.

Yours sincerely
Patrick Manson

1 Timothy Richards Lewis, (1841-1886), Assistant Professor of Pathology at the Army Medical School, Netley. He researched into cholera and leprosy with D. D. Cunningham.

Letter 241
02/309

21, Queen Anne Street,
Cavendish Square. W.
24th Oct 1908

My dear Ross,
These letters would be a feature in the tropical schools but would be lost in Col. of Surg. or Brit. Mus. Besides I don't know what I wrote or whom I slanged & would like to do a little editing before giving my share any publicity however modified.

I shall write you when you send the transcript of mine - as you so kindly promised.

Yours sincerely
Patrick Manson

Letter 242
02/310

21, Queen Anne Street,
Cavendish Square. W.
20th Jan. 1909

My dear Ross,

I have for the last fortnight been in the grip of gout & fuddled with colchicum and in consequence slothful in business. Hence the delay in acknowledging your letters.

It would be a pity to let the correspondence - especially your part of it - perish and I am very willing that my part of it (after a little editing) should be deposited in any place you might select: my idea was the Tropical School alongside of Lewis' M.S. which we already have. But I am willing to submit to your wishes in the matter provided you let us have a complete transcript of the whole correspondence for the School.

I should have liked to go to Bombay but I am not able to get away at present.[1]

Yours sincerely
Patrick Manson

1 Bombay Medical Congress 22-25 February, 1909, on which visit Ross became further alienated from the Indian malarial community. *Memoirs*, 504-5, and Bynum (1994).

Letter 243
L15/1/12

21, Queen Anne Street
Cavendish Square. W.
19th July 1909

My dear Ross,

I think Breinl the proper man for the place[1] and wrote to Martin[2] this morning to that effect. Breinl though young has had an exceptional training, is up to date, able, devoted & enthusiastic. His health is his weak point. I presume you know about this.

I will write about the letters when I get a little time but I have been frightfully rushed of late & have had to put many things aside.

I had hoped to see you at the Trop. Soc. on Friday & discuss the sending of the letters then but you did not turn up. It was a very poor meeting.

The marriage[3] went through all right but naturally we are a bit topsy turvy still.

Yours sincerely
Patrick Manson

1 A director of the new Australian Institute for Tropical Medicine in Townsville, Queensland, was being appointed. Anton Breinl, (1880-1944), director of the Runcorn Research Laboratory at the Liverpool School, took the post in 1909, remaining there until 1920.

2 Charles James Martin, (1866-1955), Director of the Lister Institute and a Member of the Royal Society Committee on Tropical Diseases, was on the selection committee which comprised representatives from the Royal Society, and the London and Liverpool Schools of Tropical Medicine.

3 Manson's daughter, Edith Margaret Manson, married Philip Manson-Bahr in 1909.

Letter 244
L15/1/16

21, Queen Anne Street,
Cavendish Square. W.
25. July 1909

My dear Ross,

I quite recognise Bancroft's[1] claims & would be glad to help him. But the object is a tropical school on modern lines & Bancroft has not, I fear, had the opportunity to get on these lines to the same extent as Breinl. I think we should nominate him as second best for the post. If local feeling is very keen for a local man they have the excuse of Breinl's trypanosome infection to supersede him in favour of Bancroft & I have written Martin that this fact about Breinl should not be suppressed.

I sent you this morning papers by Bancroft (which please send on to Rose Bradford[2]). You will see from them that Bancroft's filaria work is very thin, though I have no doubt he is an able man. Like yourself I have never met him and though the son of his father - the original Filaria Bancrofti man, I confess I think he has not quite played up to his opportunities. His age is against him as he is approaching the time at which, alas, I have long passed it, a man should be chloroformed.

Yours sincerely
Patrick Manson

1 Thomas Lane Bancroft, (1860-1933), the Australian medical naturalist, had researched into filariasis and dengue fever. He was the son of Joseph Bancroft, (1836-1894), discoverer of the worm causing filariasis (*Filaria bancrofti*).

2 (Sir) John Rose Bradford, (1863-1935), Physician to University College Hospital, London.

Letter 245
L17/1/3

21, Queen Anne Street,
Cavendish Square. W.
Nov 5th 09

Dear Ross,
I hear there will be a considerable sum of money at the disposal of the Committee, I intend to bring forward a series of suggestions, in the way of Research for the consideration of the Committee.

Any or all of these would, in my opinion, be fitting objects.

Your suggestion is a good one, & might be incorporated with those I intend to submit. The latter are as follows.

1) The possible interrelationships of the parasite of Kala-azar with that of oriental sore.
2) The completion of the life-history of Schistosomum haematobicum.
3) The etiology of Pellagra specially in its bearing on the West Indies.
4) Filaria Loa its life-history & the question of its Pathonogenicity.
5) An explanation of the absence of anophelines, from apparently favourable spots such as Barbados.
6) The bearing of sex of the tse-tse fly in relation to the trypanosome, & the possibility of hereditary transmission.
7) The explanation of the absence of malaria in certain Anopheline

haunts.

Some of these subjects are quite capable of solution at small expense.

I think we certainly could make use of our specialists in attempting to clear up the Kala-azar, the Bilharzia & the Loa questions. So that with regard to these problems the expense need not be very serious.

The malaria and trypanosome questions would cost a good deal to settle, I should think.

As regards Pellagra I am very anxious for various reasons to give *Sambon* a chance in this, for although he has many of the faults of genius, he is a genius, remarkably industrious, when he sets about a thing & full of original ideas & I am sure would struggle till he got a solution. Poor fellow he is cursed with the want of cash, which has handicapped him for years & I fear that, if we can't get him something soon, he will be lost to Tropical Medicine, & the loss, I know, would be a serious one.

He is a magnificent worker, with ideas ahead of the time, & perhaps that's the reason, or one of the reasons, why so many affect to sneer at him. Recently he has prepared a monograph of Porocephalus[1], an elaborate & perfect piece of work. His work on the Haemoprotozoa, considering his opportunities is remarkable. But everyone is down on him, because he is not like other men.

I hope if I bring this question of his working Pellagra out before the Committee, you will back me up, in trying to give Sambon a chance to show, what I know he can do.

Yours sincerely

Patrick Manson

(dictated)

PS

I am sorry I can't write myself I am laid up.

1 L. W. Sambon, 'Porocephaliasis in man', *Journal of Tropical Medicine and Hygiene*, 13 (1910), 17-24; 212-217; 258-262.

Letter 246 [copy]
58/010

9th November 1909

My dear Sir Patrick,

Many thanks for your letter of November[1] – only just received. I do not know what the cause of the delay has been. In the meantime I have already drawn up a list of what I suggest, and enclose a copy.[2] Curiously enough the 5th research on my list coincides with the 3rd of yours, and I too had Sambon in my mind when I wrote it down. I quite agree with everything you say, and we must really make an effort for him.[3] When he was here the other day we talked over the matter of Pellagra and he himself suggested going first to Italy and then to the West Indies, as I have stated in my list. I have put the price at £600 a year, but this may be too much. All the same there is another possible way of employing Sambon, that is in connection with the malaria Bureau about which I spoke to you.[4]

2. With regard to the researches on malaria. I should much like to have them here in connection with the proposed malaria Bureau, regarding which I have sent a scheme to Read.[5] This scheme ought to collect a good annual sum from local municipalities and town councils etc., in the tropics. I propose that the Bureau should bring out a Bulletin like the Sleeping Sickness one.[6] This will cost about £300 per annum for printing, and if you put aside another £300 per annum for Librarian, postage, etc., we will do nicely. With still another £250 or £200, or less, I could get a research student here who would do the work which I have been meditating for years. My routine work here occupies me for five hours a day quite, not counting meals and migrations, and I cannot do any consecutive work by myself. But I could direct a young man who could be set to work under my eye and with all my ideas. On looking through the list of malaria bearing Anophelines, and the literature concerning them I remain very dissatisfied. You know that Myssorhynchus mauritianus which was said to be malaria bearing in Mauritius proved not to be.[7] The fact is that precious little careful work has been done on this point. If therefore I could start with malaria work now in this manner, I should be ready shortly to take up your subjects Nos. 5 and 7 connected with malaria.

3. Your proposals 1, 2, 4 and 6 on Kala-azar, Schistosomum Filaria loa, and Trypanosomiasis, are all excellent, and I quite agree with you that your specialists could do the first three of these. My proposals No. 2 and 4 could be done in Liverpool at little expense, probably less than I have given. My proposal No. 7 concerning Sand-

flies in Malta might cost very little indeed. I do not think much of Boyce's suggestion for leprosy, because the matter is already being worked in Leper settlements. We want to continue our Runcorn Researches on Sleeping Sickness etc., because it would be a pity to drop them when we have got all the apparatus and the strains going.[8]

4. I have copied out your list and attached it to mine, and am sending both, merely provisionally of course, to Read, as he has asked me for mine. I also enclose them herewith for you.

5. Now again about the Malaria Bureau. If you let me have it I will charge nothing for Directorship, but a librarian or assistant director must be appointed, and I was thinking that this might be an appropriate billet for Sambon. Perhaps however the pay would be too small for him, because we could scarcely afford more than £250 a year at least to begin with. This Bureau could do an immense deal of good in many lines, and as you know, I also suggested a Bureau for general sanitation. We could also combine yellow fever with the malaria Bureau.

This is only a hurried dictated letter to keep you in touch with our ideas here.

Yours very sincerely

[R. Ross]

1 Letter 245.

2 **RA** 58/006 (see below, 'List of Researches on Tropical Diseases which may be proposed')

3 Sambon went to Italy to investigate Pellagra, *Progress Report on the Investigation of Pellagra* (London: John Bale, Sons & Danielsson, 1910), and Letter 250.

4 Ross had proposed a malaria bureau, based at the Liverpool School. Nye and Gibson (1997), 153 ff.

5 Herbert James Read, (1863-1949), Chamberlain's Private Secretary and Principal Clerk at the Colonial Office. He was one of the prime movers in the planning and execution of the London School of Tropical Medicine.

6 Established in 1908 with the support of the Colonial Office.

7 Ross had visited Mauritius in 1907 to advise on malaria (R. Ross, *Report on the Prevention of Malaria in Mauritius*, London: J. & A. Churchill, 1908). He believed that malaria had been introduced into the island in 1866, via imported *Anopheles* species.

8 Power (1998). The Liverpool School had research Laboratories at Runcorn.

Provisional [added in pencil]

List of Researches on Tropical Diseases
which may be proposed
R. Ross [added in pencil]

1. Researches on malaria to be carried out with cases in the Royal Southern Hospital at Liverpool.

(a) Studies of the urine, etc. to show the relation between ordinary malaria and blackwater fever.

(b) Estimation of the exact effect or various forms of treatment on the parasites.

(c) Cytology of the parasites and if possible their cultivation in various mosquitoes in Liverpool — this work not having yet been completed.

(d) Some experiments on Larvicides.

Expense Say £250 a year for one research student (and some small additional expenses) to work under Professor Ross.

2. Researches on *Ascaris lumbricoides* to be carried out in Liverpool with the ~~personal~~ assistance of the Health Department.

Expense Say £250 a year for one research student under Professor Ross and Dr Stephens.

3. Continued researches on Sleeping Sickness, Piroplasma, Spirochaetes etc., at Runcorn consisting of Director (£250), one assistant (£120), unqualified assistant, and two boys (£130), besides current laboratory expense.

(a) Treatment continued.

(b) Immunity of all these parasites.

(c) Life histories with special regard to carrying agents.

Note. A chemist added to the staff would be highly desirable. We possess a complete chemical laboratory, but have no one to work. Salary say £150.

4. Amoebic Dysentery in Liverpool. One research assistant under Dr. Stephens.

Expense. Say £250 a year.

5. Research on Pellagra in Italy and afterwards in the West Indies.

One student and expenses at the rate say of £600 a year.

6. Leprosy suggested by Sir R. Boyce.

Expense, say £600 a year.

7. Bionomics of Sand flies, etc. by Mr R. Newstead, during July-September in Malta.

Expense say £100.

Letter 247
02/311

21 Queen Anne St.
12th May [1910]

Dear Ross,
I am very much obliged to you for your kind letter. I had a relapse yesterday & the prospect of getting over to Ireland is very poor indeed. I want to send you your letters before we change houses at the end of June, but I cannot get up myself to find then, & my people do not know where they are. I have got some others I want to send with them, but I have been so busy or so seedy lately.

Yours sincerely
(for) Patrick Manson

Thanks for information about the malaria.[1]

1 Possibly a reference to Ross's *Prevention of Malaria*, published later that year by John Murray.

Letter 248
02/312

Royal Hotel & Baths,
Matlock Bath.
15th Oct. 1910.

My dear Ross,
Many thanks for the Apercu General sur le Travail etc etc. It is a long winded affair. Leptomonas Davidi is interesting.[1] I wonder if one of those protozoa of plants can flourish in vertebrates - just as some of the fungi can & probably do.

I am here trying to get my gouty joints to work & will not be in London till the 31st when I hope to send your letters if I can lay my hands on them. All my papers have been muddled up in the confusion of flitting to 50 Welbeck St. where I am now installed.

I was ill and away at the time of flitting & could not look after things.

I had good fishing at first in Ireland - 20 salmon & many sea & brown trout but last month there was no rain & sport tapered down to next to zero.

Yours sincerely
Patrick Manson

1 Reference untraced.

Letter 249
L17/1/14

50, Welbeck Street. W.
10th Nov 1910

Dear Ross,
Please send me the translations you refer to. Sambon says he does not know them but that other authors have referred the disease to insect bites. Sambon says you must read his report which will be sent you by the Colonial Office soon. It is in the printers hands.

At last I have got your letters which should reach you by an early post.

Yours sincerely
Patrick Manson

Letter 250
L17/1/15

11th November 1910.

Private

My dear Sir Patrick,
I enclose two of the publications on Fagopyrism in very rough translation. You will see that Raubitschek especially has proved that if white animals are fed exclusively on certain grains, such as maize and rice and are also kept in bright sunlight, they will develop a series of symptoms such as skin affections on the parts exposed to the light, and also generally poisoning, which leads to death; but that if similar animals are fed on the same diet and kept in the dark, nothing happens.[1] We have here a condition homologous to Pellagra and also perhaps beri-beri.[2] The discovery was made quite independently of researches on these diseases, and there is other literature.

Will you kindly return me the papers when you have done with them, as we shall probably begin to study the matter almost at once. Sambon could easily get the papers if you give him the references.

I have already read Sambon's report in the Journal of Tropical Medicine.[3] It seems to be another case of that old error of doctors of insufficient random sampling. He tries in effect to make out that there is a topographical correlation between the distribution of Pellagra and of sand flies. Instead of giving us any complete maps on these matters, all he does is to examine two or three places where he found Simulium together with beri beri. Of course he did not have time to make a thorough investigation; but he had no right to pretend that this very insufficient random sampling gives any real evidence. Much less had he any authority to write to the lay press stating positively that Simulium carries the disease. This sort of thing produces the worst possible impression. It is not science.

I hope you are doing quite well now as you are back in town. No hurry about this.

Yours sincerely
[R. Ross]

1 This primary photosensitivity disease, mostly of sheep and cattle, is caused by the ingestion of *Fagopyrum esculentum* (buckwheat). The specific publications have not been identified although H. Raubitschek published several papers around this date.

2 For a recent survey, with further bibliography, see Kenneth J. Carpenter, 'Nutritional diseases', in W. F. Bynum and Roy Porter (eds.), *Companion Encyclopedia of the History of Medicine*, 2 vols, (London: Routledge, 1993), i, 464-483.

3 L. W. Sambon, 'Progress report on the investigation of pellagra', *Journal of Tropical Medicine and Hygiene*, 13 (1910), 271-282; 287-300; 305-315; 319-321, reprinted as *Progress Report on the Investigation of Pellagra* (London: John Bale, Sons & Danielsson, 1910). Sambon's long report surveyed previous theories of the aetiology of pellagra, most of which implicated maize in some way. In contrast, he argued on epidemiological and clinical grounds that the disease was probably parasitic in nature, and that the parasite was probably spread through a species of the sandfly *Simulium*. He admitted (pp.290-1) that he had formed his opinions before leaving London for Italy. See, also, Daphne Roe, *A Plague of Corn: The Social History of Pellagra* (Ithaca: Cornell University Press, 1973).

Letter 251
L17/1/19

50 Welbeck Street,
Cavendish Sq,
17th November, 1910.

Dear Ross,
Herewith fagopyrism. It is very interesting but it does not explain the endemic behaviour of pellagra. I am sorry you were not at the meeting of the pellagra committee[1] last night and that you do not support Sambon who with all his failings, and they are many, has a certain capacity for research and much enthusiasm in certain directions.

Thank God I am able to hobble about again though not very actively.

Yours sincerely
Patrick Manson

1 The Pellagra Investigation of the Royal Society of Tropical Medicine consisted of twenty-four members, including many of the elites of tropical medicine and three Italians, among them the Marquis of San Giuliano, the Italian Ambassador to Britain. ('Pellagra Investigation Committee', *Journal of Tropical Medicine and Hygiene*, 13 (1910), 60-63.

Letter 252
L17/1/20

21st November 1910

Dear Sir Patrick,
Thanks for returning the papers on Fagopyrism.[1] So far as I can see the variations in the local prevalence of pellagra can easily be explained by it just as the similar variations in the case of Beri-beri can be explained by the rice theory. Cantlie appears to have omitted to have stated at the Pellagra Committee what I asked him to state, namely that I could not be present owing to the notice of the meeting having been given to me only the day before. I certainly agree with you that Sambon has a certain capacity for research and much enthusiasm and also think that he ought to be helped in some way if possible. Unfortunately judgement is also required. Medical men are too fond of accepting all kinds of hypotheses

on what is really no evidence at all. His work in Italy would have been very good, if he had added cautious conclusions to it, but he seems to have jumped at once to the idea that his hypothesis is *proved*, and this came out everywhere in the lay press. He seems to me to have scarcely sufficient evidence even for a reasonable working hypothesis in favour of pellagra being due to Simulium.

Yours very sincerely
[R. Ross].

1 Letter 250, note, 1.

Letter 253
72/236

50, Welbeck Street. W.
20th June 1911

Dear Ross,
Best congratulations on too longed delayed honours.[1] May you live long to enjoy them.

I got home from Ireland this morning to hear of your good fortunes and of poor little Boyce's death.[2] Latterly he was badly off the track but before, & for some time after, his first seizure he was an amiable and able [illegible] & I liked him.

Yours sincerely
Patrick Manson

1 Ross was made Knight Commander of the Order of the Bath in the Coronation Honours of George V.
2 Sir Rubert Boyce, Dean of the Liverpool School, died on 16 June 1911.

Letter 254
02/342

36 Harley House
Regents Park NW. 1[1]
13th December, 1920

Sir Patrick Manson, G.C.M.G., M.D.,
24a Portland Place, W.

Dear Sir Patrick Manson,
I am writing to you regarding our correspondence while I was

working on malaria from May 1895 to February 1899. You may remember that about 1905 we made an arrangement to the following effect:-

(1) That you were to send me all my letters to you to enable me to have complete copies of them made.

(2) That I should have complete copies made of your letters to me.

(3) That I was to retain the originals of my letters to you and return to you the originals of yours to me.

(4) That I was to supply you with a copy of my letters to you, and retain a copy of your letters to me.

(5) That I was free to publish my letters to you or to deposit copies in any museum should I wish, but that I was not free to deal with your letters to me.

I remember that it took a long time to have these copies made owing to the fact that all the copies had to be verified by me personally, and also because little marginal drawings in my letters to you had to be inserted into the copies. But about 1908 the work was done, and I have always believed that I sent you one copy of my letters to you and the originals of yours to me. I have a letter from you dated 21st October 1908, saying, "Your letters though long delayed are none the less welcome. When the balance arrives and if you are kind enough to give me a copy of mine I would like to deposit them in the library of the School of Tropical Medicine, etc.".[2] I think that this word "balance" refers to the originals and one copy of your letters to me, which, so far as I remember, were not sent to you with the copies of mine to you about 1908. I think that when I was starting for India about February 1909[3] I directed the typist of the Liverpool School of Tropical Medicine (or the librarian there) to send you the originals of your letters to me together with one copy of the same, and to put up the originals of mine to you together with other copies of the whole series in a packet. I was in a great hurry when leaving for India and, thinking that what I had ordered had been done I took no further interest in the matter at the time. The parcel referred to however has always been in my possession; but I did not open it until about six weeks ago, when, to my astonishment, I found the following enclosures.

(1) All the originals of your letters to me together with one set of copies of the same.

(2) Half the originals of my letters to you, namely from 1st May 1895 to 12th June 1897, the remaining half from the

latter date to the 15th February 1899 (when the correspondence closed) being missing.

(3) Three complete copies of all my letters to you, but having the marginal drawings entered only upon the best copy, the two carbon copies not having them.

I infer therefore that when I had left for India the said clerk or librarian must have made some mistake. Apparently one complete set of copies of my letters to you had been forwarded to you previously in 1908 (as I have said); but the clerk or librarian, instead of sending me the originals of yours to me, now forwarded one copy of yours to me together with half the originals of mine to you.

Will you therefore kindly inform me if you can what happened in the case? I infer that you have got one complete set of copies of the whole correspondence, together with half the originals of my letters to you. I do not possess any letter from you in 1909 acknowledging the receipt of the remaining correspondence but you may have sent a receipt to the clerk or librarian. I suppose that the clerk or librarian made a mistake as to the original letters which were to be returned to you. You had proposed to deposit your part of the correspondence at the London School of Tropical Medicine, but I gather from enquiry that those documents are not there now. I shall be very much obliged if you will kindly tell me if you have the missing half of my original letters to you. As I have never heard again from you on the matter I had always supposed that our original arrangement had been completed.

Believe me
Yours sincerely
[R. Ross]

1 Ross moved to London in 1912, though his formal association with the Liverpool School was not severed until 1917.

2 Letter 240.

3 The Bombay Medical Congress at which Ross spoke on the practice of malaria prevention.

Letter 255
02/341

24 A Portland Place
London. W.
14th December 1920

Dear Sir Ronald Ross,
Referring to your letter of yesterday's date, I regret that I have none of the correspondence you refer to with me here. All my letters are in Ireland under lock and key and I have no one whom I could trust over there to look through my papers.[1] I will, however, be in Ireland again in May when I shall be only too delighted to accede to your request. Should you not hear from me in due course, kindly remind me of your request.

Yours faithfully
Patrick Manson

1 Since the complete series of originals is now in the Library of the London School of Hygiene and Tropical Medicine, it may be assumed that Manson located the missing letters in his home in County Galway.

Biographical Appendix

Abbreviations used:

DNB	*Dictionary of National Biography*
DSB	*Dictionary of Scientific Biography*
DAB	*Dictionary of American Biography*
Munk's Roll	*Lives of the Fellows of the Royal College of Physicians of London*
Plarr's Lives	*Plarr's Lives of the Fellows of the Royal College of Surgeons of England*

These biographies are brief summaries of the careers and influence of the major personalities mentioned in the Correspondence. The index will provide further details of their part in the Ross-Manson correspondence. References are to obituaries or secondary sources where their work is discussed.

Annett, Henry Edward, (1871-1945), MD, MBE. Educated at University College, Liverpool, and the Victoria University, Annett accompanied Ross on his first trip to Freetown, Sierra Leone, in 1899. (Letters **185-187**) He directed later expeditions to Africa, the West Indies, and Uruguay. At the time of the first Freetown expedition, Annett was a demonstrator in tropical pathology at the new Liverpool School, where he remained as lecturer after becoming Professor of Comparative Pathology (1906-1911) in the University of Liverpool. He then became a Medical Officer of Health, first at Runcorn, then at Widnes, before returning to Liverpool, where he continued research on veterinary medicine and cancer.

Who was Who, 1951-60; Power (1998); Ross, *Memoirs.*

Austen, Ernest Edward, (1867-1938). Austen, educated at Rugby

School and the University of Heidelberg, spent his entire career, except for military service during the Boer War and World War I, at the British Museum of Natural History, where he finished as Keeper of Entomology. Collecting expeditions to Brazil and, with Ross, to Sierra Leone, gave him tropical experience. (Letters **185-187**) Most of his work was with mosquitoes and flies, and he served on the Royal Society Sleeping Sickness Committee. His forte was entomological taxonomy, on which he published several monographs, as well as pamphlets aimed at providing practical advice on the role of insects in the spread of disease.

William T. Stearn, *The Natural History Museum at South Kensington* (1981), 215-6.

Bignami, Amico, (1862-1929). Although Bignami was born in Bologna, his education and career were based in Rome, where in 1906 he became Professor of General Pathology. He published on a number of topics, including cerebral anatomy, acromegaly, and leucaemia. He was also a key worker in the 'Italian School' of malariology. He proposed an 'inoculation' theory of its transmission before Ross discovered the parasite in *Anopheles*, (Letter **48**) wrote an influential monograph with Ettore Marchiafava (q.v.) and, with G. B. Grassi (q.v.), Giovanni Bastianelli, and others, worked out the human transmission cycle from 1898. Although Ross reserved his greatest opprobrium for Grassi, he also painted a dark portrait of Bignami in his *Memoirs*.

Dizionario Biografico degli Italiani; Scott (1939); Harrison (1978); Ross, *Memoirs*.

Blanchard, Raphael Anatole, (1857-1919), MD. Blanchard played for French tropical medicine a similar role to that of Manson for British. He was educated at the University of Paris, where he became Professor of Medical Natural History in 1897. The name of the chair was subsequently changed to 'parasitology', and Blanchard established the *Archives de Parasitologie* in 1898, and the Institute of Colonial Medicine in 1902. He published a treatise on 'medical zoology' which Ross used in India and a monograph on mosquitoes in 1905. He was also active in issues relating to the international standardisation of zoological nomenclature. He frequently visited Britain, and was present at the BMA meeting in 1898 when Manson read out Ross's telegrams. (Letter **146**)

G. Lavier and J. Théodoridès, 'Raphael Blanchard (1857-1919), médecin, naturaliste, et fondateur de la Société Française d'Histoire de la Médecine', *Histoire de la Médecine*, 7 (1957), 75-82; *BMJ* (1 March 1919), 265-266; *Lancet* (22 Feb. 1919), 315.

Bland-Sutton, Sir John, (1855-1936), FRCS. Bland-Sutton's surgical career was associated with the Middlesex Hospital, where he acquired a good reputation as an abdominal and gynaecological surgeon. He had in addition wide scientific and cultural interests, especially in comparative pathology and in the evolutionary significance of disease. He was a competent microscopist, and this, combined with his knowledge of the diseases of animals, may have been the reason why Manson selected him, along with George Thin (q.v.) to comment on Ross's classic paper in the *BMJ*. (Letter **99**) In his later life, Bland-Sutton published several volumes of travel and autobiography.

J. Bland-Sutton, *The Story of a Surgeon* (1930); *BMJ* (2 Jan. 1937), 47-50; DNB; Plarr's Lives.

Boyce, Sir Rubert William, (1863-1911), FRS. An Irishman by birth, Boyce became interested in research while working with Victor Horsley at University College London. He was appointed to the Chair in Pathology at the University of Liverpool in 1894, and he helped create a School of Hygiene there as well as demonstrating talent in interesting local businessmen to support medical research. He was also actively involved in Liverpool public health. He published a textbook on pathological histology and was active from the first in running the new Liverpool School of Tropical Medicine. While Ross resented him to an extent as an opportunistic interloper within tropical medicine, Boyce published two volumes, *Mosquitoes or Man?* (1909) and *Yellow Fever and its Prevention* (1911) which did much to popularise the field. He suffered a stroke a few years before his early death.

BMJ (1 July 1911), 53-4; DNB; Ross, *Memoirs*; Power (1998).

Bruce, Sir David, (1855-1931), FRS. Bruce was born in Australia of Scottish parents. After a few years working in a business firm, he went to the University of Edinburgh with the intention of studying zoology. He switched to medicine instead, qualifying in 1881. He joined the Army Medical Service, where his posting to Malta gave him the opportunity of investigating an obscure local disease, 'Malta fever'. Bruce showed it to be bacterial, caused by the organism now known as *Brucella melitensis*. Following a brief period studying with

Robert Koch, Bruce then taught pathology at the Army Medical School at Netley (1889-1894). Posted to Africa, he did fundamental work on both animal and human trypanosome infections, and on the tsetse-fly which acted as the vector. There were priority disputes around discovery in trypanosomes which mirror those in malaria. During World War I, Bruce directed research on the aetiology and control of tetanus and trench fever.

DNB; DSB; *Obit. Not. Fell. Roy. Soc.*, 1 (1932-35), 79-85; Scott (1939); Maryinez Lyons, (1992); Paul Cranefield, *Science and Empire: East Coast Fever in Rhodesia and the Transvaal* (Cambridge: Cambridge University Press, 1991).

Carter, Henry Vandyke, (1831-1897), MD. Carter, whose father was an artist, also had much artistic talent, producing many of the illustrations for *Gray's Anatomy*, while he was a demonstrator of anatomy at St. George's Hospital Medical School. He had studied medicine at University College London, acquiring a University of London MD. Joining the Indian Medical Service in 1858, he was almost immediately made acting professor of anatomy and physiology at the Grant Medical College. From the mid 1860s he held various posts in hospitals and gaols, returning to Grant Medical College as its Principal in 1877. After his retirement in 1888, Carter was given the rank of Deputy Surgeon-General of the Indian Medical Service, as a token of approval of his contributions. Ross believed that this was insufficient recognition, and that he should have been made Surgeon-General during his active career. (Letters **21**, **75** and **112**) He was an extremely gifted observer and researcher who made contributions to the understanding of relapsing fever, leprosy, 'Delhi boil' and other fungal diseases of the skin, and elephantiasis. He was the first in India to appreciate the significance of Laveran's work on *Plasmodium*. Ross always singled out Carter and Cunningham (q.v.) as exceptions, in his condemnations of the lack of a research ethos within the Service. Curiously, he did not search Carter out in the early 1890s, when Ross first became interested in malaria.

BMJ (15 May 1897), 1256-7; *Indian Medical Gazette* (June 1897), 224.

Chamberlain, Joseph, (1836-1914). A radical, reforming politician with local (Birmingham) and national experience, Chamberlain became Colonial Secretary in 1895, in Lord Salisbury's government. His ambition was to strengthen the ties between Britain and the self-governing colonies, and to develop the resources in the rest of them, with the aim of increasing trade. He recognised the importance of health, and, under the influence of Manson, induced the Treasury to provide half the cost of the London School of Tropical Medicine. He also authorised the establishment of the Royal Society Malaria Committee, (Letter **141**) the enlargement of the British pharmacopoeia and the more systematic production of annual medical and sanitary reports from the Crown Colonies.

DNB; G. L. Garvin [and Julian Amery], *The Life of Joseph Chamberlain*, 6 vols. (London: Macmillan, 1932-1969); Richard Jay, *Joseph Chamberlain: A Political Study* (Oxford: Clarendon Press, 1981).

Cleghorn, James, (1841-1920), MD, CSI. Cleghorn attended the universities of Edinburgh and Vienna, took his MD at St. Andrews and entered the Army Medical Service in 1864, the Indian Medical Service then being closed. When it reopened the following year, he took the examination, along with Robert Harvey (q.v.), who succeeded him as Director General of the IMS. Cleghorn rose steadily up the ranks of the IMS, becoming Inspector-General of Civil Hospitals in the Punjab in 1891 and Director General in 1895. He held the post until 1898 and was thus the ultimate arbiter of Ross's professional fate, during the years when Ross was attempting to secure research leave.

BMJ (26 June 1920), 884.

Cobbold, Thomas Spencer, (1828-1886), MD, FRS. After a surgical apprenticeship to J. G. Crosse of Norwich, Cobbold became assistant to John Hughes Bennett at the University of Edinburgh, where he subsequently received his MD. Edward Forbes stimulated his interests in geology and natural history more generally, and in 1857 he went to London, where he lectured in botany at St. Mary's Hospital Medical School and on comparative anatomy and zoology at the Middlesex Hospital. He was forced to supplement his income with medical practice, where he consulted in cases where parasitic disease was suspected. His monographs on the parasites of human beings and domestic animals were standard during the third quarter of the century, and the Royal Veterinary College established a special chair in helminthology for him.

DNB; *Lancet* (27 March 1886), 616-617.

Crombie, Alexander, (1845-1906), MD, CB. A Scotsman, Crombie was educated at the University of Edinburgh. He entered the Army Medical Service in 1871, the Indian Medical Service being temporarily closed; but the following year it was re-opened and he was allowed to change, obtaining top marks in the Netley examinations. He arrived in India in 1872 and enjoyed a successful career there, holding surgeoncies in Rangoon, Dacca and Simla, and ending as Superintendent of the Presidency General Hospital in Calcutta. He published on a number of topics, including vaso-cardiac drugs, diarrhoea, cholera, and antipyretics, and briefly edited the *Indian Medical Gazette*. After his retirement in 1898, he became lecturer in tropical diseases at the Middlesex Hospital in London and a member of the Medical Board at the India Office.

BMJ (20 Oct. 1906), 1069-1070; *Lancet* (13 Oct. 1906), 1035.

Crosthwaite, Sir Charles Haukes Todd, (1835-1915), KCSI. Crosthwaite entered the Indian Civil Service in 1857, following graduation from St. John's College, Oxford. He held increasingly senior posts in various parts of India, including the North-Western Provinces, the Central Provinces and Burma, ending his Indian career as Lieutenant-Governor of the North-Western Provinces and Oudh. In 1895 he returned to England, as a member of the Council of India. He wrote a number of monographs on Indian topics and was a vigorous opponent of the Morley reforms.

DNB.

Cunningham, David Douglas, (1843-1914), FRS. Of Scottish origin, Cunningham received his medical education at the University of Edinburgh and entered the IMS in 1868, the year after his graduation. He topped the lists at Netley and was in consequence chosen, with Timothy Lewis (1841-1886), to study bacteriology and hygiene with Max von Pettenkofer in Germany, preparatory to an investigation of cholera in India. For ten years after their arrival in Calcutta in 1869, Cunningham and Lewis were attached as special assistants to the department of the Sanitary Commissioner, where cholera was their principal concern. In the 1880s, Cunningham had laboratories built to his specification in Calcutta, and he continued to work on a number of physiological and pathological problems, including the action of snake-venom, fungal disease, and mycetoma. His botanical interests led to his taking charge, when Sir G. King was on leave, of the Cinchona department and the Calcutta Royal Botanic Garden. He continued his natural historical work after he retired to England in 1898. Ross characterised him, along with Lewis and Vandyke Carter, as one of the few officers actually pursuing experimental medical work in India during the nineteenth century.

DNB; *Proc. Roy. Soc. London*, 84, 1917, xv-xx; Isaacs (1998).

Daniels, Charles Wilberforce, (1862-1927), FRCP. Son of a clergyman, Daniels studied medicine at Cambridge University and the London Hospital. He entered the Colonial Medical Service in 1890, where postings took him to the Fiji Islands and British Guiana. In the latter location, his work with filaria brought him into correspondence with Manson, who arranged his appointment as the Royal Society Malaria Committee representative to join Ross in Calcutta. (Letter **162** onwards) He then went to Africa, where S. R. Christophers and J. W. Stephens were. Daniels briefly became superintendent of the London School of Tropical Medicine before going to Kuala Lumpur in 1903 as director of a new Institute for Medical Research there. On his return to London, he lectured on tropical diseases at several London medical schools, and succeeded Manson as medical advisor to the Colonial Office. He published a three volume survey, *Tropical Medicine and Hygiene* (1907-12), although this never secured a niche in the field. Ill health forced his retirement in 1920.

Lancet (13 Aug. 1927), 361; *BMJ* (13 Aug. 1927), 287-288; Munk's Roll; Wilkinson and Hardy (1998).

Fayrer, Sir Joseph, (1824-1907), FRS, FRCS, FRCP. Fayrer's long and colourful life included experiences in the Sicilian revolution (1848), survival of the siege of Lucknow (1857), and travelling with the Prince of Wales on his grand tour of India (1875). Originally destined for engineering, Fayrer became interested in medicine while in Bermuda, where an outbreak of yellow fever occurred. He trained at Charing Cross Hospital (where he was a contemporary of T. H. Huxley) and went to India as an assistant surgeon in 1850. His career there flourished and in 1859 he became professor of surgery at the Medical College, Calcutta. He was a prolific author on surgical, medical and natural historical topics, including a monumental treatise on the poisonous snakes of India. Although Fayrer certainly considered himself a scientific clinician, he had some trouble completely assimilating the implications of germ theory, and his resistance to Ross's work on malaria (Letter **68**) (even while exerting influence to help Ross (Letters **109-114**)) reflected his lingering fondness for earlier climatological formulations of Indian fevers to which he had contributed.

DNB; Munk's Roll; Plarr's Lives; *BMJ* (25 May 1907), 1277-1281; J. Fayrer, *Recollections of my Life* (Edinburgh; London: W. Blackwood, 1900).

Fielding-Ould, Robert, (1872-1951), MD, MRCP. Educated at Oxford, Fielding-Ould was briefly a lecturer in the Liverpool School of Tropical Medicine, following field work, mostly on malaria and leprosy, in Africa (1900-1902). He then settled in London, where he became a consultant at the Mount Vernon Hospital for Diseases of the Chest. He was in Macedonia during World War I and subsequently acted as a consultant to the Ministry of Pensions. He was also a barrister and involved in medico-legal work.

Who was Who, 1951-1960.

Giles, George Michael James, (1853-1916), FRCS. The son of a Naval Captain, Giles studied medicine at St. Mary's Hospital Medical School and after a couple of years as a civil surgeon in South Africa, he entered the Indian Medical Service in 1880, retiring with the rank of Lieutenant Colonel in 1901. He served for some years as Surgeon Naturalist on the *Investigator*, and also worked in the civil branch of the IMS in the Central Provinces and the United Provinces. He wrote an early report on kala-azar (1890), which established a framework to which Leonard Rogers (q.v.) and Ross subsequently responded, and published the first systematic monograph on Indian mosquitoes (1900) in the post-Ross period. Ross remarked rather testily (*Memoirs*, 330) that Giles unfortunately chose a non-malaria bearing mosquito to name after him (*Anopheles rossi*).

Plarr's Lives; *BMJ* (23 Sept. 1916), 442.

Golgi, Camillo, (1843-1926). Born in Corteno (now Corteno Golgi), Golgi studied medicine at the University of Pavia, where he became interested in histology, and where he spent most of his career. He is best remembered for his work on the fine structure of the nervous system, for the study of which he developed a new stain. It was for his neurohistological research, and its implications for the neurone theory, that Golgi shared with Santiago Ramón y Cajal the 1906 Nobel Prize for medicine and physiology. However, from 1885 to about 1893, Golgi did important work in malariology, in particular demonstrating the existence of different species of *Plasmodia*, showing that these different species cause different varieties of disease (quartan, tertian, etc.), and that the onset of fever corresponds to the release of spores, in the asexual part of the organism's life cycle. In the Ross-Manson correspondence, Golgi figures principally as a name which Manson incorrectly wrote instead of Grassi. (Letters **215** and **234**)

DSB; *BMJ* (30 Jan. 1926), 221; Scott (1939); Harrison (1978); Leonida Santamaria, 'Camillo Golgi as clinical pathologist: epicritical reading of Golgi's works on malaria', *Medicina nei secoli*, 6 (1994), 581-608; Paolo Mazzarello, *La Struttura Nascosta: La Vita di Camillo Golgi* (Bologna: Cisalpino, 1996).

Grant, Allan Ewan, (1862-1904). Grant's father was in the Indian Army, so service in India was an obvious choice for him. He entered the Indian Medical Service in 1888, after graduating from the University of Edinburgh. After a couple of years active service, chiefly in Burma, Grant became Second Physician to the General Hospital in Madras, and Professor of Hygiene in the Medical College there. He acquired an excellent reputation as a teacher of hygiene and published a treatise on the subject, *The Indian Manual of Hygiene* (1894). He had almost completed the second volume when he developed diabetes and was forced to return to England, where he died prematurely. At the time he left India in 1902, he had become Acting Sanitary Commissioner with the Government of Madras.

BMJ (6 Feb. 1904), 340-341.

Grassi, Giovanni Battista, (1854-1925). Born in Rovellasca, Grassi studied medicine at Pavia, and then spent several years in Heidelberg, where he worked with the zoologist Otto Bütschli and the anatomist Carl Gegenbaur. He taught zoology and comparative anatomy for twelve years in Catania before being obtaining the chair in comparative anatomy in Rome, where he remained for rest of his life. He did important work across a wide zoological and pathological terrain, including entomology, helminthology, and protozoology. He received the Darwin Medal of the Royal Society for his monumental work on termites, and in the 1880s he discovered that flies could spread a number of pathogenic organisms and instituted anti-fly campaigns. He also did important work on insect pests of grapes. It was his investigations on filaria and malaria which brought him most into contact with the British community. He had contributed much to the knowledge of malaria before 'Mosquito day' (20 August 1897), including the important identification of *Proteosoma praecox*, one of the organisms of bird malaria. However, his attempts to transmit malaria by mosquito bites failed until August 1898. Between then and 1898, Grassi and his colleagues worked out the basic facts of the human cycle, including the identification of female *Anopheles* species as the vector. He was as tenacious as Ross in his claims of priority, and the feud between these two strong-willed men lasted until their deaths. It was intensified by the sole award of the 1902 Nobel Prize for Medicine and Physiology to Ross.

DSB; *Rivista di Biologia*, 19 (1935), 1-46; Ernesto Capanna, ed., 'Battista Grassi, Uno zoologo per la malaria', *Parassitologia*, 38 Supplemento 1 (1996); Scott (1939); Harrison (1978); Ross, *Memoirs*.

Haffkine, Waldemar Mordecai Wolfe, (1860-1930), CIE. Haffkine, a Russian Jew, came under the influence of Elie Metchnikoff (q.v.) as a student at the University of Odessa. After a few years in marginal positions in Odessa (regular posts were closed to him because he refused to convert to Russian Orthodoxy) he joined Metchnikoff at the Pasteur Institute. He there developed a cholera vaccine, which in 1893 he tried out in India, with significant if modest success. In 1895, he caught malaria and went to England to recover, returning to India the next year, when plague was rife. First in Calcutta, then in Bombay, he worked on a vaccine against bubonic plague, which in January 1897 he had injected into himself. It was subsequently used to some effect and his Bombay laboratories became famous. In 1902, in the Punjab, a contaminated batch resulted in the deaths of nineteen people from tetanus, and Haffkine was widely blamed. Ross took up his case in England, and although Haffkine himself was ultimately exonerated, his career was damaged. He spent the last years of his life primarily involved in Jewish affairs, but he lived to see the Plague Research Institute in Bombay renamed in his honour.

DAB; *BMJ* (8 Nov. 1930), 801-802; Selman A. Waksman, *The Brilliant and Tragic Life of W. M. W. Haffkine, Bacteriologist* (New Brunswick: Rutgers University Press, 1964); Löwy (1992); Eli Chernin, 'Ross defends Haffkine: the aftermath of the vaccine-associated Mulkowal Disaster of 1902', *Journal of the History of Medicine and Allied Sciences*, 46 (1991), 201-218; Ross, *Memoirs*.

Hankin, Ernest Hanbury, (1865-1939), ScD. Hankin was educated at University College London and St. Bartholomew's Hospital Medical School. He obtained a fellowship at St John's College, Cambridge and did post-graduate work in Koch's laboratory in Berlin and at the Pasteur Institute. Hankin then went to India where he became director of a bacteriological laboratory at Agra. He was associated with Haffkine's (q.v.) work on vaccines against cholera and plague, and himself contributed to methods to isolate the causative organisms of typhoid and cholera. His most important contribution was of a practical nature, showing how to disinfect wells by the use of potassium permanganate. He published books on cholera and plague, and, after his retirement to England, on prehistoric man.

BMJ (22 April 1939), 850-851; *Lancet* (15 April 1939), 904; Ross, *Memoirs*.

Harvey, Robert, (1842-1901), CB, MD, FRCP. Son of a professor of materia medica at Aberdeen, Harvey took his medical degrees there. Along with Cleghorn (q.v.), he entered the re-opened ranks of the Indian Medical Service in 1865. He immediately saw active service in the Bootan war of 1865-66 and then held various civil and military posts before becoming professor of midwifery in the Calcutta Medical College. He developed a large and successful obstetric practice before deciding to return to active medical military duty, whence he was rapidly promoted through the ranks, from Inspector-General of Civil Hospitals in Bengal, to Surgeon-General of the Punjab Command, before becoming Director-General of the IMS in 1898. In addition to his obstetrical work, Harvey was noted for his medico-legal expertise. Ross had a low opinion of his abilities, but this was softened when Harvey visited Ross in Liverpool in 1901 and offered him a research post back in India. (Letter **179**)

BMJ (14 Dec. 1901), 1775-1776; *BMJ* (28 Dec. 1901), 1876; *Lancet* (14 Dec. 1901), 1705-1706; Munk's Roll; Ross, *Memoirs*.

Hehir, Sir Patrick, (1859-1937), KCIE, FRCPEd, FRSE. An Irishman, Hehir received his medical education at the Calcutta Medical School and the University of Edinburgh. He joined the Indian Medical Service in 1886 and immediately saw active service in Burma and Tirah. He later had senior medical posts in Burma, Bombay and Simla and was active in the Near East during World War I, where he was captured by the Turks at the fall of Kut. Hehir was a prolific author, though his work displayed more industry than originality. He published monographs on sanitation, cholera, medical jurisprudence in India and malaria. His books on malaria were not written until after Ross's Indian work, but they pay appropriate tribute to Ross and contain valuable summaries of the malaria situation on the Sub-Continent in 1910 (*Prophylaxis of Malaria in India*) and 1927 (*Malaria in India*). The latter was written after his retirement to England.

BMJ (22 May, 1937), 1100; *Lancet* (8 May 1937), 1139; Ross, *Memoirs*.

Jones, Sir Alfred Lewis, (1845-1909), KCMG. A Welshman by birth, Jones spent most of his life in Liverpool, where he worked his way up from an apprenticeship to become one of the most successful shipping magnates of his era. By the late 1870s he had become the leading player in the Elder Demster line. He was an exceptionally shrewd businessman, quickly expanding the firm and absorbing other shipping firms. His base also grew to include the Canaries and the West Indies, in addition to West Africa. He used his position in shipping as a springboard for other activities, such as holiday and hotels, banana importation, banking and manufacturing. He had the ear of Joseph Chamberlain (q.v.) and was the principal philanthropist behind the foundation of the Liverpool of Tropical Medicine.

DNB; Power (1998); Peter N. Davies, *Sir Alfred Jones: Shipping Entrepreneur Par Excellence* (London: Europa Books, 1978).

Lankester, Sir Edwin Ray, (1847-1929), FRS. Son of a distinguished doctor and medical officer of health, Lankester acquired his father's love of microscopy, but opted instead to study natural sciences at Oxford, where his brilliance was recognised. This was followed by Continental work and the Jodrell Chair of Zoology at University College London, in 1874. After a stint as Linacre Professor of Comparative Anatomy at Oxford (1891-98), he returned to London as director of the British Museum (Natural History). Lankester was a zoologist of international reputation whose work touched many areas, from embryology to ichthyology and palaeontology and the comparative cerebral anatomy of primates. He also wrote a number of popular books on evolution and other aspects of the natural sciences. It was his work on parasitic protozoa which was of especial use to Ross, however, both when Ross was still in India and after his return, when he used Lankester as a valued consultant.

DNB; Lester (1995).

Laveran, Charles Louis Alphonse, (1845-1922). If 'Mosquito Day' was 20 August 1897, 'Malaria Day' was 6 November 1880, when Laveran first saw the causative parasite of malaria in a blood smear. Like Ross, he was a military medical man, having studied medicine in Strasbourg and, after a competitive examination, become *professeur agrégé* at the French military medical college, *Val de Grâce*. At the time he made his discovery, he was serving in Algeria. He described several of the forms the parasite assumes but did not get very far in relating these to its life-cycle. It took several years for Laveran's 'germ' to be accepted by the scientific community (as the Ross-Manson correspondence amply documents), and Laveran himself believed that his military superiors had no appreciation of the importance of his work. From 1884 until 1896 he occupied various teaching and administrative posts in France; retiring from the army he based himself at the Pasteur Institute, where he did important work on trypanosomiasis, kala-azar and other parasitic infections. He received the 1907 Nobel Prize for Medicine and Physiology for his discovery of the *Plasmodium*.

DSB; Daniel M. Fox, Marcia Meldrum and Ira Rezak (eds), *Nobel Laureates in Medicine or Physiology: a Biographical Dictionary* (New York: Garland, 1990); Marie Phisalix, *Alphonse Laveran, sa Vie et son Oeuvre* (Paris: Masson et cie, 1923).

Lawrie, Edward, (1846-1915). Lawrie was educated at Edinburgh University (MB, CM, 1867) and also studied briefly in Paris. He entered the Indian Medical Service in 1872 and rose through the ranks to become surgeon lieutenant-colonel in 1892. During his time in India, he held various academic positions in Calcutta and Lahore, and became in 1885 the Resident surgeon at Hyderabad, one of the most desirable posts in the Service. His role in the Ross-Manson correspondence is an unfortunate one, since he wasted a considerable amount of talent and energy attacking the mosquito-transmission theory. (Letters **25**, **26**, **32**, **35**, **44** and **158**) Even his obituarists admitted that his zeal sometimes outran his judgement, and that he had difficulty seeing issues in their fullness. Much of his professional activity was spent attempting to prove that chloroform was the safest anaesthetic, a proposition he absorbed as a house-surgeon in Edinburgh, when he had worked with James Syme. He instigated an Indian Chloroform Commission in 1889 and performed an impressive series of experiments on monkeys in his attempt to convince the members of the Commission that chloroform deaths resulted from respiratory failure rather than heart problems. (Letter **90**) Later work showed that he was mistaken.

BMJ (28 Aug. 1915), 350; *Lancet* (4 Sept. 1915), 581; *Lancet* (11 Sept. 1915), 624; *Lancet* (25 Sept. 1915), 712; Lawrence (1992).

Leslie, J. T. W., (1861-1911), CIE. Leslie graduated from the medical school at Aberdeen University and immediately entered the Indian Medial Service. He saw active service in Burma, and after a period in Rangoon became Acting Chemical Examiner for the Government, as well as successfully teaching chemistry. He became Secretary to the Director-General of the Indian Medical Service and Sanitary Commissioner in 1893. He was Ross's main point of contact with the IMS when he attempted to secure his research appointment, but Leslie was also much involved with the plague epidemic in the later 1890s. Ross maintained that Leslie always opposed his ideas, but he participated in the formation of Indian malaria policy in the post-Ross period. He died prematurely, of a heart condition, in the process of being invalided home.

BMJ (8 April 1911), 848-849; Ross, *Memoirs.*

Low, George Carmichael, (1872-1952), MD, FRCP. Low graduated with first-class honours in medicine from Edinburgh in 1897, and then proceeded to London, to study with Manson. Following a brief period in Europe, where he learned newer techniques of microscopical slide preparation, he returned to London, where he was soon able to show, contrary to Manson's beliefs, that the parasite of filaria is transmitted through the bite of the mosquito. (Letter **199**) With L. W. Sambon (q.v.) and Signor Terzi, Low lived for three months from August 1900 in the highly malarious Roman Campagna, where the three successfully used anti-mosquito measures to protect themselves from getting the disease. (Letter **201**) In the early years of the new century, Low worked in British Guiana and in Uganda, the latter as part of the Royal Society's Sleeping Commission investigations. (Letter **228**) Low then became superintendent of the London School of Tropical Medicine, and henceforth his career was based there as a teacher and physician to the Hospital of Tropical Diseases. He was one of the founders of the Royal Society of Tropical Medicine and Hygiene (1907) and a sophisticated ornithologist.

BMJ (9 Aug. 1952), 341-2; *Lancet* (9 Aug. 1952), 296-297; Munk's Roll.

MacCallum, William George, (1874-1944), MD. MacCallum, a Canadian, was educated at the University of Toronto and the Johns Hopkins University School of Medicine. His discovery of the sexual phase of *Halteridium* reproduction was made at his home in the summer after his graduation from medical school. (Letter **105**) He communicated his findings to the British Association for the Advancement of Science, which happened to be meeting in Toronto in 1897. Lord Lister proposed the vote of thanks. He subsequently held the chair in pathology at Columbia University and, from 1917, Johns Hopkins, in succession to his mentor W. H. Welch. He worked on a variety of pathophysiological problems, including the independent functions of the thyroid and parathyroid glands, and valvular heart disease. His *Textbook of Pathology* (1916) went through seven editions during his lifetime.

DAB; Harrison (1978).

Maitland, John, (1853-1908), MD. Maitland attended the medical school at the University of Edinburgh and shortly after entered the Indian Medical Service, where his father had also served. Most of his career was spent in Madras, where he became in 1896 Senior Surgeon to the Madras General Hospital. He did original work on filariasis, including its surgical treatment. His last three years in Madras were spent as Principal of the Medical College and Senior Administrative Officer of the hospital. He was always actively involved in the meetings of the South Indian Branch of the British Medical Association, where Ross had most contact with him. He died prematurely, shortly after his retirement.

BMJ (11 Jan. 1908), 122.

Mannaberg, Julius, (1860-1941), MD. Born in Budapest, Mannaberg studied medicine in Vienna, where he remained for the rest of his career, serving as the head of the outpatient department of internal medicine for more than three decades (1898-1930). In addition to his monographs on malaria, he also published on kidney diseases. Ross had a high opinion of *The Malaria Parasites* (Mannaberg, 1894), especially since it argued that the flagellum was a vital part of the parasite's life-cycle, instead of a part of its death-struggles.

Erna Lesky, *The Vienna Medical School of the 19th Century* (Baltimore: Johns Hopkins University Press, 1976), 289; Ross, *Memoirs*.

Marchiafava, Ettore, (1847-1935). Except for a short period of postgraduate study with Robert Koch, Marchiafava spent his whole career at the University of Rome, as student and, from 1883, professor of pathological anatomy. He made contributions to the understanding of a number of diseases, including meningitis, haemolytic anaemia, glomerulonephritis and myocardial infarction. He also did early pioneering work in malariology, much of it in collaboration with Angelo Celli or Amico Bignami (q.v.). Laveran (q.v.) demonstrated 'his' parasite to Marchiafava and Celli in 1882, and for the next decade, Marchiafava studied the pathophysiological development of the parasite in the human erythrocyte, and the relation between parasite species and clinical forms. Marchifava's monograph on 'aestivo-autumnal' fever, (the Italian name for malignant, i.e. falciparum, malaria) with Bignami, was translated by the New Sydenham Society and provided Ross with a synopsis of Italian work up to 1892. (Marchiafava and Bignami, 1894). His *La Infezione Malarica* (1902), also with Bignami, long remained a standard work.

DSB; *Transactions of the Society of Tropical Medicine and Hygiene*, 29 (1935-36), 425-426; Scott (1939); Harrison (1978).

Marchoux, Émile, (1862-1943). Described by one obituarist as 'the first Pastorian in Africa', Marchoux had a long and distinguished career, working, in addition to Senegal, in the Orient and in Brazil, where his researches (with P-L Simond, q.v.) on yellow fever were especially important. He was educated in Paris and had a lifelong friendship with Émile Roux, with whom he worked at the Pasteur Institute in the 1890s. In addition to yellow fever, Marchoux investigated a number of other diseases, including typhoid, paratyphoid, pneumonia and leprosy. He also had a lifelong interest in malaria, and, with Charles Grall, published a large monograph in 1910. He was active on the League of Nations Malaria Committee during the inter-war years.

Annales de l'Institut Pasteur, 70 (1944), 1-6; *Bulletin de l'Académie de Médecine*, 127 (1943), 586-592; Ilana Löwy, 'Yellow fever in Rio de Janeiro and the Pasteur Institute Mission (1901-1905): the transfer of science to the periphery', *Medical History*, 34 (1990), 144-163.

Maynard, Frederic Pinsent, (1864-1921), FRCS. Maynard was educated at St. Bartholomew's Hospital Medical School and Durham University, where he graduated. He entered the Indian Medical Service in 1887. After six years of military duty, he became medical officer to the Baluchistan-Afghanstan Boundary Commission, following which he went into civil employment in Bengal. In 1905, he was appointed Professor of Ophthalmic Surgery at the Medical College, Calcutta. He published on botany and was also the author of two monographs on ophthalmic surgery. He was acting editor of the *Indian Medical Gazette* in 1898. Ross described him as 'among the first students of the *Plasmodia* in India in 1895 or before'.

BMJ (20 Oct. 1921), 724; *Indian Medical Gazette* (Dec. 1921), 460; Plarr's Lives; Ross, *Memoirs.*

Metchnikoff, Elie, (1845-1916). Although Metchnikoff is most commonly associated with the Pasteur Institute, where he worked for the last third of his life, he had had a varied career before, in his native Russia, as well as Italy and Germany. His approach to biological problems was always comparative and evolutionary, and he was equally adept at invertebrate embryology, protozoology and parasitology. His discovery of the phenomenon he called 'phagocytosis' was of course known to Ross (and was the main reason why Metchnikoff shared the 1908 Nobel Prize with Paul Ehrlich), and Metchnikoff was familiar with ongoing work on Plasmodia. His knowledge of protozoan taxonomy was such that he was a natural expert for Ross and Manson to appeal to. In 1887, he had classified the malaria parasite (which he named *Haematophyllum malariae*) with coccidia. (Letter **137**)

DSB; Alfred I. Tauber and Leon Chernyak, *Metchnikoff and the Origins of Immunology: From Metaphor to Theory*, (New York: Oxford University Press, 1991).

Nuttall, George Henry Falkiner, (1862-1937), MD, FRS. Nuttall was born in San Francisco, of a Scottish father and American mother. He grew up in Europe, where he acquired several languages, and returned to University of California for his medical training. After a brief period at the Johns Hopkins University, he went in 1886 to Germany, where he remained for the majority of the next thirteen years, at Breslau, Göttingen and Berlin. In 1899, he was invited to Cambridge to give a course in bacteriology, and the following year a post was established there for him. He was appointed Quick Professor of Biology in 1906, and in 1921 he became director of the newly-established Molento Institute for Research in Parasitology in Cambridge. He founded and edited two journals, *Journal of Hygiene* (1901) and *Parasitology* (1908). His research touched many areas of parasitology and immunology, including insect vectors and the distribution of British Anophelines. Nuttall's knowledge of the Continental scene made him as especially valuable contact for Ross and Manson.

Obit. Not. Fell. Roy. Soc., 2 (1936-38), 493-499; DNB.

Rogers, Sir Leonard, (1868-1962), FRCS, FRCP, FRS. Described by one obituarist as the 'most outstanding member' of the IMS, Rogers entered the Service in 1893, after his medical training at St. Mary's Hospital Medical School, London. He was especially concerned to relate the findings of the pathology laboratory to the understanding and treatment of disease at the bedside. Rogers rose rapidly in the IMS, becoming professor of pathology in Calcutta in 1900. During the main period of the Ross-Manson correspondence, Rogers investigated kala-azar, which he considered to be a form of chronic malaria, (Letters **79**, **123** and **124**) and his relatively late conversion to the mosquito-transmission theory of malaria led Ross and Manson to undervalue his scientific potential. He made fundamental contributions to the treatment of cholera with intravenous hypertonic saline solutions, to the role of *Entamoeba histolytica* in the causation of liver abscesses and its treatment with emetine, and to the differentiation of tropical 'fevers'. After his retirement from the IMS in 1920, he became a physician to the Hospital for Tropical Diseases, London, and a lecturer at the LSHTM. He was a driving force behind the British Empire Leprosy Relief Association and investigated the drug treatment of leprosy and tuberculosis.

DNB; *BMJ* (29 Sept. 1962), 862-863; L. Rogers, *Happy Toil* (1950); Power (1993).

Sambon, Louis Westenra, (1865-1931), MD. One of the colourful characters of the golden age of tropical medicine, Sambon was of mixed English and French parentage, and received his preliminary medical education at St. Bartholomew's Hospital Medical School before proceeding to the University of Naples, where he graduated MD. He worked on the Italian cholera epidemic of 1884 and developed an epidemiological approach to the study of this and other diseases. He also was an outspoken critic of older climatological theories of tropical diseases. He acquired the patronage of Manson and, with George Carmichael Low (q.v.) and Signor Terzi, participated in the famous experiment in the Roman Campagna. (Letter **201**) He lectured for many years at the London School of Tropical Medicine. He later worked on sleeping sickness and pellagra, where his work failed to satisfy Ross's scientific standards. (Letter **250**) During his later years, he developed a parasitic model of cancer, based on its distribution and epidemiology.

BMJ (12 Sept. 1931), 514-5; *Lancet* (12 Sept. 1931), 613; Wilkinson and Hardy (1998).

Sibthorpe, Charles, (1847-1906), CB, FRCPI. An Irishman and ardent Freemason, Sibthorpe was born and educated in Dublin. He entered the Indian Medical Service in 1870 and in 1875 became Resident Surgeon at the Madras Hospital and Professor of Ophthalmology at the Medical College there. He subsequently taught anatomy and general surgery and produced a *Clinical Manual* for student use which went through four editions. He possessed good organisational abilities, which led to his appointment as Principal Medical Officer to the Rangoon District and, then, to the Secunderabad District. In 1894, he became civil Surgeon-General with the Government of Madras. Ross wanted more support from him in his efforts to secure research leave, but points out in his *Memoirs* that the opposition came mostly from the military side of the Service. Sibthorpe retired in 1900 and died in Dublin.

BMJ (26 May 1906), 1257-1258; Ross, *Memoirs*.

Simond, Paul-Louis, (1858-1947). Simond's medical education in Bordeaux directed him towards the French Naval Medical Corps, and as part of his training he spent two years in French Guyana, where he investigated leprosy. After qualification, he returned abroad, this time to China and Indo-China, where he first encountered plague. He was in Paris in 1895, where he attended Pasteur's funeral and was encouraged by Emile Marchoux (q.v.) to join the staff of the Pasteur Institute. It was from here that he published his 1897 paper, which showed that the flagellum of coccidians was the male element in the sexual cycle of their reproduction. (Letters **99** and **101**) In the same year, he went to India, to undertake field work on Alexandre Yersin's anti-plague serum. He worked in Bombay and Karachi, and in the latter place in April 1898 performed his experiment which offered suggestive evidence that the plague bacillus is transmitted via the rat-flea. Manson was more prescient about the importance of Simond's flagellum work for Ross's own malaria researches, and Ross managed to get Simond's name wrong in his *Memoirs*.

Edward A. Crawford, Jr., 'Paul-Louis Simond and his work on plague', *Perspectives in Biology and Medicine*, 39 (1996), 446-458; Hirst (1953); Harrison (1978); J. Voelckel, 'La vie et l'oeuvre de P. L. Simond', *Médecine Tropicale*, 29 (1969) 429-41.

Smyth, John, (1857-1927). An Irishman, Smyth received his medical education at Queen's College, Belfast and joined the Indian Medical Service in 1881. He saw a good deal of active service and was wounded while serving with the Indian Army in the Sudan campaign of 1885. When Ross knew him, he was professor of pathology at Madras Medical

College and editor of the *Transactions of the South Indian Branch of the British Medical Association*; he subsequently became surgeon to the Maharajah of Mysore, and in 1904, sanitary commissioner and inspector-general of jails in Mysore. He retired from the Service in 1919.

BMJ (16 July 1927), 117.

Sternberg, George Miller (1838-1915), MD. Son of a clergyman, Sternberg graduated from the College of Physicians and Surgeons (later Columbia University) in 1860. He joined the US Army shortly after the outbreak of the Civil War and rose eventually to become (in 1893) its Surgeon-General. He had an eventful medical officer's life, being captured at Bull Run (1863), serving in the Indian Wars in the American West, and surviving a serious attack of yellow fever. Although largely a self-taught medical scientist, he was regarded as the pre-eminent American bacteriologist of his generation. In addition to investigating yellow fever in New Orleans and Havana, he formally enquired into the competing claims of Laveran and Klebs and Tommasi-Crudeli about the nature of the causative organism of malaria. He reported that the *Bacillus malariae* played no part in the disease and in 1885 was the first American to demonstrate Laveran's *Plasmodium*. Independently of Louis Pasteur, he cultivated the pneumococcus. His *Manual of Bacteriology* (1892) was the first systematic American treatise on the subject, and his monograph on *Malaria and Malarial Diseases* (1884) provided an up-to-date summary of the disease as it was then understood.

DAB; John M. Gibson, *Soldier in White. The Life of General George Miller Sternberg* (Durham: Duke University Press, 1958).

Thayer, William Sydney, (1864-1932), MD. Educated at Harvard College and Harvard Medical School (MD, 1889), Thayer studied briefly in Berlin and Vienna. In November 1890, he joined (Sir) William Osler at the Johns Hopkins Hospital, where he remained, as resident physician, professor of clinical medicine, and, eventually, physician-in-chief. He was reputed to be a superb diagnostician and published on many clinical topics, including leucaemia, typhoid, heart murmurs, bacterial endocarditis, and malaria. The latter was still common in Baltimore. His clinico-pathological conferences, run jointly with W. G. MacCallum (q.v.) became legendary, and Thayer exemplified the attributes of the scientific clinician which the Johns Hopkins Medical School so prized.

DAB; DSB.

Thin, George, (1839-1903), MD. Thin was educated at the University of Edinburgh and after a short time in practice in Scotland he went to Shanghai, where he worked for seven years. Returning to Europe, he pursued postgraduate study in dermatology in Paris and Vienna. In his London practice in Harley Street, dermatology gradually gave way to consultations on tropical cases. He also advised banks, businesses and shipping lines doing business in the Far East. He published widely in both areas, including an influential book on sprue and numerous articles on ringworm. He was a competent microscopist and respected participant in the malaria debates on the late 1890s. Although Manson and Ross believed that he undervalued British contributions to medical science, the fact that Manson chose him, along with Bland-Sutton (q.v.) to comment on Ross's important paper (Letter **99**) is indicative of his standing among London doctors.

BMJ (23 Jan. 1904), 221; *BMJ* (13 Feb. 1904), 412; *Lancet* (13 Feb. 1904), 474.

Bibliography

Square brackets around an author's name or [————] indicates that the article was published anonymously. Publication dates are given after the author's name only when they have been so referenced in the notes to the correspondence.

[Anon] 'Resolution regarding the reorganisation of the Sanitary Department in India', *Indian Medical Gazette* (Dec. 1895), 506-508.

[Anon] 'A discussion on the parasite of malaria', *Proceedings of the Royal Medical and Chirurgical Society* , 3rd ser. 8 (1896), 118-151.

[Anon] *How to collect mosquitoes (Culicidae).* London: British Museum, Department of Natural History (1898).

[Anon] 'D. D. Cunningham', *Proceedings of the Royal Society, London*, Series B, 89 (1917), xv-xx.

Adami, J. G. 'On the bactericidal functions of the liver and the etiology of progressive hepatic cirrhosis', *BMJ* (22 Oct. 1898), 1215-1218.

Aitken, William *The Science and Practice of Medicine.* 2 vols. 5th ed. London: Charles Griffin and Company (1868).

Allbutt, Thomas Clifford (ed.) *A System of medicine.* 8 vols. London: Macmillan and Co. Limited (1896-99).

[Annett, H. E.] 'The "malaria" expedition to the West coast of Africa', *Lancet* (9 Sept. 1899), 743; (16 Sept. 1899), 806; (30 Sept. 1899), 912; (14 Oct. 1899), 1041-2.

Arnold, David *Colonizing the Body: State Medicine and Epidemic Disease in Nineteenth-Century India.* Berkeley: University of California Press (1993).

[B, L. F.] 'Review of W. S. Thayer *Lectures on Malarial Fevers* (New York: D. Appleton & Co, 1897)', *Bulletin of the Johns Hopkins Hospital*, 8 (December 1897), 265-267.

Bartrip, P. W. *Mirror of Medicine: A History of the British Medical Journal.* Oxford: Clarendon Press (1990).

———— *Themselves Writ Large. The British Medical Association 1832-1966.* London: BMJ Publishing Group (1996).

Bastianelli, G. and Bignami, A. 'Sullo sviluppo dei parassiti della terzana nell' anopheles claviger', *Bollettino della reale Accademis Medica di Roma*, 25 (1899). A translation was carried out by the Liverpool School, *On the development of tertian parasites in the "Anopheles Claviger"*, **RA** 09/005.

Beaumont, B. E. 'Sir Ronald Ross: A Bio-Bibliography'. MA Thesis: Queen's University, Belfast (1974).

Bignami, Amico, 'Le ipotesi sulla biologica dei parassiti malarici fuori dell' uomo (a proposito di un recente scritto del dott. P. Manson', *Policlinico*, (15 July, 1896), 320-329.

——— 'Hypothesis as to the life-history of the malarial parasite outside the human body. (Apropos of an article by Dr Patrick Manson)', *Lancet* (14 Nov. 1896), 1363-1367; (21 Nov. 1896), 1441-1444. (translation of the above article)

——— 'The inoculation theory of malarial infection', *Lancet* (3 Dec. 1898), 1461-1463; (10 Dec. 1898), 1541-1544.

——— 'On the structure of the semi-lunar and flagellate bodies of malarial fever' *Lancet* (17 Dec. 1898), 1620-1621. (an appendix to the above article)

Blanchard, Raphael *Traité de Zoologie Médicale*. 2 vols. Paris: J.-B. Ballière (1889-1890).

——— 'Instructions à l'usage des médecins, des naturalistes et des voyageurs, rédigées au nom de la Commission du Paludisme', *Bulletin de l'Académie de Médecine, Paris*, 3rd ser. 44 (1900), 6-58.

Bosc, F. J. *Le Cancer*. Paris: Georges Carré et C. Naud (1898).

Boyce, R., Ross, R. and Sherrington, C. S. 'Note on the discovery of the human trypanosome', *Lancet* (22 Nov. 1902), 1426.

Brown, E. Harold 'A Report on *Kala Dukh*, a form of fever met with in the North-East portion of the district of Purnea', *Indian Medical Gazette* (Sept. 1898), 324-330.

Bruce-Chwatt, L. J. (ed.) *The Great Malaria Problem and its Solution* (London: The Keynes Press, 1988).

——— 'History of malaria from prehistory to eradication', in Walther H. Wernsdorfer and Ian McGregor (eds) *Malaria: Principles and Practice of Malariology*. 2 vols. Edinburgh: Churchill Livingstone (1988), i, 1-59.

Bynum, W. F. 'An experiment that failed: malaria control at Mian Mir', *Parassitologia*, 38 (1994), 107-120.

Calandruccio, Sauveur [Salvatore] 'Unicuique suum, Prof. J.[sic] B. Grassi', *Journal of Tropical Medicine*, 4 (1901), 214-221.

Carpenter, Kenneth J. 'Nutritional diseases', in W. F. Bynum and Roy Porter (eds), *Companion Encyclopedia of the History of Medicine*.

2 vols. London: Routledge (1993), i, 464-483.

Carter, H. V. 'Note on some aspects and relations of blood organisms in ague', *Scientific Memoirs by Medical Officers of the Army of India* (1887 part III), 139-167.

Chernin, Eli 'Sir Ronald Ross, malaria, and the rewards of research', *Medical History*, 32 (1988), 119-141.

———— 'Sir Patrick Manson: physician to the Colonial Office, 1897-1912', *Medical History*, 36 (1992), 320-331.

Conyers, J. H. 'Cassava poisoning', *British Guiana Medical Annual and Hospital Reports*, 7 (1895), 91-94.

Cook, G. C. *From the Greenwich Hulks to Old St. Pancras: A History of Tropical Disease in London*. London: Athlone Press (1992).

———— 'Correspondence from Dr George Carmichael Low to Dr Patrick Manson during the first Ugandan sleeping sickness expedition', *Journal of Medical Biography*, 1 (1993), 215-229.

———— 'Dr Patrick Manson's leading opposition in the establishment of the London School of Tropical Medicine: Curnow, Anderson, and Turner', *Journal of Medical Biography*, 3 (1995), 170-177.

Councilman, W. T. and Lafleur, H. A. 'Amoebic dysentery', *The Johns Hopkins Hospital Reports*, 2 (1890-91), 395-548.

Crawford, D. G. *History of the Indian Medical Service, 1600-1913*. London: W. Thacker, (1914).

Crombie, Alexander 'Presidential address in medicine and pathology', *Indian Medical Gazette* (Jan. 1895), 8-14.

———— 'Scientific Research on India', *Indian Medical Gazette* (Mar. 1895), 116-119.

———— 'Treatment of malarial fever', *Indian Medical Gazette* (Feb. 1896), 41-42.

Daniels, C. W. 'The demonstration of malarial organisms', *BMJ* (27 April 1895), 920.

———— 'Discovery of the parental form of a British Guiana blood worm', *BMJ* (16 April 1898), 1011-1012.

———— 'Development of "crescents" in the "small dark" Anopheles prevalent in British Central Africa', *Reports to the Malaria Committee of the Royal Society*, 5th ser. (1901), 41-44.

[———— Waddell, L. A. and Ross, R.] 'A new fashoda incident: the Italian flag hoisted on the mosquito-theory', *Indian Medical Gazette* (Jan. 1899), 15-16.

Dantec. A. le *Précis de Pathologie Exotique: Maladies des Pays Chauds et des Pays Froids*. Paris: Octave Doin (1900).

Fedchenko, Aleksiei Pavlovich [On the structure and reproduction of Filaria medinensis L.] *Izvest. Imp. Obsh. Liub. Estes. (Mosk.)*, 8

(1869-70), 71-82; translated in *American Journal of Medicine*, 20 (1971), 511-23.

Ghosh, Amitav *The Calcutta Chromosome*. London: Picador (1997).

Gibson, G. A. (ed.) *Textbook of medicine*. 2 vols. Edinburgh & London: Young J. Pentland (1901).

Gibson, Mary E. *The Ross Archives Catalogue*. London: London School of Hygiene and Tropical Medicine (1983).

——— 'The Ross/Osler correspondence', *Journal of Medical Biography*, 1 (1993), 117-124.

——— 'Ronald Ross and India', *Indian Journal of Malariology*, 34 (1997), 56-70. *See also Nye and Gibson.*

Giles, G. M. *A Report of an Investigation into the Causes of the Diseases known in Assam as Kálá-azár and Beri-beri*. Shillong: Printed at the Assam Secretariat Press (1890).

——— 'Kala-azar', *BMJ* (26 Mar. 1898), 861.

Grassi, [G.] B. (1900a), *Studi di Uno Zoologo sulla Malaria*. Roma: Tipografia della R. Accademia dei Lincei. (1900).

——— (1900b), 'Per la storia delle recenti scoperte sulla malaria', *Policlinico*, 7 (1900), 593-600.

——— 'Replica del prof. Grassi', *Policlinico*, 8 (1901), 284-288.

——— *Documenti Riguardanti la Storia della Scoperta del Modo di Trasmissione della Malaria Umana*. Milan: A. Racanti (1903).

——— 'Twenty-five years after: a chronicle of the discoveries relating to the transmission of human malaria', *Parasitology*, 16 (1924), 355-64.

——— 'The transmission of human malaria', *Nature*, 113 (1924), 304-7.

——— and Noè, G. 'The propagation of the filariae of the blood exclusively by means of the puncture of peculiar mosquitoes', *BMJ* (3 Nov. 1900), 1306-1307.

Harrison, Gordon *Mosquitoes, Malaria and Man: A History of the Hostilities since 1880*. London: J. Murray (1978).

Harrison, Mark *Public Health in British India: Anglo-Indian Preventive Medicine, 1858-1914*. Cambridge: Cambridge University Press (1994).

Hart, Ernest 'An address on the medical profession in India. Its position and its work', *BMJ* (29 Dec. 1894), 1496-1474.

——— 'Public health legislation and the needs of India', *BMJ* (3 Aug. 1895), 287-291.

Haynes, Douglas 'From the Periphery to the Center: Patrick Manson and the Development of Tropical Medicine as a Medical Specialty in Britain, 1870-1900'. PhD Thesis: University of California, Berkeley (1992).

Hehir, Patrick 'The amoeba coli; its relations to dysentery and tropical supurative hepatitis', *Indian Medical Gazette* (Nov. 1892), 321-323.

———— 'Microscopical observations on the blood and excreta in cases of cholera', Special supplement to the *Indian Medical Gazette* (1892).

———— 'Plasmodium malariae, its importance in the diagnosis of tropical diseases', *Indian Medical Record,* 8 (1895), 326-328.

———— 'The haematozoon of malaria and its discovery in water and soil', *Lancet* (28 Nov. 1896), 1514-1518; (5 Dec. 1896) 1589-1595; also published as *The Haematozoon of Malaria and its Discovery in Water and Soil.* Hyderabad (1896).

———— and Gribble, J. D. B. *Outlines of Medical Jurisprudence for India.* 4th ed. Madras: Higginbotham (1898).

Hirst, Leonard Fabian *Conquest of Plague.* Oxford: Clarendon Press (1953).

Hughes, A. J. 'Some points relating to sanitary polity in India', *Transactions of the First Indian Medical Congress, 24th to 29th December 1894.* Calcutta: Caledonian Steam Printing Works (1895), 227-230.

Isaacs, Jeremy D. 'D D Cunningham and the aetiology of cholera in British India, 1869-1897', *Medical History,* 42 (1998), 279-305.

James, Lawrence *Raj: The Making and Unmaking of British India.* London: Little, Brown and Co. (1997).

Jenner, Louis 'A new stain for rapidly fixing and staining blood', *Lancet* (11 Feb. 1899), 370.

Johnston, Christopher 'Auditory apparatus of the culex mosquito', *Quarterly Journal of Microscopical Science,* O.S. 3 (1855), 97-102.

Kaminsky, Arnold *The India Office, 1880-1910.* London: Mansell (1986).

Kelsch, A. and Kiener, P.-L. *Traité des Maladies des Pays Chauds: Région Prétropicale.* Paris: Ballière (1889).

Kennedy, Dane *The Magic Mountains. Hill Stations and the British Raj.* Los Angeles: University of California Press (1996).

Koch, R. *Gesammelte Werke von Robert Koch.* 2 vols. in 3 parts. Leipzig: Verlag von Georg Thieme (1912).

———— 'Reiseberichte über Rinderpest, Bubonenpest in Indien und Afrika, Tsetse- oder Surrakrankheit, Texasfieber, tropische Malaria, Schwarzwasserfieber', in *Gesammelte Werke von Robert Koch.* 2 vols in 3 parts. Leipzig: Verlag von Georg Thieme (1912), 2, ii, 688-742.

Kumar, Deepak *Science and the Raj, 1857-1905.* Delhi: Oxford University Press (1995).

Labbé, A. 'Sur les coccidies des oiseaux', *Comptes Rendus Hebdomadaires de Séances de L'Académie des Sciences,* 116 (1893), 1300-1303.

——— 'Recherches zoologiques et biologiques sur les parasites endoglobulaires du sang des vertébrés', *Archives de Zoologie Expérimentale et Générale*, 3rd ser. 2 (1894), 55-258.

——— 'Recherches zoologiques, cytologiques et biologiques sur les coccidies', *Archives de Zoologie Expérimentale et Générale*, 3rd ser. 4 (1896), 517-654.

Lankester, E. Ray 'Protozoa', *Encyclopaedia Britannica*. 9th ed. Edinburgh: Adam & Charles Black (1875-89), vol. xix, 830-866.

——— 'Note on the morphological significance of the various phases of haemamoebidae', *Quarterly Journal of Microscopical Science*, 43 (1900), 581-588.

Laveran, A. *Traité des Fièvres Palustres avec la Description des Microbes du Paludisme*. Paris: Octave Doin (1884).

——— 'Des trypanosomes parasites du sang', *Arch. de Méd. Expér. et d'Anat. Path, Paris*, 4 (1892), 257-269.

——— *Paludism* translated by J. W. Martin. London: New Sydenham Society (1893).

——— *Traité d'Hygiène Militaire*. Paris: G. Masson (1896).

——— *Traité de Paludisme*. Paris: Masson & Cie. (1898).

——— 'Sur un travail de M. le Dr. Ronald Ross, intitulé: Note pour l'histoire du parasite du paludisme en dehors de l'organisme humaine', *Bulletin de l'Académie de Médecine*, 3rd ser. 41(1899), 153-161.

——— and F. Mesnil, *Trypanosomes et Trypanosomiases*. Paris: Masson (1904).

Lawrence, Christopher 'Experiment and experience in anaesthesia: Alfred Goodman Levy and chloroform death, 1910-1960', in Christopher Lawrence (ed.) *Medical Theory, Surgical Practice*. London: Routledge (1992), 263-294.

Lawrie, Edward 'An address on the cause of malaria', *Lancet* (16 May 1896), 1334-1338.

——— (1897a), 'Chloroform and the heart', *BMJ* (17 July 1897), 131-132.

——— (1897b) 'Partial anaesthesia with chloroform', *BMJ* (31 July 1897), 271-272.

——— 'The mosquito and the malaria "parasite"', *Lancet* (3 Dec. 1898), 1468-1469.

Léger, Louis 'Le cycle évolutif des coccidies chez les arthropodes', *Compt. Rend. Acad. de Sc., Paris*, 124 (1897), 966-969.

Lester, Joe *E. Ray Lankester and the Making of Modern British Biology*. Farringdon: British Society for the History of Science (1995), 147-149.

Leuckart, Rudolf *The parasites of Man and the Diseases which Proceed from them*, translated by William E. Hoyle. London: Young J. Pentland (1886).

Lingard, Alfred *Report on Horse Surra*. 2 vols. Bombay: Government Central Press (1993; 1898-99).

Liverpool School of Tropical Medicine Historical Record. Liverpool: The University Press of Liverpool (1920).

Low, G. C. 'A recent observation on filaria nocturna in culex: probable mode of infection', *BMJ* (16 June 1900), 1456-1457.

Löwy, Ilana 'From guinea pigs to man: the development of Haffkine's anticholera vaccine', *Journal of the History of Medicine and Allied Sciences*, 47 (1992), 270-309.

Lyons, Maryinez *The Colonial Disease: A Social History of Sleeping Sickness in Northern Zaire, 1900-1940*. Cambridge: Cambridge University Press (1992).

MacCallum, W. G. 'On the flagellated form of the malarial parasite', *Lancet* (13 Nov. 1897), 1240-1241.

———— (1898a), 'Notes on the pathological changes in the organs of birds infected with haemocytozoa', *Journal of Experimental Medicine*, 3 (1898), 103-116.

———— (1898b), 'On the haematozoan infections of birds' *Journal of Experimental Medicine*, 3 (1898), 117-136.

McGuire, William (ed.) *The Freud/Jung Letters: The Correspondence between Sigmund Freud and C. G. Jung*, translated by Ralph Manheim and R. F. C. Hull. London: Hogarth Press (1974).

Maitland, J. 'Removal of adult filariae in cases of lymphangitis', *BMJ* (2 Oct. 1897), 903.

Mannaberg, Julius *The malarial parasites. A description based upon observations made by the author and other observers*, translated by R. W. Felkin. London: New Sydenham Society (1894).

Manson, Patrick 'Diseases of the skin in tropical climates' in A. Davidson (ed.), *Hygiene and diseases of warm climates*. Edinburgh and London: Young J. Pentland (1893), 928-95.

———— 'A Malaria Chart', *BMJ* (1 Dec. 1894), 1252-1254.

———— 'A clinical lecture on the parasite of malaria and its demonstration', *Lancet* (6 Jan. 1894), 6-9.

———— 'The annual oration, 1894. Malaria and its associated parasite', *Hunterian Society Transactions*, 76th session (1894-1895), 19-50.

———— 'Malarial parasites in the blood', *BMJ* (10 Aug. 1895), 394.

———— 'On the guinea worm', *BMJ* (30 Nov. 1895), 1350-1.

———— (1896a), 'The Goulstonian Lectures on the life history of the malaria germ outside the human body', *BMJ* (14 March 1896)

641-646; (21 March, 1896) 712-717; (28 March 1896) 774-779.
——— (1896b), 'The malarial parasite', *BMJ* (30 May, 1896), 1355.
[———] (1896c), 'The microscopic diagnosis of malaria', *BMJ* (1 Feb. 1896), 293.
[———] (1897a) 'A neglected responsibility of empire', *BMJ* (30 Jan. 1897), 289.
——— (1897b) 'A method of staining the malaria flagellated organism', *BMJ* (10 July 1897), 68-70.
——— (1897c), 'The necessity for special education in tropical medicine', *BMJ* (9 Oct. 1897), 985-989.
——— (1897d), 'On certain new species of Nematode Haematozoa occurring in America', *BMJ* (25 Dec. 1897), 1837-1838.
——— (1897e) 'Malarial fever' in Allbutt (ed.) (1896-99), vol. viii, 941-950.
[———] (1897f) 'A malaria problem', *BMJ* (18 Dec. 1897), 1805-1806.
——— (1898a), *Tropical Diseases: A Manual of the Diseases of Warm Climates*. London: Cassell (1898); 2nd edition, London: Cassell (1900).
——— (1898b), 'Surgeon-Major Ronald Ross's recent investigations on the mosquito-malaria theory', *BMJ* (18 June 1898), 1575-1577.
——— (1898c), 'The mosquito and the malaria parasite', *BMJ* (24 Sept. 1898), 849-853.
——— (1898d), 'An exposition of the mosquito-malaria theory and its recent developments', *Journal of Tropical Medicine*, 1 (1898), 4-8.
——— (1898e) 'Appearance of pigmentation in lymphocytes', *BMJ* (24 Sept. 1898), 881.
——— (1898f), 'A clinical lecture on the sleeping sickness', *BMJ* (3 Dec. 1898), 1672-1677.
——— 'The need for special training in tropical disease', *BMJ* (7 Oct. 1899), 922-926.
——— 'Experimental proof of the mosquito-malaria theory', *BMJ* (29 Sept. 1900), 949-951.
——— 'Malaria and malarial disease' in Gibson (1901) vol. i, 290-316.
——— 'Professor Grassi's recent pamphlet', *Lancet* (28 Mar. 1903), 923.
Manson-Bahr, Philip *History of the School of Tropical Medicine in London, 1899-1949*. London: H. K. Lewis (1956).
——— and Alcock, A. *The Life and Work of Sir Patrick Manson*. London: Cassell (1927).
Marshall, Robert J. 'The malaria parasite', *Lancet* (24 Oct. 1896), 1187.

———— and Thin, G. 'The parasite of malaria as observed in the malarial fevers of the south of Spain', *Medico-Chirurgical Society Transactions*, 79 (1896), 101-141.

Marchiafava, E. and Bignami, A. *On Summer-Autumn Malarial Fevers*, translated by J. Harry Thompson. London: The New Sydenham Society (1894).

———— 'Malaria' in Thomas L. Stedman (ed.) *Twentieth Century Practice: an International Encyclopedia of Modern Medical Science*. 20 vols. London: Sampson, Low, Marston, (1895-1900), 19, 1-522.

Maynard, F. P. 'Notes on the examination of malarial blood', *Indian Medical Gazette* (November 1895), 412-420.

Murray, J. 'Notes on the malarial parasite as observed in the blood during life, and in the tissues post-mortem, at Lahore, Punjab', *Scientific Memoirs by Medical Officers of the Army in India*, 10 (1897), 29-52.

Neumann, L. G. *A Treatise on the Parasites and Parasitic Diseases of the Domesticated Animals*, translated and edited by George Fleming. London: Ballière & Co. (1892).

Noè, Giovanni 'Sul ciclo evolutivo della Filaria bancrofti (Cobbold) e della Filaria immitis (Leidy)' *Recherche fatte nel Laboratorio di Anatomia normale della R. Università di Roma ed in altri Laboratorî Biologici'*, 8 (1900-1901), 275-353.

Nuttall, George H. F. 'Die Mosquito-Malaria Theorie', *Centralblatt für Bakteriologie, Parasitenkunde und Infektionskrankheiten*, 25 (1899), 161-170; 209-217; 245-247; 285-296; 337-346.

Nye, Edwin R. and Gibson, Mary E. *Ronald Ross: Malariologist and Polymath. A Biography*. Basingstoke: Macmillan (1997).

Opie, E. L. 'On the haemocytozoa of birds', *Journal of Experimental Medicine*, 3 (1898), 79-101.

Osler, W. 'Malarial fever' in Allbutt (ed.) (1896-99), vol. ii, 721-742.

Pandit, C. G. and Rao, K. Someswara *Indian Research Fund Association and Indian Council of Medical Research, 1911-1961*. New Delhi: Indian Council of Medical Research (1961).

'Pellagra Investigation Committee', *Journal of Tropical Medicine and Hygiene*, 13 (1910), 60-63.

Power, Helen J. 'Sir Leonard Rogers FRS (1868-1962): Tropical Medicine in the Indian Medical Service'. PhD thesis: University of London (1993).

———— *Tropical Medicine in the Twentieth Century: A history of the Liverpool School, 1898-1990*. London: Kegan Paul (1998).

Power, Henry and Sedgwick, Leonard W. *The New Sydenham Society's*

Lexicon of Medicine and the Allied Sciences. 5 vols. London: New Sydenham Society (1882).

Rho, Filippo *La malaria secondo i più recenti studi*. Torino: Rosenberg & Sellier (1896).

Roe, Daphne, *A Plague of Corn: The Social History of Pellagra*. Ithaca: Cornell University Press (1973).

Rogers, Leonard 'The etiology of malarial fever with special reference to the ground water level, and the parasite', *Indian Medical Gazette* (February 1896), 49-55.

——— (1897a) 'On the influence of variations of the ground-water level on the prevalence of malarial fevers', *Scientific Memoirs by Medical Officers of the Army in India*, 10 (1897), 53-58.

——— (1897b) *Report of an Investigation of the Epidemic of Malarial Fever in Assam, or Kala-azar*. Shillong: Assam Secretariat Printing Office (1897).

——— 'The relation of variations in the level of the ground-water to the incidence and seasonal distribution of malarial fevers in India', *Transactions of the Epidemiological Society of London*, 17 (1897-98), 60-77.

——— 'Abstract of a paper on the relationship of drinking-water; - water-logging and the distribution of anopheles mosquitoes, respectively to the prevalence of malaria north of Calcutta', *Indian Medical Gazette* (Sept. 1900), 345-349.

——— 'A reply to Major Ross's criticism', *Indian Medical Gazette* (Dec. 1900), 463.

——— *Happy Toil. Fifty-five Years of Tropical Medicine*. London: Frederick Muller (1950).

Romanowsky, Dimitri 'On the question of parasitology and therapy of malaria', in B. H. Kean, Kenneth E. Mott and Adair J. Russell, (eds) *Tropical Medicine and Parasitology: Classic Investigations*. 2 vols. Ithaca: Cornell University Press (1978), i, 35-44.

Ross, Ronald *The Child of Ocean*. London: Remington (1889).

——— (1893a) 'The true nature of the plasmodium and the malaria parasite', *Indian Medical Gazette* (Oct. 1893), 329-336.

——— (1893b) 'Some objections to haematozoic theories of malaria', *The Medical Reporter*, 2 (1893), 65-71.

——— (1893c) 'Nodulated and vacuolated corpuscles, and the solution of corpuscles mistaken for parasites', *Indian Medical Record*, 4 (1893), 213-214.

——— 'The third element of the blood and the malaria parasite', *Indian Medical Gazette* (Jan. 1894), 5-14.

——— 'Some observations on the crescent-sphere-flagella

metamorphosis of the malaria parasite within the mosquito', *Transactions of the South Indian Branch of the British Medical Association*, (17 Dec. 1895), 334-350, reprinted in the *Indian Medical Gazette* (March 1896), 109-113.

——— (1896a) 'Observations on malaria parasites', *BMJ* (1 Feb. 1896), 260-1.

——— (1896b), 'Some practical points respecting the malaria parasite', *Indian Medical Gazette* (February 1896), 42-49; (March 1896), 86-88.

——— (1896c), 'Surg. Lt. Col. Lawrie and the parasite of malaria', *Indian Lancet* (1 Oct. 1896).

——— (1896d), 'Some experiments in the production of malarial fever by means of the mosquito', *Transactions of the South Indian Branch of the British Medical Association* (Dec. 1896), 93-106.

——— (1896e) *The Spirit of Storm. A romance.* London: Methuen & Co. (1896).

——— (1897a) 'Observations on a condition necessary to the transformation of the malaria crescent', *BMJ* (30 Jan. 1897), 251-255.

——— (1897b) 'Surgeon-Captain Hehir and the parasite of malaria', *Lancet* (20 Feb. 1897), 551-552.

——— (1897c) 'The cause of malaria', *Pioneer* (6 May 1897).

——— (1897d) 'Notes on some cases of malaria, amoeba coli and cercomonas', *Indian Medical Gazette* (May 1897), 172-175.

——— (1897e) *Letter to the Secretary of the United Planters' Association of Southern India.* Madras: Addison & Co (1897).

——— (1897f) 'On some peculiar pigmented cells found in two mosquitos fed on malarial blood. (With a note by Surgeon-Major Smyth, M.D., I.M.S.)', *BMJ* (18 Dec. 1897), 1786-1788.

——— (1897g) 'Further observations on the transformation of crescents', *Transactions of the South Indian Branch of the British Medical Association*, 7 (1897), 118-123.

——— (1898a) 'Pigmented cells in mosquitos', *BMJ* (26 Feb. 1898), 550-551.

——— (1898b) *Report on the Cultivation of Proteosoma, Labbé, in Grey Mosquitos.* Calcutta: Government Printing (1898), reprinted in the *Indian Medical Gazette* (Nov. 1898), 401-408; (Dec. 1898), 448-451.

——— (1899a) *Report on the nature of kala-azar.* Calcutta: Office of the Superintendent of Government Printing (1899).

——— (1899b) 'Extermination of Malaria', *Indian Medical Gazette* (July 1899), 231-232.

——— (1899c) 'The possibility of extirpating malaria from certain localities by a new method', *BMJ* (1 July 1899), 1-4.
——— (1899d) 'An outbreak of fever attributed to mosquitos', *BMJ* (22 July 1899), 208.
——— (1899e) 'Life-history of the parasites of malaria', *Nature* (3 Aug. 1899), 322-4.
[———] (1899f) 'The malaria expedition to Sierra Leone' *BMJ* (9 Sept. 1899) 675-676; (16 Sept. 1899) 746; (30 Sept. 1899) 869-871; (14 Oct. 1899) 1033-1035.
[———] (1899g) *Instructions for the Prevention of Malarial Fever, for the Use of Residents in Malarious Places.* Liverpool: The University Press of Liverpool (1899).
——— (1899h) 'Mosquitos and malaria. The infection of birds by mosquitos', *BMJ* (18 Feb. 1899), 432-433.
——— (1900a) 'Malaria and mosquitoes', *Nature* (29th March 1900), 522-527.
——— (1900b) 'Malarial Fever', *The Medical Annual and Practitioners Index.* Bristol: John Wright & Co (1900), 342-357.
——— (1900c) 'Captain Rogers' recent investigation on malaria', *Indian Medical Gazette* (Dec. 1900), 461-462.
——— (1900d) 'Le scoperte del prof. Grassi sulla malaria', *Policlinico*, 7 (1 Nov. 1900), 550-552.
——— 'Le scoperte del prof. Grassi', *Policlinico*, 8 (1901) 274-284.
——— *First Progress Report of the Campaign against Mosquitoes in Sierra Leone.* Liverpool: University Press (1901).
——— (1902a) 'Some recent chicanery in science', *Lancet* (13 Sept. 1902), 775.
——— (1902b), *Malarial fever, its cause, prevention and treatment.* Liverpool: University Press (1902).
——— (1902c)'Malarial disease', in H. Montague Murray (ed.) *Quain's Dictionary of Medicine.* 3rd ed. London: Longmans, Green & Co (1902), 947-958.
——— 'An improved method for the microscopical diagnosis of intermittent fever', *Lancet* (10 Jan. 1903), 86.
——— *Researches on Malaria being the Nobel Medical Prize Lecture for 1902.* Stockholm: P. A. Norstedt & Soner (1904).
——— 'Parasites of mosquitoes found in India between 1895 and 1899', *Journal of Hygiene*, (April 1906), 101-108.
——— *Report on the Prevention of Malaria in Mauritius.* London: J. & A. Churchill (1908).
——— *The Prevention of Malaria.* London: John Murray (1910).
——— *Memoirs with a Full Account of the Great Malaria Problem and its*

Solution. London: John Murray (1923).
——— 'The transmission of human malaria', *Nature*, (8 March 1924), 353.
——— *Studies on Malaria*. London: John Murray (1928).
——— (ed.) *Letters from Rome on Certain Discoveries Connected with Malaria* ([1929]).
——— *Memories of Sir Patrick Manson*. London: Harrison (1930).
——— Annett, H. E. and Austen, E. E. *Report of the Malaria Expedition of the Liverpool School of Tropical Medicine and Medical Parasitology*. Liverpool: The University Press (1900).
——— and Fielding-Ould, R. 'Diagrams illustrating the life-history of the parasites of malaria', *Quarterly Journal of Microscopical Science*, 43 (1900), 571-579.

Russell, Paul F. *Man's Mastery of Malaria*. London: Oxford University Press (1955).

Sambon, L. W. 'Remarks on the life-history of *Filaria bancrofti* and *Filaria immitis*', *Lancet* (16 Aug. 1902), 422-426.
——— 'Progress report on the investigation of pellagra', *Journal of Tropical Medicine and Hygiene*, 13 (1910), 271-282; 287-300; 305-315; 319-321, reprinted as *Progress Report on the Investigation of Pellagra*. London: John Bale, Sons & Danielsson (1910).

[Sceptic], 'The cause of malaria', *Pioneer*, (25 Apr. 1897), 7.

Schneidemühl, Georg *Die Protozoen als Krankheitserregen des Menschen und der Hausthiere*. Leipzig: Wilhelm Engelmann (1898).

Scott, H. H. *A History of Tropical Medicine*. 2 vols. London: Edward Arnold (1939).

Simond, P.-L. (1897a), 'Recherches sur les formes de reproduction asporulée dans le genre coccidium', *Compt. Rend. Soc. Biologie*, (1 Mai 1897), 425-428.
——— (1897b), 'L'évolution des sporozoaires du genre coccidium', *Annales de l'Institut Pasteur*, 11 (1897), 545-581.

Simpson, W. J. 'The need of a sanitary service for India', *Transactions of the First Indian Medical Congress, 24th to 29th December 1894*. Calcutta: Caledonian Steam Printing Works (1895), 222-227.

Smith, Frederick and Taylor, M Logan 'Two cases of Blackwater fever', *Lancet* (21 Sept. 1901), 776-777.

Stephens, J. W. W. and Christophers, S. R. 'The malarial and blackwater fevers of British Central Africa', *Reports to the Malaria Committee of the Royal Society*, Report No 2. London: Harrison and Sons (1900), 12-42.

Thayer, William Sydney and Hewetson, John *The Malarial Fevers of Baltimore: An Analysis of 616 Cases of Malarial Fever with Special*

Reference to the Relations Existing Between Different Types of Haematozoa and Different Types of Fever. Baltimore: Johns Hopkins Press (1895).

Taylor, M. Logan *Second Progress Report of the Campaign against Mosquitoes in Sierra Leone*. Liverpool: University Press (1902).

Thin, George 'The parasite of malaria and malarial fevers', *Lancet* (6 July 1895), 12-19.

——— 'The etiology of malarial fever', *BMJ* (5 Aug. 1899), 349-354.

Thomas, Henry Sullivan *Tank Angling in India*. Madras: Higginbotham & Co (1887).

Thomson, J. C. 'The prevalence of mosquitoes and malaria in the colony of Hong-Kong', *Lancet* (12 Jan. 1901), 126-127.

Vincent, M. H. 'Contribution à l'étude du processus leucocytaire dans la malaria', *Annales de l'Institut Pasteur*, 11 (1897), 891-908.

Waller, August D. *An Introduction to Human Physiology*. 3rd ed. London: Longmans, Green (1896).

Weatherstone, John *The Pioneers 1825-1900: The Early British Tea and Coffee Planters and Their Way of Life*. London: Quiller Press (1986).

White, P. Carr 'A short note on the change the malarial parasite undergoes in the mosquito', *Indian Medical Gazette* (April 1896), 121.

Wilkinson, Lise and Hardy, Anne *Prevention and Cure: The London School of Hygiene and Tropical Medicine, a 20th Century Quest for Global Public Health*. London: Kegan Paul (1998).

Index

Note: Commonly occurring entries such as Ross, Manson, *BMJ*, mosquitoes and malaria have not been indexed.

D

E

F

G